NURSING ADMINISTRATION

Strategic Perspectives and Application

With 21 Cases and Applications

EDITED BY

Jacqueline A. Dienemann, RN, PhD
Associate Professor
Coordinator, Nursing Administration
School of Nursing
George Mason University
Fairfax, Virginia

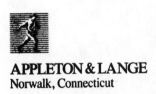

APPLETON & LANGE
Norwalk, Connecticut

0-8385-6999-4

90 91 92 93 94 / 10 9 8 7 6 5 4 3 2 1

Prentice Hall International (UK) Limited, *London*
Prentice Hall of Australia Pty. Limited, *Sydney*
Prentice Hall Canada, Inc., *Toronto*
Prentice Hall Hispanoamericana, S.A., *Mexico*
Prentice Hall of India Private Limited, *New Delhi*
Prentice Hall of Japan, Inc., *Tokyo*
Simon & Schuster Asia Pte. Ltd., *Singapore*
Editora Prentice Hall do Brasil Ltda., *Rio de Janeiro*
Prentice Hall, *Englewood Cliffs, New Jersey*

Library of Congress Cataloging-in-Publication Data

Nursing administration strategic perspectives and application/edited by
Jacqueline A. Dienemann.
    p.   cm.
    ISBN 0-8385-6999-4
    1. Nursing services—Administration.   I. Dienemann, Jacqueline A.
    [DNLM: 1. Administrative Personnel.   2. Nursing Services-
organization & administration.   WY   105 N9737]
RT89.N768 1990
362.1'73'068—dc20
DNLM/DLC
for Library of Congress   89-6834
                                                                 CIP

Production Editor: Amanda D. Egan
Designer: M. Chandler Martylewski
Cover Designer: Michael J. Kelly

PRINTED IN THE UNITED STATES OF AMERICA

Dedication

To my students who develop and test new case applications daily in their nursing administration practice.

REVIEWERS

Carol A. Brooks, RN, DNSc
Vice President for Nursing
Long Island Jewish Medical Center
New Hyde Park, New York

Olive Y. Burner, RN, PhD
Assistant Professor
Graduate Program in
  Nursing Administration
School of Nursing
University of California, Los Angeles
Los Angeles, California

Catherine Ecock Connelly, RN, DNSc
Associate Dean for Research,
  Graduate School
Associate Professor
School of Nursing
George Mason University
Fairfax, Virginia

Barbara Conway, RN, MSN
Assistant Director of Nursing,
  Clinical Services
Sibley Memorial Hospital
Washington, D.C.

Veronica Feeg, PhD, RN
Associate Professor
School of Nursing
George Mason University
Fairfax, Virginia
Editor, *Pediatric Nursing*

Susan B. Gantz, RN, MS
Executive Director
Self Care Institute
George Mason University
Fairfax, Virginia

Nan Goddard, RN, MSN
President
Goddard Management Resources
Houston, Texas

Barbara Happ, RN, MS
Consultant, Health Care Practice
Federal Consulting and Systems
American Management Systems, Inc.
Arlington, Virginia

Helen Jenkins, RN, PhD
Associate Professor
School of Nursing
George Mason University
Fairfax, Virginia

Richard Magenheimer, MBA
Vice President of Finance
Inova Health Systems
Falls Church, Virginia

Margaret Fisk Mastal, RN, MSN
Administrative Director
Professional Development and Research
Washington Hospital Center
Washington, D.C.

Virginia Millonig, PhD, CPNP
President
Health Leadership Associates
Potomac, Maryland

Joan Roche, RN, PhD
Director
Department of Nursing Education
  and Research
Fairfax Hospital
Falls Church, Virginia

Gail Dempsey Russell, RN, MSN
Vice President, Nursing
Potomac Hospital Corporation
Woodbridge, Virginia

Kitty S. Smith, RN, MSN
Associate Professor
School of Nursing
George Mason University
Fairfax, Virginia

Dorothy Jean Walker, RN, PhD, JD
Professor
School of Nursing
George Mason University
Fairfax, Virginia

CONTRIBUTORS

Alice Biache, RN, MSN
Vice President
Goodwin House
Alexandria, Virginia

Jennifer Burks, RN, MSN
Nursing Consultant
J.B. and Associates
Germantown, Maryland

Brenda S. Cherry, RN, PhD
Dean
College of Nursing
Harbor Campus
University of Massachusetts-Boston
Boston, Massachusetts

Katrina Clark, MPH
Director
Fair Haven Community Health Clinic
New Haven, Connecticut

Roberta M. Conti, RN, MSN, FAAN
Assistant Professor
School of Nursing
George Mason University
Fairfax, Virginia

Barbara A. Conway, RN, MSN
Assistant Director of Nursing,
 Clinical Services
Sibley Memorial Hospital
Washington, D.C.

Jean Cross, RN, MPH
Section Chief, Director of School
 Health Services
Dennis Avenue Health Center
Montgomery County Health Department
Silver Spring, Maryland

Emilie M. Deady, RN, MSN
Executive Director
Visiting Nurse Association
Arlington, Virginia

Margaret R. Dear, RN, PhD
Professor and Director of Nursing
 Research and Faculty Development
School of Nursing
George Mason University
Fairfax, Virginia

Lloyd M. DeBoer, PhD
Special Assistant President for
  Community Relations
Dean Emeritus
School of Business Administration
George Mason University
Fairfax, Virginia

Jacqueline A. Dienemann, RN, PhD
Associate Professor
Coordinator, Nursing Administration
School of Nursing
George Mason University
Fairfax, Virginia

R. Douglas First, PhD
Senior Research Associate
Office of Institutional Planning and
  Research
George Mason University
Fairfax, Virginia

Theodore Gessner, PhD
Associate Professor
Department of Psychology
George Mason University
Fairfax, Virginia

Eric Goplerud, PhD
Assistant Professor
Department of Psychology
George Mason University
Fairfax, Virginia

Patricia J. Graham, RN, MSN
Assistant Administrator
Mount Vernon Hospital
Alexandria, Virginia

James W. Harvey, PhD
Assistant Professor
Department of Marketing
School of Business Administration
George Mason University
Fairfax, Virginia

Janet Heinrich, RN, DPH
Director, Division of Extramural Programs
National Center for Nursing Research
National Institutes of Health
Department of Health and Human
  Services
Bethesda, Maryland

Harold L. Hirsh, MD, JD
Distinguished Visiting Professor
Department of Health Services
  Administration
George Washington University
Washington, D.C.

Mary Suzanne Hudec, RN, MSN
Chief, Nursing Service
Veterans Administration Medical Center
Washington, D.C.

Raymond D. Hylton, RN, MSN, CNAA
Acting Associate Chief Nurse
Acute Psychiatric Hospital
St. Elizabeth's Campus
D.C. Commission on Mental
  Health Services
Washington, D.C.

Joyce E. Johnson, RN, DNSc
Vice President
Division of Nursing
Washington Hospital Center
Washington, D.C.

Phillipa Ferguson Johnston, RN, MSN
Assistant Administrator
Capitol Hill Hospital
Washington, D.C.

Joanne M. Jorgenson, RN, MSN
Director of Nurses
Fairfax County Health Department
Fairfax, Virginia

Karen J. Kelly, RN, MSEd
Associate Director of Nursing for
  Education and Research
Center for Nursing Education
Greater Southeast Community Hospital
Washington, D.C.

Elizabeth Magenheimer, FNP, CNM
Director of Nursing
Fair Haven Community Health Clinic
New Haven, Connecticut

Julianne G. Mahler, PhD
Associate Professor
Department of Public Affairs
George Mason University
Fairfax, Virginia

Margaret Fisk Mastal, RN, MSN
Administrative Director
Professional Development and Research
Washington Hospital Center
Washington, D.C.

Mary Jo Moran, RN, MGA, CNA
Assistant Administrator
Nursing Systems
Washington Hospital Center
Washington, D.C.

Carol M. Ondeck, DBA
Associate Professor of Management
School of Business and Economics
Towson State University
Towson, Maryland

Carol A. Patney, RN, MSN, CS
Director of Clinical Intake
Psychiatric Institute of Washington
Washington, D.C.

Georgine M. Redmond, RN, EdD
Assistant Dean, Student Affairs
School of Nursing
George Mason University
Fairfax, Virginia

Joyce Richardson, RN, MSN
Assistant Chief Nurse and Major,
  U.S. Army Nurse Corps
Fox Army Community Hospital
Huntsville, Alabama

Gertrude L. Rodgers, RN, MSN
Associate Administrator/Nursing
Fairfax Hospital
Falls Church, Virginia

Stephen R. Ruth, PhD
Professor
Department of Decision Sciences
School of Business Administration
George Mason University
Fairfax, Virginia

Mary Cipriano Silva, RN, PhD, FAAN
Professor and Director, Center for
  Nursing Ethics
School of Nursing
George Mason University
Fairfax, Virginia

Susan Simms, RN, MPS, CNAA
Assistant Administrator/Nursing
Fresno Community Hospital and
  Medical Center
Fresno, California

Kitty S. Smith, RN, MSN
Associate Professor
School of Nursing
George Mason University
Fairfax, Virginia

Patricia Snyder, RN, MSN, CNA, RNC
Director of Nursing
HCA Dominion Hospital
Falls Church, Virginia

Wayne P. Thomas, PhD
Associate Professor
Department of Education Leadership and
  Human Development
College of Education and Human Services
George Mason University
Fairfax, Virginia

Mary S. Tilbury, RN, EdD, CNAA
Vice President, Administration
Director of Nursing Practice
Rochester General Hospital
Rochester, New York

James D. Vail, RN, DNSc
Associate Professor
School of Nursing
George Mason University
Fairfax, Virginia

Mary Dowling Willigan, RN, MSN
Nurse Manager
Memorial Sloan-Kettering Cancer Center
New York, New York

Leigh Wintz, RN, MSN
Executive Director
General Federation of Womens Clubs
Washington, D.C.

CONTENTS

Preface   *xvii*

Introduction   *xix*

**PART I   EXTERNAL FORCES INTERACTING WITH
            NURSING ADMINISTRATION**

  1 Ethical Frameworks Shaping Health Care Delivery............................ **3**
     Mary Cipriano Silva

       Moral Reasoning and Justification 3   /   Classical Ethical Theories 4   /
       Ethical Principles 11   /   Interrelationship of Ethics and Law 15   /
       Standards of Care as Ethical Choices 17

       Application 1-1:
       Moral Reasoning in Personnel Decisions 21
       Patricia Snyder

  2 Legal Aspects of Nursing Administration....................................... **29**
     Harold L. Hirsh

       Nursing Practice: Legal Liability 29   /   Administrative Law 40   /
       Labor-Management Laws 43   /   Health Care Employment Laws 49

       Application 2-1:
       Managing Unionized Nurses 55
       Mary Suzanne Hudec, Mary Dowling Willigan

       Application 2-2:
       Designing a Nursing Risk Management System........................... 61
       Leigh Wintz

3 Health Policy **71**
James D. Vail

Historical Review 72 / Forces Shaping Health Policy 75 /
Reorganization of Health Care Delivery 79 / The Future 85

Case 3-1:
The Role of ANA in Legislative Reform
of Nursing Homes 1986–1987 .... **92**
Janet Heinrich

4 Nurse Administrators as Women Managers **99**

Section 1:
Stereotyping **99**
Carol M. Ondeck

Stereotyping Theory 99 / Attribution Theory 100 / Combining
Sex Role Stereotypes and Expectations 101 / A Sex-Segregated
Occupation 101 / Professional Practice 102 / Administrative
Change 102

Section 2:
Successful Women Administrators **105**
Georgine M. Redmond

Personal Profiles of Women Executives 106 / An Organizational
Perspective 109 / Characteristics of Successful Women
Administrators 110 / Role Models, Mentors and Networks 112

Case 4-1:
Head Nurse Preceptor Program
at a Community Hospital **116**
Barbara A. Conway

Case 4-2:
Feminist Management at a Community
Health Clinic **124**
Katrina Clark, Elizabeth Magenheimer

PART II ORGANIZATIONAL STRATEGIES

5 Organizations as Decision Making Systems **133**
Julianne G. Mahler

Methods of Decision Making 134 / Comparisons and
Recommendations 143

Case 5-1:
A Decision Trail for Implementing a
Policy Change **148**
Margaret Fisk Mastal

6 Strategic Planning in Health Care Organizations............................ 153
Eric Goplerud

Response to Rapid Change 153 / Effectiveness 154 / Strategic
Planning Process 154 / Looking Inward: Assessing Internal
Strategic Capacities 157 / Looking Outward:
Competitive Analysis 158 / Formulating a Plan 162 /
Implementation: Avoiding the Pitfalls 163 /
Evaluation and Control 165

Case 6-1:
Strategic Plan of the Nursing Education
Department in a Community Hospital.. 172
Karen J. Kelly

Case 6-2:
Strategic Implementation: Some Practical
Aspects of Opening a New
Continuing Care Retirement Center 179
Alice Biache

7 Integrating Marketing into Health Care Organizations..................... 185
James W. Harvey

Overview of Marketing 185 / Marketing's Role in Strategic
Planning 193 / The Marketing Plan 202 / Applying Marketing
to Recruitment and Retention 203

Case 7-1:
Marketing Principles Applied by Nurses
in an Outpatient Psychiatric Service....................................... 208
Carol A. Patney

Case 7-2:
Initiating Marketing in a County
Health Department 219
Joanne M. Jorgenson

PART III   STRUCTURING HEALTH CARE ORGANIZATIONS

8 Organizations as Open Systems 229
Jacqueline A. Dienemann

Open Systems Models 229 / Systems Model 231 / Congruence
Model 234 / Professional Bureaucracy Model 236 /
Contingency Model 239 / Life Cycle Stages of Organizations 241 /
Using Open Systems Models 244

Application 8-1:
Management Consultation 247
Kitty S. Smith

Case 8-1:
Changes in Medicare Reporting: Its Impact
on a Home Health Agency.. 254
Emilie M. Deady

9   Organizations as Financial Systems 263
Lloyd M. DeBoer

Interpreting Financial Statements 263 / Financial Analyses 271 /
Cost Concepts and Controls 277 / Budgeting 283

Case 9-1:
Nursing Assuming Financial Control
in a Tertiary Hospital 289
Gertrude L. Rodgers, Joyce Richardson

10   Organizations as Information Systems 299
Stephen R. Ruth

Information Systems in Health Care 299 / Management
Information Systems 300 / Automation
of Routine Work 304 / Selection 308 / Future Directions 311

Case 10-1:
Automating a Patient Classification System
Nurse-Vendor Collaboration.. 316
Raymond D. Hylton, Joyce E. Johnson, Mary Jo Moran

11   Organizations as Work Flow Systems.. 329
Theodore Gessner

Job Analysis 329 / History of Systematic Job Design 330 /
Job Design in Nursing 336 / Implementing Job Design 339

Application 11-1:
Decentralizing a Nursing System 344
Phillipa Ferguson Johnston

PART IV   NURSING ADMINISTRATION

12   The Organization of Nursing Care Delivery................................. 353
Roberta M. Conti, Jennifer Burks

Placement of Nursing in the Overall Structure 353 / Organizing
Nursing Care Delivery at the Unit Level 359 / Roles in Nursing
Administration 362 / Costing Nursing Resources 363

Case 12-1:
Nursing Administration in a Product
Line Environment.. 370
Patricia J. Graham

Case 12-2:
Delineation of Nursing Services
in a Community Health Agency 378
Jean Cross

13 **Professional Development** **385**
Brenda S. Cherry

Purposes of Professional Development Programs 385 / Nurses as
Adult Learners 388 / Centralization versus Decentralization
of Professional Development Departments 392 / Creative Linkages
Between Service and Education 394

Application 13-1:
Guidelines for Establishing a Clinical
Nursing Research Program in a Medical Center
Teaching Hospital.. 402
Margaret R. Dear

14 **Performance Appraisal** **409**
R. Douglas First

Purposes of the Performance Appraisal 410 / Components of the
Performance Appraisal 412 / Methods to Evaluate Performance 416 /
Validity and Reliability 421

Case 14-1:
Goal Setting by Staff Nurses in a
Community Hospital... 424
Susan Simms

15 **Program Evaluation** **437**
Wayne P. Thomas

Evaluation: A Closer Look 438 / Major Characteristics of Evaluation
Models 441 / Evaluation Models: Paradigms for Evaluation 444 /
Efficiency Models 448 / Quality Assurance 450

Case 15-1:
Maintaining JCAHO Accreditation 455
Mary S. Tilbury

INDEX **463**

PREFACE

Health care organizations are becoming increasingly complex. Accompanying this complexity is health care's shift from a community service orientation to a service business orientation. Nurse administrators, together with all other health administrators, are stretching themselves to gain more business skills while maintaining their human relation skills gained from nursing practice and sustaining the values that originally attracted them to nursing.

This book recognizes the need for nurse administrators at all levels to draw on information from business, psychology, education, and other related fields to practice more effectively. It differs from other nursing administration books in two respects. One, the authors represent multiple disciplines. Each chapter presents concepts derived from the research and theory established in a specific topical area that is essential for nurse administrators. Each chapter is accompanied by a case example or suggested application written by a nurse administrator that illustrates the usefulness of this information. The second unique characteristic of this book is its perspective of an organization as a whole. For example, Chapter 14: "Performance Appraisal," examines the design of a system rather than emphasizing the managerial behaviors to implement the system. The focus is on understanding the external factors interacting with an organization, the infrastructures supporting an effective organization, and nursing care delivery systems that create an environment for holistic nursing practice.

Using an open systems perspective no actions are prescribed. The authors assume there is no one right way to act; rather, nurse administrators must assess their situations and choose their actions accordingly. They also assume that nurse administrators must view their situations from a whole organization perspective in order to act in congruence with organizational goals and strategic plans. To do this they need knowledge of the language and perspectives of their colleagues in departments throughout the organization.

This book is intended for graduate students in nursing administration and nurse administrators. Nurse administrators at all levels can use this book as a guide to integrating information from related disciplines into their administrative practice. Nurse executives are increasingly represented within the organization's executive management team. They need to be knowledgeable of business practices and management theory in the health care arena. Nurse middle managers, as designers of the systems to implement strategic plans and the managers of multiple departments, also need a macro perspective supported by organization theory. Nurse department managers require an understanding of their department's contribution to the goals of the whole organization in order to comprehend higher administration's responses to their innovative ideas and requests for resources.

The major lesson to be learned from this book is that nurse managers need theory and information from many perspectives in order to develop a macro perspective in resolving administrative problems. It is only by moving to this broader perspective that nurse administrators will gain the competencies necessary to gain power and become leaders administering the health care delivery organizations of the future.

As with any endeavor of this magnitude, I am indebted to many people. The one responsible for urging me for over a year to create a book using a macro perspective was Rita Carty, Dean of the School of Nursing, George Mason University. Once committed to such a venture it was Susan Gantz and Veronica Feeg who listened, read outlines, and generally kept me focused. My greatest debt is to my husband Paul who, as an experienced writer, offered guidance and a macro view of the purpose of this effort.

Finally, I must recognize the major contribution of the faculty of George Mason University and the nurse administrators of metropolitan Washington, the source of most of my authors and volunteer reviewers. All were committed to a book that clearly communicates important information relevant to the daily practice of nurse administrators. They graciously accepted my guidance through many revisions and conferences. Thank you.

Jacqueline A. Dienemann

INTRODUCTION

Health care organizations are in the midst of a significant transformation. Health care administration texts are moving from how to control and direct others to how to lead others and shape environments for professional practice. It is more difficult to create a climate of excellence than to manage an organization. This book recognizes that there is no "one minute solution" to administering a health care organization in today's environment. It directs you to look ahead—to focus on the future you want to create. It offers no solutions, only the information and tools to make wise choices.

The book is organized into four parts: External Forces Interacting With Nursing Administration; Organizational Strategies; Structuring Health Care Organizations; and Nursing Administration.

Part I examines selected forces and how they interact with the American health care delivery system. The selected forces include: Ethics, Law, Health Policy and Women in Management. They are chosen as being representative of the many forces contributing to the American definition of health care and how it is delivered. The authors do not offer a simplified, single point of view based on their interpretation of primary sources. Rather, they present a synthesis of several theories, suggest further reading, and provide illustrative case applications for analysis and personal application. They assume that there are many paths to the same action and there is no inherently "right" action. This approach assists nurse administrators to hone their critical thinking skills in order to better analyze uncertain situations where there is no right answer.

Part II provides information and guidance in methods of decision making, strategic planning, and marketing. All three are related disciplines with well developed applications in health care and nursing. Together they assist the nurse administrator to develop transformational leadership and vision.

Together, these two sections provide the theoretical underpinnings for nurse administrators to develop a macro perspective in analyzing managerial dilemmas and recognizing the importance of boundary spanning activities such as political action, competitor analysis, professional association leadership and community service.

Part III examines systems which may support effective and efficient management. Views of organizations as open systems, financial systems, management information systems, and work systems enrich the nurse administrator's understanding of how structure and processes must mesh for effective coordination of the work of both managers and care providers.

Nursing is the primary service offered by inpatient facilities and home health agencies. In a hospital with a functional division of labor, nursing is the largest and most widely dispersed department. With any structure nurses are the largest occupational group. Part IV focuses on the design, support, and evaluation of nursing care delivery systems which support the professional practice of nurses.

Nurse administrators at any level of management who master the ideas presented in this book shall become more aware of the ramifications of their actions for the whole organization. This understanding will change the thrust of their energies from nursing to the entire organization and its environment. They will act for nursing by political action, community involvement, and networking throughout their organization to influence decisions that involve nursing's interests.

They will possess the business skills and speak the language used outside nursing by other health care managers. They will use this language to better articulate nursing's needs to board members and administrators who have no clinical background. They will also be better prepared to collaborate with non-nurses to clarify the clinical implications of financial and marketing decisions. To implement these collaborative decisions they must also work within nursing to widen other nurse's appreciation of the financial and marketing implications of clinical decisions.

Acting with this world view, nurse administrators will gain power and their careers will encompass wider responsibilities. This trend is already evident as many of the case examples and suggested applications describe dramatic changes in nurse administrators responsibilities over time. Nurse administrators, using a macro view and increased political and business sophistication will lead others in the creation of a more humanistic and financially sound health care system.

PART I

External Forces Interacting with Nursing Administration

PART 1

1

Ethical Frameworks Shaping Health Care Delivery

Mary Cipriano Silva

Despite the proliferation of literature on health care ethics, I have been able to locate only a handful of references that specifically focus on ethics in nursing administration. This situation is puzzling in light of the frequency and complexity of ethical dilemmas faced by nurse administrators. Therefore, in this chapter, to help nurse administrators cope with these ethical dilemmas, I will provide the reader with knowledge related to (1) moral philosophy, (2) the interrelationships of ethics and law, and (3) how standards of care affect ethical choices in nursing administration.

MORAL REASONING AND JUSTIFICATION

When talking about ethical frameworks, one is concerned with two components: process and content. Process refers to moral reasoning; content refers to moral justification. Both are essential to and interdependent in making a sound moral decision. Moral reasoning is a way of thinking; in particular, it is a way of thinking in which a person's deliberations about what is morally right or wrong are justified by appeals to moral reasons such as ethical theories, principles, and rules. Such appeals to moral reasons, then, constitute moral justification.

The essence of moral decision making is:

1. Moral reasoning is a systematic and reflective process of deliberation by which moral judgments are justified.
2. Justification means that an individual has sufficient moral reasons for claiming that a judgment is morally right or wrong.

Preparation of this chapter was supported by the Division of Nursing, Health Resources and Service Administration, Public Health Service, Department of Health and Health Services Special Project Grant DIO NU23091.

3. The moral reasons give appeal to an independent standard outside of oneself.
4. An independent standard validates or justifies what is claimed to be correct.
5. The independent standards used to validate one's claim may be ethical judgments, rules, principles, or theories.

According to Beauchamp (1982, pp. 308–309), moral reasons can be arranged in a hierarchy, as shown in Table 1–1. The levels in Table 1–1 are often linked, thus a judgment can be justified in terms of a rule, which in turn can be justified in terms of a principle, which in turn can be justified in terms of a theory. Coverage of a decision or an act at all four levels of the hierarchy provides the strongest moral justification. Such a justification of adherence to standards of care could be outlined as follows:

- Judgment
  This nurse administrator upholds standards of care.
- Principle
  Nurse administrators ought to treat clients with respect.
- Theory
  Nurse administrators respect clients because it is their moral duty to do so. The act that the nurse administrator is morally obligated to follow is the one that is done for the sake of duty.

The hierarchy, however, also has some limitations: (1) clear cut distinctions are not always possible among the four levels; (2) all forms of justifying reasons are not depicted in the schema; and (3) sometimes singular justifications may be inappropriate because many judgments may be governed by many rules rather than a singular judgment being governed by a singular rule. Nevertheless, the content of ethics provides moral justification, and the highest level of this justification is ethical theory.

CLASSICAL ETHICAL THEORIES

Viable ethical theories meet certain standards. According to Mappes and Zembaty (1986, pp. 5–6), the two most important standards are congruency and guidance. Congruency means an ethical theory that makes sense out of the

TABLE 1-1. LEVELS OF MORAL JUSTIFICATION

Ethical theory
Principle
Rule
Judgment

moral life by making visible, without holding sacrosanct, the structure of common moral thinking. Guidance means an ethical theory that provides a framework for determining morally right from morally wrong actions. When two or more ethical theories compete, one must decide which theory best meets the preceding criteria.

Two major classes of ethical theory dominate Western normative ethics (Veatch and Fry, 1987). One class of consequentialism focuses on consequences; the other, nonconsequentialism, focuses on features of acts that make the acts right or wrong. To highlight these classes of ethical theories, I now describe a consequentialist theory (utilitarianism), a nonconsequentialist theory (deontology), and a mixed theory (theory of prima facie duties).

Utilitarianism

The consequentialist theory of utilitarianism has been substantially derived from the writings of David Hume (1711–1776), Jeremy Bentham (1748–1832), and John Stuart Mill (1806–1873). Utilitarianism may be summarized as follows:

1. No acts are right or wrong outside of the consequences produced by the acts.
2. Desired consequences maximize what is intrinsically valuable, that is, what is good in and of itself. (According to philosophers, intrinsic values include, for example, happiness, pleasure, freedom from pain, truth, beauty, and knowledge.)
3. Undesirable consequences diminish what is intrinsically valuable.
4. The right act is the one that leads to the greatest possible balance of good consequences (or to the least possible balance of bad consequences) for all persons affected, or most affected, by the act. This is known as the principle of utility, which is the underlying, and only, principle of utilitarianism.

There are two types of utilitarianism: act and rule. In act utilitarianism, appeals are made directly to the principle of utility based on the thesis: *A person ought to act in accord with the action that, if followed in a specific situation, would produce the greatest balance of good over evil, everyone considered.* The emphasis is on the greatest general good in a specific situation, even if in that particular situation a general moral rule must be violated. The act utilitarian does not discount acting in accord with moral rules if the rules maximize utility; however, if the breaking of the moral rule produces more utility than disutility, the act utilitarian breaks a rule.

Act utilitarians determine what they ought to do as follows (Mappes & Zembaty 1986):

1. Determine alternative paths of action.
2. Project the short-term and long-term consequences of each alternative action.

3. Evaluate the consequences in each specific situation and weigh the good against the bad while taking into consideration the impact of the action on everyone affected by it.
4. Carry out the act that is most likely to produce the greatest balance of good consequences over bad consequences in a particular situation.
5. If confronted with actions that cause only bad consequences, carry out the act that brings about the fewest bad consequences.

By contrast, those who ascribe to rule utilitarianism consider moral rules important because of their significance to society. Rule utilitarians make indirect appeals to the principle of utility based on this thesis: *A person ought to act in accordance with the rule that, if generally followed, would produce the greatest balance of good over evil, everyone considered.* Moral assessment of individual acts are carried out only in reference to established moral rules and to the consequences of following such rules.

Rule utilitarians determine what they ought to do as follows (Mappes & Zembaty, 1986, pp. 12–14):

1. Determine alternative courses of action.
2. Articulate a set of moral rules that enhance utility (e.g., do not lie; do not steal; do not kill).
3. Incorporate exceptions into the rules when these exceptions maximize utility (e.g., do not kill except in self-defense).
4. Determine the consequences of following a rule or of following a rule with exceptions.
5. Carry out the act that is most often likely to produce the greatest possible balance of good consequences over bad consequences for persons affected, or most affected, by the act.

In summary, utilitarianism is a major consequentialist ethical framework whose proponents ascribe to the premise that the rightness or the wrongness of an act is determined by its consequences. Act utilitarians appeal directly to the principle of utility in determining right actions, whereas rule utilitarians first appeal to moral rules and then to the principle of utility in determining right actions.

Deontology

The nonconsequentialist theory of deontology has been substantially derived from the writings of Immanuel Kant (1724–1804). A summary of the key points of deontology are:

1. Persons must act out of a good will.
2. Duty is central to a good will.

3. Duties are derived from the supreme principle of morality known as the *categorical imperative*.

According to Kant (1785/1981, pp. 7–12), the highest good in the world is a good will. In assessing the total worth of our actions, a good will holds first place; all other considerations follow from it. Because a good will is good in itself, its goodness does not depend on consequences or on what it accomplishes or affects. Rather, a good will is uncompromising in its motivation to carry out its duty. Thus, an act is right only when it is done for the sake of duty.

From what basis are duties derived? According to Kant, duties are derived from the categorical imperative. The categorical imperative is complex; Kant formulated it in five different ways. The formulation that is significant for nursing is, in Kant's (1785/1981) words, "Act in such a way that you treat humanity, whether in your own person or in the person of another, always at the same time as an end and never simply as a means" (p. 36). Kant views violation of the end in itself as wrong because when a person is treated as a mere means, respect for that person is diminished. There can be no moral double standard— one standard for oneself and one for others. One can integrate the preceding Kantian concepts of good will, duty, and end in itself as follows: The highest good is a good will; a good will acts for the sake of duty and only the sake of duty; the right act is the one that is done for the sake of duty; a good will acting for the sake of duty would treat persons as ends in themselves and never as mere means to ends.

Not all philosophers with a deontological orientation view rightness as conservatively as did Kant. Variations take these forms: (1) Features of acts other than, or in addition to, duties (e.g., conscience, intuition, faith, rights, motives, virtues) may determine the rightness or wrongness of an act and (2) consequences may be relevant to deontological thinking but are not the sole or final determiner of such thinking. Within this more liberal perspective, deontology is defined as follows: Deontology is a moral theory whose proponents endorse the premise that features of acts other than, or in addition to, their consequences determine the rightness or wrongness of an act.

As with utilitarianism, there are two types of deontology: act and rule. In act deontology, appeals are made directly to, for example, conscience, intuition, or faith to determine what is right or obligatory in a given situation. Act deontologists do not rely on rules. Because they view each situation as unique, they stress the changing nature of moral experience. If rules are used, they serve only as guidelines that can be broken if one has good reason based on conscience, intuition, or faith.

Conversely, in rule deontology, moral rules incur binding obligations that transcend individual situations. Courses of action, then, are right or wrong because of their adherence or nonadherence to one or more rules or principles. Rule deontologists assess how the rules enhance their ability to act from duty (or some other relevant characteristic), thus enabling them to do what is right.

Rule deontology, however, does not provide direction to resolve the dilemma presented when two or more absolute rules conflict.

Prima Facie Duties

The theory of prima facie duties was conceptualized by W. D. Ross (1930), an English philosopher, to determine one's duty when moral rules conflict. He did not agree that moral rules were absolute. Prima facie means valid on first appearance. Therefore, a prima facie duty is one that is always binding unless it conflicts with equal or stronger duties. One ought always to keep promises unless keeping a promise competes with a stronger duty such as the duty to prevent harm to another. A nurse administrator may break a promised luncheon commitment with a colleague if, during that promised time, the nurse administrator must assist a head nurse in preventing a patient's suicide. When a prima facie duty conflicts with an equal or stronger duty, the prima facie duty may be overridden. The duty that is actually carried out (in this case, preventing harm to a patient) is called one's actual duty or duty proper. One's actual duty is determined by assessing the various weights of the competing duties.

According to Munson (1983),

> Ross offers us two principles to deal with cases of conflicting duty. The first principle is designed to handle situations in which just two prima facie duties are in conflict. This is the principle: That act is one's duty which is in accord with the more stringent prima facie obligation.
>
> The second principle is intended to deal with cases in which several prima facie duties are in conflict: That act is one's duty which has the greatest balance of prima facie rightness over prima facie wrongness. (p. 24)

Ross (1930, p. 21) considered the following duties to be prima facie: duties of fidelity, reparation, justice, gratitude, self-improvement, beneficence, and nonmaleficence. This list of duties may not be complete or precise enough to define all aspects of the duty; nevertheless, his theory is helpful in reflecting on what one ought to do when moral rules compete.

Based on Ross's theory of prima facie duties, I offer the following framework for the assessment of an ethical dilemma:

1. Identify the ethical problem.
2. List relevant ethical rules or principles.
3. For each anticipated course of action, determine which, if any, ethical rules or principles are in conflict.
4. For each anticipated course of action, determine which duties (rights, virtues, etc.) emerge from the ethical rules or principles.
5. For each anticipated course of action, determine which duties (rights, virtues, etc.) are in conflict with equal or stronger duties.
6. If a conflict exists, determine which duties (rights, virtues, etc.) derived from moral rules and principles generate the more stringent prima facie

obligation, or the greatest balance of prima facie rightness over prima facie wrongness. Choose the course of action that is consistent with those duties.

7. If no conflict exists, choose the duty and course of action that are consistent with ethical rules and principles.

In summary, as depicted in Table 1–2, four perspectives on ethical theory have been presented: act utilitarianism, rule utilitarianism, act deontology, and rule deontology.

Based on Table 1–2, we examine the situation of four nurse executives faced

TABLE 1–2. UTILITARIAN AND DEONTOLOGICAL ETHICAL THEORIES

Utilitarian Theory
The rightness and wrongness of an act is based on the goodness and badness of the consequences resulting from the act.

Act Utilitarianism	*Rule Utilitarianism*
The morality of an action depends on the relationship between a particular situation or circumstance and the principle of utility. That is, a person ought to perform that act whose consequences produce the greatest balance of good over evil for everyone affected by the act in a particular situation even if a moral rule must be violated. (Focus is on good and evil *consequences in a particular situation.*)	The morality of an action depends on the relationship between moral rules and the principle of utility. That is, a person ought to perform that act based on moral rules that, if generally followed, would produce the greatest balance of good over evil for everyone affected by the act. (Focus is on good and evil *consequences of moral rules that apply generally.*)

Deontological Theory
The rightness and wrongness of an act is determined by features of an act other than, or in addition to, their consequences.

Act Deontology	*Rule Deontology*
The morality of an action depends on an immediate grasp of a particular situation without strict reliance on moral rules or on consequences as the final determiners of rightness or wrongness. That is, a person ought to perform that act that best accords with, for example, conscience, intuition, faith, duties, rights, motives, and/or virtues. (Focus is primarily on *features of acts* other than consequences *in a particular situation.*)	The morality of an action depends primarily on the relationship between moral rules and features of acts other than consequences. That is, a person ought to perform that act based on moral rules that, if generally followed, enables the person to act from, for example, conscience, intuition, faith, duty, etc. (Focus is primarily on *moral rules that apply generally* without any, or sole, reference to consequences.)

with a common ethical dilemma that affects nursing administration policy: whether or not to restrain confused or combative patients.

- *Act utilitarianism.* The nurse administrator using act utilitarian thinking would assess the positive and negative consequences to all persons involved in a *specific situation if a given patient* were restrained or not restrained. The administrator would choose a *policy* that would produce the *greatest balance* of good consequences over bad consequences for all persons involved *in that situation.*
- *Rule utilitarianism.* The nurse administrator using rule utilitarian thinking would identify a rule or rules that maximize utility regarding the use or nonuse of restraints (e.g., prevent patients from harming themselves). The administrator would choose a *policy based on the moral rule that,* if *generally followed* in this and similar situations, would produce the greatest balance of good consequences over bad consequences for everyone considered. Put another way, the consequences of following the rule are better than the consequences of allowing confused or combative patients to harm themselves.
- *Act deontology.* The nurse administrator using act deontological thinking would determine a *policy* of whether or not to restrain a given patient in a *specific situation based on conscience, intuition, faith, duty, or some other feature of an act* other than, or in addition to, consequences. The administrator would choose a policy that best accords with the relevant feature (e.g., duty) in a particular situation.
- *Rule deontology.* The nurse administrator using rule deontological thinking would *identify a rule* or rules relevant to the use of restraints (e.g., prevent patients from harming themselves) that would enable the administrator to act from, for example, conscience, faith, or duty in the formulation of the policy. The nurse administrator would choose a policy that would *support choice of that act based on the moral rule* that, if *generally followed* in this and similar situations, would enhance one's ability to act from duty (or another relevant moral characteristic).

Each of the preceding four approaches could lead to the same or to different actions, depending on the nature of the moral reasoning and justification. For example, in the preceding situation, a person using act utilitarian thinking and a person using rule utilitarian thinking could arrive at the same decision—to restrain a patient. On the other hand, a person using act utilitarian thinking could arrive at a decision *not* to restrain the patient, whereas another person using rule utilitarian thinking could arrive at a decision *to* restrain the patient. Furthermore, *two persons using any one of the four theories may not necessarily arrive at the same decision.* This discrepancy may occur because of differences of opinions over, for example, what consequences of an act maximize utility, or what duties derived from moral rules generate the more stringent prima facie obligation. Thus, use of one theoretical perspective does not denote a particular action; the action to be taken is determined by the *processes* of moral reasoning and moral justification.

ETHICAL PRINCIPLES

In addition to moral reasoning and ethical theory, ethical principles also help shape health care delivery. In this section I describe briefly three such principles: the principle of respect for autonomy, the principle of beneficence, and the principle of justice.

Ethical Principle of Respect for Autonomy

The ethical principle of respect for autonomy incorporates the concepts of (1) respect for persons and (2) autonomy. The *concept of respect for persons* encompasses both empathy and lack of exploitation. Empathy means listening to and understanding another person in such a way that one is able to put oneself in that other person's position. Lack of exploitation means that other persons should not be used as mere means to one's own or other's ends. The goal of respect for persons, then, is to appreciate and give due weight to other persons' capacities, beliefs, and perspectives (Jameton, 1984, p. 125).

The *concept of autonomy* deals less with other persons than with oneself. Autonomy can mean self-determining capacities or self-determining actions, or both. Put another way, to a substantial degree, autonomous persons (1) have the capability of self-governance, (2) operate from a stable and internalized set of principles, and (3) view themselves as capable of implementing autonomous actions (Faden & Beauchamp, 1986, pp. 235–237).

Persons engaging in self-determining actions must act (1) with intention, (2) with understanding, and (3) without controlling influences (Faden & Beauchamp, 1986, p. 238). Autonomous administrators not only know what they intend when they act, but they also understand the relevant aspects of a situation to carry out a decision. Note that this definition does not demand a perfect grasp of all aspects of a situation; instead, it demands an *adequate* grasp of *relevant* aspects. Thus, nurse administrators must find a balance between acting with too little knowledge or not acting at all in the hopes of attaining a perfect grasp of a situation. Finally, to be a self-determining action, an act must be free of controlling influences. This means administrators essentially are not affected by external pressures such as threats, monetary incentives, promises of (or withdrawal of) love, affection, or power.

How do "respect for persons" and "autonomy" interrelate to formulate the ethical principle of respect for autonomy? This ethical principle is: One should treat autonomous others in such a way that they are allowed to choose and act without controlling constraints placed on them. The principle of respect for autonomy focuses on *how* autonomous persons should be treated—an attitude of respect or with an attitude of noninterference regarding their autonomous actions. This principle constrains the administrator from manipulating or coercing others.

Ethical Principle of Beneficence

Frankena (1973) identified the following four components of the ethical principle of beneficence:

1. One ought not to inflict evil or harm (what is bad).
2. One ought to prevent evil or harm.
3. One ought to remove evil.
4. One ought to do or promote good. (p. 47)

The first component, not inflicting harm on others (nonmaleficence) or putting them at risk of harm, is often summed up as "do no harm." Harm can come to others through acts of omission or commission and can take the form of impairments, injuries, disabilities, damages, or death.

In addition to do no harm, other aspects of the principle of beneficence include the prevention of harm, the removal of harm, and the promotion of good. Prevention of harm means that a person proactively takes advanced measures against some probable harmful event (e.g., an administrator, anticipating a nurses' strike, plans in advance for the safe care of patients during the strike). Removal of harm means a person eliminates existing situations where injury or damage has occurred (e.g., an administrator fires an employee who has injured patients through incompetence). Promotion of good means a person contributes to the welfare of others (e.g., an administrator establishes an AIDS information hot line for the community). Prevention of harm, removal of harm, and promotion of good are sometimes referred to collectively as the principle of positive beneficence (Beauchamp & Childress, 1983, p. 149).

Two questions, however, arise in regard to the preceding three components: (1) What ought one to do if one cannot produce benefits without causing harm? (2) What ought one to do when a person's actions would be harmful to oneself? The first question can be addressed in terms of the principle of balancing benefits and harm. As with the other ethical principles, the principle of balancing benefits and harm is prima facie. Thus, it is morally permissible to perform an action if the risks are reasonable, when compared with the anticipated benefits.

The second question of "what ought one to do when a person's actions would be harmful to oneself?" brings us to the topic of paternalism. In ethics, paternalism means that a person's intended actions are overridden for beneficent reasons without the person's consent. Under what conditions, if any, nurse administrators or other health care providers should engage in paternalistic interventions are controversial. To help clarify this controversy, Beauchamp and Childress (1983) recommend that paternalism can only be justified if:

1. The harms prevented from occurring or the benefit provided to the person outweighs the loss of independence or the sense of invasion suffered by the interference.
2. The person's condition seriously limits his or her ability to choose autonomously.
3. It is universally justified under relevantly similar circumstances always to treat persons in this way (p. 172).

For example, suppose a health team asks a nurse administrator to support ethically their decision to deny a patient's request for discharge from a hospital. To gain the nurse administrator's ethical support, the team must first demonstrate that the anticipated harms being prevented are greater than the anticipated liberties being sacrificed. Second, the team must show evidence that the patient's competency is in question. And third, the team must convince the nurse administrator that similar patients in similar situations would also be refused discharge from the hospital. If the latter criterion is not met, issues of justice arise.

Ethical Principle of Justice

Justice means giving a person his or her due, or that which a person deserves or can legitimately claim. What a person deserves may be burdens, rewards, or punishments. There is a common basic principle of justice, attributed to Aristotle, that asserts that persons who are equals ought to be treated equally, and persons who are unequal ought to be treated unequally. For example, within a given institution, nurse administrators of equal position, work load, education, experience, and merit should receive comparable salaries; nurse administrators of lesser power position, education, merit, or so forth, should not receive salaries comparable to the preceding administrators. Either violation is an injustice. Frankena (1973) summarizes injustice well: "The paradigm case of injustice is that in which there are two similar individuals in similar circumstances and one of them is treated better or worse than the other" (p. 49).

Although the formal principle of justice is useful, it is not comprehensive of all situations. For example, it does not specify who is equal and who is unequal, nor does it specify morally relevant differences among persons for distributing benefits and burdens. To overcome these problems, philosophers offer material principles of justice for determining what a person is due. In particular, material principles of justice specify on what basis social benefits and burdens should be allocated. Examples of materials principles of justice are as follows (Silva, 1984):

1. To each person according to effort.
2. To each person according to societal contribution.
3. To each person according to merit.
4. To each person equally.
5. To each person according to . . . (state other morally relevant characteristics).

To take the preceding example of what should constitute a fair salary for a nurse administrator, one could base the decision on one or more of the preceding morally relevant characteristics (e.g., to each administrator according to effort or merit). Differences of opinion about this salary may occur because persons do not always agree on which material principles of justice should dominate. In organizations, policies often delineate the material principles of justice used to determine performance merit raises. When an administrator's and an organization's viewpoints about the basis for merit pay differ, the administrator may experience dissatisfaction and a feeling that injustice is present.

Typically, one holds one of several perspectives about distributive justice (Silva, 1984):

- *Libertarian perspective.* Libertarians focus primarily on economic benefits and burdens in free market or capitalist systems. Libertarians ascribe to the viewpoint that they may enter and withdraw from economic arrangements freely and in accord with their own interests, as long as their collective self-interests benefit the larger society. Libertarians believe that individuals who produce more should receive more economic benefits than individuals who produce less, even if this arrangement leads to inequalities of wealth in a society. Libertarians, thus, place a high value on autonomy and the ethical principle of respect for autonomy. Because of this orientation, they tend to ascribe to material principles of justice such as "to each person according to merit."
- *Utilitarian perspective.* Utilitarians, as noted in the ethical theory of utilitarianism, consider the intrinsic value of consequences for all persons involved to be the morally relevant factor that determines an act's right-making or wrong-making characteristics. The action that ensures the best consequences is the right one. Because utilitarians hold the doing of good and the prevention of harm as central concepts, they place a high value on the ethical principle of beneficence. Because of this orientation, such persons tend to ascribe "to each person according to the greatest good for the greatest number."
- *Egalitarian perspective.* Egalitarians focus primarily on equality as the morally relevant characteristic in allocating resources. According to Veatch (1981), justice requires the "equality of net welfare for individuals" (p. 265). Egalitarianism demands comparability, not necessarily uniformity. In other words, all persons in a society would not have to receive the exact same benefits and burdens. Some persons could receive great benefits and great burdens; other persons could receive an average amount of both, but over time benefits and burdens would be balanced. Because egalitarians value equality highly, they place a high value on the ethical principle of justice as equality. Thus, persons with egalitarian perspectives tend to ascribe to material principles of justice such as "to each person an equal (or comparable) share."

- *Need based perspective.* The moral rationale for specifying need as relevant to distributive justice is that a person would be harmed if a need (usually interpreted to mean a basic or fundamental need) was denied. Examples of fundamental or basic needs include nutrition, health care, education, and freedom from environmental harms. The needs viewpoint about justice, imposes an obligation to provide whatever is necessary to meet the need. For example, if a nurse works in a state where continued licensure is dependent on continuing education, then the state must provide opportunities by which this requirement can be met. Persons who ascribe to the needs viewpoint of justice place a high value on the ethical principle of nonmaleficence. Persons with a needs perspective would tend to ascribe to material principles of justice such as "to each person according to basic needs."

Because persons who ascribe to each of the preceding four frameworks use different perspectives as a rationale for a just decision, we can begin to see why nurse administrators and other policy makers may disagree on the morality of what constitutes just allocation of resources. Being aware of various viewpoints, nurse administrators can better understand their own and other persons' positions on distributive justice.

So far in this chapter I have been describing content from moral philosophy that is relevant to health care. Now I shift focus and examine how ethics and law are related and affect administrative roles.

INTERRELATIONSHIP OF ETHICS AND LAW

Ethics is a systematic process of reflection in which issues of what one morally ought to do are analyzed, determined, and evaluated through moral reasoning. The goal of ethics is to clarify what is right and wrong or good and evil in human conduct or character. In contrast with ethics, law is "a system of principles and processes by which people who live in a society attempt to control human conduct in an effort to minimize the use of force as a means of resolving conflicting interests" (Rhodes & Miller, 1984, p. 1). Neither ethics nor law is an exact science; thus, neither ethicists nor lawyers always are able to predict with precision what the outcome of an ethical or a legal conflict may be. Both, however, are sensitive to established, sanctioned, and sometimes changing rules that are culturally transmitted.

How, then, do ethics and law interface in nursing practice and administration? According to Smith and Davis (1980), there are four situations in which ethics and law interface:

1. That which is ethical is legal (e.g., informed consent).
2. That which is ethical is illegal (e.g., some would say euthanasia).

3. That which is unethical is legal (e.g., some would say abortion).
4. That which is unethical is illegal (e.g., involuntary medical treatment in nonemergency situations).

Two of the preceding situations are congruent and two are in conflict. These latter two situations often produce conflict for the nurse administrator.

Although there is no easy answer on how to resolve the preceding conflicts, the following statements serve to put the two in perspective:

1. The conflict between ethical and illegal and unethical and legal will probably always be with us. Ethics cannot be bound by the law when ethical considerations override legal ones. Law cannot be held hostage to ethics in the sense that a law cannot be enacted to control every immoral act. Therefore, the nurse administrator must expect this tension between ethics and law.

2. The role of the institutional lawyer and that of the nurse administrator may conflict. A primary purpose of institutional lawyers is to protect the institution and the people who work therein from legal entanglements. The primary purpose of the nurse administrator is to ensure that patients receive the best possible care. Therefore, a nurse administrator might reduce this conflict by recommending that a health care institution hire additional lawyers as advocates for patients. This other legal opinion would be helpful in achieving a balanced perspective between the needs of the institution and those of the patient.

3. Lawyers use basic tenets of ethics in formulating laws, and ethicists use laws or court decisions as part of their database in arriving at morally justified decisions. Ethics, however, is not the final determinant of law, and law is not the final determinant of ethics. According to Curtin (1982, p. 61), although the action decided on to resolve an ethical dilemma may be swayed by legal requirements, legal requirements are extrinsic to ethical reasoning and should not be confused with right or wrong.

4. If a conflict about resolution of an ethical dilemma exists among lawyers and nurses, then both should consider how the decision will affect those persons most affected by it. Sometimes one must stand alone but, at other times, reasonable compromise or acquiescence to a majority decision may be in the overall best interest of all (Curtin, 1982, p. 63).

As advances in science and technology precipitate more ethical and legal dilemmas, nurse administrators need greater understanding of the relationship between law and ethics. Pellegrino (1986) puts it well:

Defining relationships between law and ethics is crucial as more and more ethical conflicts are litigated. It is easy to forget that establishing legal procedures does not settle substantive ethical disputes. Health professionals are accountable moral agents. . . . Law and ethics are separate realms of necessity in constant interaction. A proper balance between them is essential to a just society, as is the maintenance of the integrity of both. (p. 2)

STANDARDS OF CARE AS ETHICAL CHOICES

Standards of care help nurse administrators ensure that they are creating and maintaining a professional nursing system within their health care institutions. Standards of care are not static; they reflect changing social, technological, and professional shifts. Nursing's reflection of these changing shifts, however, must always be responsible ones that ultimately are accountable to ethics, law, and the social contract between nursing and society. Regarding law and ethics, the American Nurses' Association's (ANA) Commission on Nursing Services (1982) says,

> Nursing policies and practices . . . [should be] congruent with the ANA *Code for Nurses*, the ANA *Standards for Organized Nursing Services*, the ANA *Standards of Nursing Practice*, the state nursing practice act, the standards of the voluntary accrediting body appropriate to the agency, and the requirements of the regulatory body appropriate to the agency. (p. 9)

Regarding the social contract between nursing and society, the Commission (1982) says, "The social contract between society and the nursing profession grants authority to the profession over functions vital to society and in return expects the profession to act responsibly through self-regulation" (p. 2). The ANA's Commission on Nursing Services (1982) has seven standards of care for organized nursing services, which are shown in Table 1–3.

How, then, do these standards reflect ethics and, thus, ethical choice? Standard I, with its emphasis on high quality nursing care and appropriate methods for the resolution of nursing practice issues, is compatible with the ethical principle of beneficence. Concern with quality care reflects the desire of nurse administrators to provide an atmosphere where patients and families are neither harmed nor placed at risk of harm. High quality care also reflects the commitment of nurse administrators to go beyond lack of harm to the promotion of good. Likewise, appropriate means for resolving nursing practice issues benefit patients.

Standard II, with its emphasis on a nurse executive who is qualified, is compatible with the ethical principles of beneficence and justice. According to criteria defining this standard, only persons who are registered nurses knowledgeable in nursing practice and administration and who have been appropriately educated and certified should serve as nurse administrators. Why? Prepared nurse administrators are more likely to implement the mechanisms needed to ensure quality care than unprepared ones. Thus, less harm and more good will come to patients. In addition, qualified nurse administrators are better prepared to handle fiscal matters. Management of funds to ensure fair allocation of available resources is consistent with the ethical principle of distributive justice.

TABLE 1-3. ANA STANDARDS FOR ORGANIZED NURSING SERVICES

Standard I	The division of nursing has a philosophy and structure that assure the delivery of high quality nursing care and provide means for resolving nursing practice issues throughout the health care organization. (p. 3)
Standard II	The division of nursing is administered by a qualified nurse executive who is a member of corporate administration. (p. 4)
Standard III	Policies and practices of the division of nursing provide for equality and continuity of nursing services that recognize cultural, economic, and social differences among patients of the health care organization. (p. 4)
Standard IV	The division of nursing ensures that the nursing process is used to design and provide nursing care to meet the individual needs of patients/clients in the context of their families. (p. 5)
Standard V	The division of nursing provides an environment that ensures the effectiveness of nursing practice. (p. 6)
Standard VI	The division of nursing assures the development of educational programs to support the delivery of high quality nursing care. (p. 6)
Standard VII	The division of nursing initiates, utilizes, and participates in research studies or projects for the improvement of patient care. (p. 7)

From American Nurses' Association Commission on Nursing Services. (1982). Standards for organized nursing services. *Kansas City, MO: American Nurses' Association.*

Standards III and IV, with their emphasis on recognizing individual differences, are compatible with the ethical principle of respect for persons. Respect for persons means that nurse administrators have the ability to feel empathy for patients and families and to formulate policies and practices that treat patients and families as ends and never as mere means to ends. In addition, Standard IV, with its emphasis on needs, highlights the following material principle of justice: "to each patient according to basic need."

Standards V and VI, with their emphasis on an environment that ensures effective nursing practice, are consistent with the ethical principles of beneficence and justice. Whereas Standards III and IV focus on care of patients and families, Standards V and VI reflect the commitment of nurse administrators to promote good by contributing to the welfare of their employees. In addition, one criterion for Standard V specifies that the performance of the nurse should be recognized. This criterion is compatible with the material principle of justice that specifies "to each person according to merit."

Finally, Standard VII, with its emphasis on advancement of nursing practice through research, is consistent with the ethical principle of respect for autonomy. Criteria for the standard make clear that the rights of human subjects in research should be protected. Usually this protection is ensured through an enformed consent. Essential components of an informed consent include adequate disclosure of study purpose, procedures, risks and benefits, and sufficient understanding of them. To the extent that these criteria are met without controlling constraints, the research subject is free to decide whether or not to participate in research.

In summary, standards of care reflect underlying ethical concepts and principles (and vice versa). Although I have highlighted only a few of these relationships, nurse administrators should be able to see that, to the degree that they organize nursing services around these standards, they have made a choice for the ethical integrity of nursing in their institutions. On the other hand, to the degree that nurse administrators ignore or violate these standards, they have compromised the ethical integrity of nursing in their institutions. The choice is up to the nurse administrator.

BIOGRAPHICAL SKETCH

Mary Silva received her BSN and MS from the Ohio State University and her PhD from the University of Maryland. In addition, as a Kennedy Fellow in Medical Ethics for Nursing Faculty, she undertook postdoctoral study in ethics at Georgetown University. Recently, she was a Visiting Scholar at The Hastings Center, Briarcliff Manor, New York. Since 1984, Dr Silva has served as Project Director on a Special Project Grant funded by the Division of Nursing on ethical decision making for nurse executives. She is a Professor and Director, Center for Nursing Ethics, George Mason University, Fairfax, VA, and a Fellow in the American Academy of Nursing.

SUGGESTED READING

Codes

American Nurses' Association. (1985). *Code for nurses with interpretive statements.* Kansas City, MO: American Nurses' Association.

American Nurses' Association. (1985). *Human rights guidelines for nurses in clinical and other research.* Kansas City, MO: American Nurses' Association.

International Council of Nurses. (1973). *Code for nurses: Ethical concepts applied to nursing.* Geneva, Switzerland: International Council of Nurses.

Bibliographies

American Nurses' Association. (1982). *Ethics references for nurses.* Kansas City, MO: American Nurses' Association.

Pence, T. (1986). *Ethics in nursing: An annotated bibliography* (2nd ed.). New York: National League for Nursing.

Walters, L. (Ed.). (1975–1980). *Bibliography of bioethics* (Vols. 1–6). Detroit, MI: Gale Research.

Walters, L. (Ed.). (1981–1983). *Bibliography of bioethics* (Vols. 7–9). New York: Free-Press, Macmillan.

Walters, L., & Kahn, T. J. (1984–1986). *Bibliography of bioethics* (Vols. 10–12). Washington, D.C.: Kennedy Institute of Ethics.

Encyclopedia

Reich, W. T. (Ed.). (1978). *Encyclopedia of bioethics* (4 vols.). New York: Free-Press, Macmillan.

General Source of Bioethics Information

Goldstein, D.M. (1982). *Bioethics: A guide to information sources*. Detroit, MI: Gale Research.

Books

Beauchamp, T.L. (1982). *Philosophical ethics: An introduction to moral philosophy*. New York: McGraw-Hill.

Beauchamp, T.L., & Childress, J.F. (1983). *Principles of biomedical ethics* (2nd ed.). New York: Oxford University Press.

Benjamin, M., & Curtis, J. (1986). *Ethics in nursing* (2nd ed.). New York: Oxford University Press.

Cranford, R.E., & Doudera, A.E. (Eds.). (1984). *Institutional ethics committees and health care decision making*. Ann Arbor, MI: Health Administration Press.

Mappes, T.A., & Zembaty, J.S. (1986). *Biomedical ethics* (2nd. ed.). New York: McGraw-Hill.

Thompson, J.E., & Thompson, H.O. (1985). *Bioethical decision making or nurses*. Norwalk, CT: Appleton-Century-Crofts.

Veatch, R.M., & Fry, S.T. (1987). *Case studies in nursing ethics*. Philadelphia: Lippincott.

Wright, R.A. (1987). *Human values in health care: The practice of ethics*. New York: McGraw-Hill.

Computerized Data Base

Bioethicsline is an automated data base containing over 10,000 references on bioethics. It is developed and maintained at the Center for Bioethics, Kennedy Institute of Ethics, Georgetown University, Washington, D.C. Bioethicsline is available via the National Library of Medicine's MEDLARS system.

Videoseries

Ethics in Nursing is a 5-unit videoseries on ethics in nursing administration that is presented by Mary Silva, Professor, George Mason University and Tom L. Beauchamp, Senior Research Scholar, the Kennedy Institute of Ethics. The videoseries contains content on moral justification, ethical theories, ethical principles, and allocation of scarce resources. For more information, call *Nursing Economic$* at (609) 589-2319.

REFERENCES

American Nurses' Association Commission on Nursing Services. (1982). *Standards for organized nursing services*. Kansas City, MO: American Nurses' Association.

Beauchamp, T.L. (1982). *Philosophical ethics: An introduction to moral philosophy.* New York: McGraw-Hill.

Beauchamp, T.L., & Childress, J.F. (1983). *Principles of biomedical ethics* (2nd ed.). New York: Oxford University Press.

Curtin, L. (1982). No rush to judgment. In L. Curtin & M.J. Flaherty (eds.), *Nursing ethics: Theories and pragmatics.* Bowie, MD: Brady, pp. 57–63.

Faden, R.R., & Beauchamp, T.L. (1986). *A history and theory of informed consent.* New York: Oxford University Press.

Frankena, W.K. (1973). *Ethics* (2nd ed.). Englewood Cliffs, NJ: Prentice-Hall.

Jameton, A. (1984). *Nursing practice: The ethical issues.* Englewood Cliffs, NJ: Prentice-Hall.

Kant, I. (1981). *Grounding for the metaphysics of morals* (J.W. Ellington, Trans.). Indianapolis: Hackett. (Original work published 1785.)

Mappes, T.A., & Zembaty, J.S. (1986). *Biomedical ethics* (2nd ed.). New York: McGraw-Hill.

Munson, R. (1983). *Intervention and reflection: Basic issues in medical ethics* (2nd ed.). Belmont, CA: Wadsworth.

Pellegrino, E.D. (1986). Controversy looms at the intersection of law and ethics. *Kennedy Institute of Ethics Newsletter, 1*(5), 1–2.

Rhodes, A.M., & Miller, R.D. (1984). *Nursing & the Law* (4th ed.). Rockville, MD: Aspen.

Ross, W.D. (1930). *The right and the good.* Oxford: Oxford University Press.

Silva, M.C. (1984). Ethics, scarce resources, and the nurse executive. *Nursing Economic$, 2*(1), 11–18.

Smith, S.J., & Davis, A.J. (1980). Ethical dilemmas: Conflicts among rights, duties, and obligations. *American Journal of Nursing, 80,* 1462–1466.

Veatch, R.M. (1981). *A theory of medical ethics.* New York: Basic Books.

Veatch, R.M., & Fry, S.T. (1987). *Case studies in nursing ethics.* Philadelphia: Lippincott.

APPLICATION 1–1

Moral Reasoning in Personnel Decisions
Patricia Snyder

Biomedical ethics, allocation of scarce resources, and standards of care all come immediately to mind as areas of continual concern to the nurse administrator, which at times present extremely difficult ethical choices. Obviously, the need of patients for nursing care that meets accepted standards is the overriding issue. Complicating the problem of achieving this goal, however, are competing needs and rightful claims that must be reconciled with each other and with the patient care mission of the organization.

Decisions must be made in light of nurse administrators responsibility to their organization's goals and objectives which are essential to organizational stability and growth. Nurse administrators must also look at their responsibility to honor the contract between the nursing profession and society, to promote the public good in provision of health care, and to meet societal demands for conservation of resources and control of costs. In some situations these two responsibilities may conflict.

In addition to the organization itself, patients and their families, and society as a whole, nurse administrators must also be cognizant of ethical considerations involved in the management of one especially valuable resource—nursing personnel who staff the health care facility. The response of nurse administrators to this last constituency, and the issues that arise in regard to it, are the primary focus of this discussion.

Ethical dilemmas present themselves in all areas of personnel management. Patient care delivery issues notwithstanding, the staff has a legitimate claim on the nurse administrator for decisions that acknowledge their individual needs and rights as well as their responsibilities to their patients, their profession, and the organization that employs them.

Decision making in personnel management is most commonly discussed in relation to the organization's need to secure adequate numbers of motivated staff who are qualified and competent to carry out their responsibilities and to use this staff in a manner that maintains costs within budgeted limits. Legal and risk management considerations involved in employer–employee relationships are also given considerable attention. Another dimension of the issue is the right of the nurses in the ethical consideration of their welfare as individuals and their need for growth as professionals through their association with the health care organization.

Maintaining conditions of employment that promote high standards of practice is clearly identified as one ethical responsibility of nurses by the American Nurses' Association Code for Nurses (1985). Structuring the organization to permit autonomous practice is one manifestation of the efforts to achieve this goal. The supervisory relationship with each nurse affects all aspects of growth as a nurse and as an individual and is, therefore, another perhaps more profound manifestation. Whether the issue is selection, orientation and staff development, promotion, performance appraisal, discipline, or the components of the reward system, a clear understanding of the ethical principles involved is critical to the consideration of each nurse's rights as an individual with inherent dignity.

Ethical dilemmas encountered in management of personnel are exacerbated by the recent emphasis on cost containment and careful use of all types of resources in the health care industry. As organizations have acted to reduce costs in relation to benefits received, slack resources have shrunk, sometimes into nonexistence. At times, decreases have resulted in levels of expenditures viewed by individual practitioners as not only lean but inadequate. At such times, creativity and wisdom is required on the part of nurse administrators to respond to competing rightful claims for the allocation of available resources.

Simultaneously, administrators find themselves with fewer options in making ethical choices in personnel management. As slack resources have disappeared, the number of solutions available to respond to employee needs, both as individuals and in groups, has also shrunk, making the choices more problematic.

We have recently become more acutely aware of the importance of ethical decision making in personnel matters as we struggle to manage in the face of the growing nursing shortage. Its influence is felt in a myriad of ways within the organization as priorities are set and decisions made. Long-term conservation of nursing resources becomes an even more pressing concern as we strive to create an environment that responds to nurses' professional satisfaction. As we address this issue some of the more common responses to other personnel management problems demand reexamination.

In doing so, we become more aware of some of the ethical principles that must be applied in relationships with employees as well as patients: confidentiality; justice; autonomy, defined as independent decision making; nonmalfeasance (avoidance of harmful actions); and beneficence. Acknowledgment of the employee's dignity as an individual and truthfulness also must apply.

As a stimulus to clarification of some of the ethical dilemmas that apply to personnel management a number of situations are described. Each is common—or at least far from unique—in health care settings.

Consider this first example: a nurse is observed by her supervisor, two hours after the beginning of an evening shift, to be displaying marked symptoms of alcohol intoxication. She is confronted in private about the situation and acknowledges tearfully that she has, in fact, been ingesting alcohol. She is replaced on the unit by another nurse, calls a family member to provide transportation home, and is instructed to return the following day for a meeting with the supervisor.

At that time, she is referred to the employee assistance service where she indicates her willingness to accept treatment. A referral is made to an intensive outpatient program as she refuses inpatient care. Because she is in treatment she is permitted to return to work. Several days later she again reports to work intoxicated.

In considering a decision on her next action, the unit nurse manager knows that the staff has recently been reorganizing after heavy turnover and they are stressed by an especially demanding patient population. No one is able to assume another's burden. The staff on each shift needs to know that each member can "pull their own weight." And certainly, the nurse manager must be able to rely on the ability of those assigned to report punctually and ready to work so that all patients will be safely cared for.

But the nurse in question is an individual suffering from a disease with a right to treatment and assistance in seeking it. Should she be placed on a leave of absence? She could not be replaced by another regular employee and her peers would be burdened by working with less productive temporary staff—an eventuality that may do them harm—and that may impact negatively on patient care. Should the nurse be discharged or requested to resign? What impact would such an action have on her ability to accept treatment? What impact will any of these actions by the nurse manager have on a staff group that is not yet soundly cohesive?

All of the above questions can be viewed from an organizational behavior viewpoint and in legal terms. In addition, the thoughtful nurse manager will want to consider the impact of her choices based on the ethical principles described earlier. An action that avoids harm to one party in the situation may well be seen as harmful to another. Which has the greatest claim? And how will the nurse administrator who supervises the unit manager guide her in exploring the situation?

The conflict between the needs of the work group and the organization and the individual can be seen as well in the following situation. The nurse administrator selects a new unit nurse manager who is a talented clinician and has shown promise as a manager in a charge nurse role. She is provided with an orientation to her new position and receives ongoing supervision. But, as often happens, she is faced early on with difficult problems. She works energetically to master her new role but finds it very hard to remove herself sufficiently from direct patient care involvement and her former place in the staff group. As time goes by, the nurse administrator recognizes deterioration in the unit's functioning and is forced to the conclusion that the promotion may have been an inappropriate one. She recognizes that intervention is indicated.

For how long, and how intensively, does justice demand that additional training and support be provided to maintain the new nurse manager in her role? On the other hand, to what extent can the staff justly be expected to function in a troubled situation? Removing her from her position must be considered. But when—to minimize harm to all concerned? What of the nurse manager herself? She has accepted her role in good faith and tried hard to fill it but is apparently not well suited to it. What impact does leaving it feeling unsuccessful have on her personally and professionally? How can she be helped to feel competent to pursue another course better suited to her talents? The nurse administrator is concerned with justice to all but also with doing good to a professional whose efforts have been energetic and well-motivated, if ineffective. She must also consider the need of society and the profession to preserve this individual as a valuable asset in another area of practice. All of these considerations may make intervention more complex and demanding of time and energy than a less thoughtful resolution of the problem might. Also, the nurse administrator must decide how much of the organization's resources can rightly be invested in this effort, balancing the claims of all.

The issue of the organization's duty to an employee can be studied further through exploration of another example with some similar themes. An inexperienced nurse manager is faced with several staff vacancies and is struggling to cover the unit with too few resources. She makes an impulsive decision in hiring a psychiatric technician, discounting indications obtained in the interview that he may not be well suited to care for the patient population in question. In addition, because the unit is short-staffed, his orientation is hasty and superficial. The initial employment period is marked by erratic performance and a decision must be made about his continued employment.

The moral responsibility the organization has in relation to the employee's predicament and the impact that it should have on the decision that is made about him must be determined. Did the organization fail him by placing him in an impossible situation through a flawed selection process? Did he accept a position knowing he was ill-equipped to perform well? Does that influence the organization's obligations to assist him in succeeding? The nurse manager needs to decide if there is reasonable hope of his performance improving and what resources are required to accomplish this goal. Are they available or must they be used in another way? The nurse administrator will want to assess the adequacy of the supervision given the unit manager during the selection process. Should this be considered in the decision? And the other staff? How much assistance, for how long, can they be rightfully expected to provide in an effort to continue his employment? Very careful assessment of the situation is required to ensure that such a troubled employee receives just treatment but that others' needs are met as well.

At times, an individual may, by her own unethical activity seem to compromise her claims on the organization, although legal constraints may still apply. Consider the case of a powerful informal leader in a staff group who is discharged for cause. Her right to confidentiality precludes informing the staff group of the circumstances surrounding this disciplinary action and the events leading to it are unknown to the others. The discharged employee gives members of the staff group a highly distorted account of the events. Because of her powerful influence with the group members, and the fact that she has for some time assumed an adversarial stance in relation to the unit manager, she is able to portray her situation as being the result of punitive action by the manager. Turmoil erupts and the unit manager finds herself the recipient of considerable anger that is having a deleterious effect on the staff's ability to accomplish its work.

What actions can she ethically take to restore equilibrium? Must the discharged employee's confidentiality be maintained at all costs? The staff group's need to function smoothly in the interest of completing their patient care mission might be viewed as the overriding value. What part does the staff's responsibility to respond to their environment in a mature, thoughtful manner play in the choice of a course of action? Can they be led to assume a problem-solving approach to the situation while confidentiality is still maintained? And if not, what of the nurse manager herself? To what extent must she subject herself to untruthful accusations to protect one who has behaved unethically? How much of the organization's resources should rightfully be invested in an effort to maintain the former employee's confidentiality?

Ethical decision making for the nurse administrator in personnel matters frequently extends to groups as well as to individuals. This is an area that is becoming particularly troublesome as the shortage of nurses increases.

One nurse administrator—who is undoubtedly far from alone in her dilemma—finds herself faced with an unacceptably high vacancy rate. Clearly recruitment and hiring practices must change drastically as more conservative measures have not produced sufficient improvement.

Her organization serves a disadvantaged patient population that often only seeks medical care when acutely ill and frequently has multiple, complex problems. In the past, she has avoided hiring newly graduated nurses because she judged the work situation to be too demanding for their limited skills. Staff development resources are very limited in her organization and she has not felt that she can provide adequate orientation and ongoing training. Faced with rising costs for temporary personnel and increasing inconsistency in providing patient care, she develops a plan of action. Staff development personnel are diverted from usual activities to organize an intensive orientation for new graduates and two senior staff nurses are removed from an already lean complement to act as preceptors. The nurse administrator is still not sure that new graduates can be given adequate supervision and support for a long enough time to become independent and self-confident. She worries that some may find themselves overwhelmed and leave, perhaps even leave the profession.

Has she behaved ethically? Has she taken unwarranted risks that jeopardize the development of new practitioners? Are these risks justified given the fact that her facility meets a community need for services not available elsewhere and protection of its long-term stability is important? Has she too severely compromised current patient care delivery to improve the long-term situation by detailing the senior staff nurses to staff development? Is the overriding concern protection of the need of society to have scarce nursing resources preserved whenever possible, even at the expense of more immediate demands for patient services?

Reaching ethical conclusions in dilemmas such as these requires the use of a sound theoretical base. The nurse administrator's understanding of the principles involved must be coupled with a firm grasp on the moral reasoning underpinning ethical systems. So armed, administrators will be equipped to fulfill their responsibility to honor the rightful claims of those who are affected by these decisions—the patient, the nursing staff, and the organization.

Nurse administrators will find, at the same time, that the beneficial outcomes of using an ethical approach to decision making will extend beyond the individual dilemmas to which it is applied. One important responsibility of nurse administrators in leading staff to achieve high standards of professional practice is to assist them to incorporate ethical dimensions into all aspects of their practice, not only those that are currently receiving wide attention as ethical and moral issues.

Achieving this goal requires development of a certain sensitivity to the presence of ethical concerns, as well as an ability to think in ethical terms. Nurse administrators will find that including ethical principles in a clear and explicit manner in their rationale for the decisions they make will have a positive influence on the ability of the staff to do likewise. Role modeling, the process of including ethical principles in problem-solving, especially in personnel matters, will demonstrate with the special clarity gained through personal experiences the salutary effect of acting in accordance with an ethical theory framework. Having experienced it themselves, and having it taught as an inherent part of the philosophy of the nursing department, staff members will be prepared to grow in their ability to respond to ethical demands in their own area of practice.

BIOGRAPHICAL SKETCH

Patricia Snyder is Director of Nursing at Dominion Hospital in Falls Church, VA, an acute care facility providing treatment to psychiatric and chemical dependency patients. She has held a variety of positions in both public and private psychiatric hospitals. She received her BSN from Duquesne University, Pittsburgh, PA and an MSN in Nursing Administration from George Mason University. She is a member of Sigma Theta Tau, the American Organization of Nurse Executives and is active in the Virginia Nurses Association.

2

Legal Aspects
of Nursing Administration

Harold L. Hirsh

The nurse administrator needs to be cognizant of four major areas of law: nursing practice, administration, labor–management, and employment, especially regarding professional workers. This chapter discusses the issues and current practices in each of these areas.

NURSING PRACTICE: LEGAL LIABILITY

Scope of Nursing Practice

The scope of nursing practice is defined in each state by its "nurse practice act" and common law. In recent years many states have changed their acts to reflect more clearly current practice. A problem area has been the definition of the nurse's role in diagnosis, evaluation, or assessment, particularly as differentiated from the physician's role (Cohn, 1984). Clearly there is overlap, particularly involving the nurse practitioner. Some states have resolved this issue by defining nurses as able to screen and identify and physicians as additionally able to prescribe the course of treatment.

Nurse practice acts and common law define three types of nurses: licensed practical nurse, registered nurse, and nurse practitioner. These practice acts vary widely in: (1) establishing educational and examination requirements, (2) providing for licensing or regulation of individuals who have met the requirements, and (3) defining the functions of each type of nurse in general and in specific terms. They also set up public boards of nursing examiners to administer the practice acts.

Boards of Nursing Examiners

The licensing board in each state is responsible for licensing nurses and for suspending or revoking the licenses for just cause. Suspension is temporary denial of the right to practice nursing. Revocation is permanent withdrawal of permission to practice nursing. Most nurse practice acts provide that nursing licenses can be revoked if obtained through fraud or the practitioner is found guilty of gross immorality, illegal activity, or malpractice. All nurse practice acts provide for the loss of license for *unprofessional conduct*. Few, however, define what this constitutes, making it very difficult for courts to decide appeals other than those stemming from drug or alcohol misuse or addiction.

The Nurse and Corporate Liability

Recent judicial decisions have imposed the doctrine of corporate liability on hospitals. Corporate liability has grown with the hospital's deepening involvement in patient care. Hospitals are now responsible for credentialing and recredentialing members of the medical staff, monitoring the competence of care delivered within their institutions, and actively and affirmatively intervening on behalf of the patient when the care is substandard. This is achieved largely through medical employees, particularly nurses. Therefore, to speak of the hospital's increasing responsibility is to speak of the nurse's expanding duties as well. Nurses are now health care providers in their own right. Nurses have assumed the role of guardian or ombudsmen for the patient. (Creighton, 1984).

The nurse must take action to eliminate any real or perceived danger to the patient. Merely notifying the immediate supervisor, if the nurse knows this will not eliminate the danger, is not enough. The nurse's duty extends to reporting incompetent, unethical, or illegal practice to the appropriate authority within the institution. If the practice is not corrected within the employment setting, then it is the nurse's duty to report it to an appropriate professional organization or legally constituted licensing body. Failure to carry out the mandate may render the nurse or the employing institution, or both, liable for resultant injuries (Hirsh, 1981).

As employees, nurses often have a false sense of security about their responsibilities and liabilities. This has been fostered by the legal doctrines of *respondeat superior* and *vicarious liability*, which allow a patient to sue the employer if the nurse deviates from the standard of care. Respondeat superior translated means "let the master answer" and refers to the legal principle that an employer is legally responsible for the wrongful acts of the employees.

Vicarious liability comes about when employees are under the immediate direction, supervision, and control of the employer while carrying out their job. This doctrine, however, does not preclude the nurse from being sued separately, in addition to the employer. It does not protect the nurse when the employer or insurance carrier sues the nurse for damages they have incurred due to his or her practice. Some hospitals offer liability insurance to nurses as a benefit. Nurses should be aware if they have liability coverage (Fiesta, 1983).

Malpractice

Malpractice has been defined as any professional misconduct, unreasonable lack of skill or fidelity in professional or fiduciary duties, evil practice, or illegal or immoral conduct. Malpractice suits generally come from angry patients who have poor results from treatment. Friendly patients who feel that nurses and doctors have done their best are not as likely to sue.

Most malpractice suits against nurses are *torts*, which are private civil wrongs committed by one individual against another. Torts are predicated on the duty one person owes another, either to do something for the person or not to do something that will hurt the person. The law imposes greater legal burdens on nurses because of their greater, unique knowledge, training, and expertise. Thus, the nurse–patient relationship is legally based on fiduciary duty rather than contract. Most malpractice actions brought against nurses usually involve negligence but increasing numbers charge assault and battery, invasion of privacy, false imprisonment, fraud, deceit, or defamation (Wiemerslage, 1983). These are discussed later.

Because malpractice involves matters outside general knowledge, these criteria must generally be established by an acceptable medical expert such as a nurse or a physician. This means that the patient must find an expert or demonstrate "res ipsa loquitur."

Res ipsa loquitur means "the thing speaks for itself." Three conditions are necessary before this rule may be applied: (1) that in the ordinary course of affairs the accident would not have occurred if reasonable care had been used; (2) that the thing that caused the accident was under the exclusive control of the nurse; and (3) that the patient did not contribute to the occurrence of the accident. When the patient proves that these conditions exist, it is regarded in some states as circumstantial evidence of negligence, which judge or jury may accept or reject. In other states, it creates a presumption of negligence, which must be accepted (Guarriello, 1982, Philpott, 1985).

Assault and Battery

Assault and battery are two words we often hear together, but they have separate meanings. Assault is the unjustifiable attempt to touch another person or the threat to do so in such circumstances as to cause the other reasonably to believe that it will be carried out. Battery involves an intentional act that is a harmful or offensive touching of another without that person's consent. Medical care and treatment without informed consent that involves the touching of another person has been held to constitute a battery. The lack of consent or privilege is an important part of the meaning of assault and battery. If a nurse goes beyond the limits to which a patient consented, the nurse may be liable (RNs, 1982).

Privacy and Confidentiality

Privacy is a patients' right to have peace of mind regarding the exposure and revelation of their body or depictions thereof to unauthorized persons. Confidentiality is the identical right to privacy of records. Patients' right to privacy and confidentiality has one of the highest priorities in our legal system. Nurses are duty-bound to protect that right.

The courts have limited access to both the patient's body and records to "charter members" of the health care team: attending physicians, assigned house officers, all nursing personnel, technicians, orderlies, ward clerks, therapists, social service workers, and patient advocates.

Consultants, students in the health professions, and chaplains are not charter members of the health care team. Patients must be informed of their involvement and given the opportunity to agree or reject them. Ward rounds, patient examinations, and conferences may be attended only by charter members, unless the patient has given prior consent.

The administration of the health care institution is entitled to review the patient's record without consent for three purposes only: statistical analysis, staffing, and quality of care review. When the patient is discharged, only the attending physician retains the right to review the record in perpetuity, unless the consent of the patient or surrogate is obtained.

Health care institutions are charged with responsibility of continuity of care. Therefore, no patient should suffer when moved from one facility to another. Adequate information should be transferred with the patient to ensure continuity of care. A transfer agreement between the discharging and receiving institutions is a good solution to this problem. Such an agreement could specify the exchange of information necessary for continuity of care. Although theoretically the patient's consent is not needed, it is better to secure it.

In this country, the relationship between physician and patient generally enjoys the protection of *privileged communications* in civil, but not criminal, matters. Privileged communication is a statutory rule forbidding physicians from disclosing information learned in the course of treating a patient, unless the patient permits it. It is a rule for the protection of patients so they may feel free to be open and frank about their condition or history.

A few states have extended the protection of privileged communications to the nurse as the primary care provider. In these states, nurses cannot disclose patient information obtained during the course of care, unless such information relates to the commission of a crime. The same rule applies if the nurse receives the information concurrently with the physician.

Defamation

Defamation consists of the verbal or written communication about someone to another that injures that person's reputation. *Slander* is oral defamation; *libel* is written defamation. Because slander is less weighty than libel, slander is usually not actionable unless actual damage is proved by the plaintiff. The information must be believed by the third party who then acts to the detriment of the defamed party. Truth is a defense to suits for defamation.

The administration can reduce the probability of defamation among health care providers by establishing an effective process by which any caregiver can register complaints about the quantity or quality of patient service rendered by another in an objective, confidential, and effective fashion. Each health institution should have a policy and procedure for these situations (Greenlaw, 1980).

Many hospitals have been sued for libel or slander by former staff members based on statements in unfavorable evaluations, termination notices, and responses to inquiries from prospective employers. The law, depending on the jurisdiction, extends a *qualified or absolute privilege* to such communications and there is no liability as long as the administrator was reporting what she believed was true without intending malice.

False Imprisonment

False imprisonment occurs when there is an intentional and unprivileged nonconsensual confinement of an individual. It is the unlawful restraint of an individual's personal liberty. A reasonable fear of force, rather than confinement itself, is all that is required. The tort of false imprisonment has been found in cases where patients have been detained in a hospital for failure to pay their bills, or when a patient who is not a danger to self or others was prevented from signing out against medical advice. Restraining a patient unnecessarily or with excessive or unnecessary force may constitute false imprisonment and possibly battery.

Damages and the Statute of Limitations

Under our system of law, patients who have suffered calculable harm from treatment by health care providers may sue to be made "whole" again economically. More often than not, it is impossible to completely alleviate scars or pain. To that end, our courts award the victim money damages to compensate for the injury. There are three types of damages: nominal, compensatory, and punitive.

Occasionally, an injured person has suffered essentially no loss. Under these circumstances the trier of fact, jury and judge, may award the plaintiff *nominal damages*. The claimant receives merely a token sum, one cent or one dollar, depending on the jurisdiction. The plaintiff receives the satisfaction of having the claim vindicated. Financially the losing defendant has to pay court costs, which are often significant, and sometimes at the judge's discretion, the plaintiff's attorney's fees.

When the injury has resulted in significant harm, the claimant is awarded *compensatory damages*. There are two types of compensatory damages: special and general. *Special damages* are reimbursement for actual economic loss. These include payments for medical care, physician, hospital, and nursing care fees, medicine, transportation incurred in recovering from the injury, and loss of wages. These must be shown to be usual, customary, and reasonable charges actually incurred.

General damages are awarded for emotional injury including pain and suffering, indignation associated with the injury, mental anguish including anxiety, tension, and nervousness, grief, and other related symptoms or complaints. Their existence, severity, duration, and future impact must be established by expert testimony. Our legal system allows the jury and judge to set monetary awards for these injuries based on the proof that the plaintiff, through their lawyer, can establish. In the last two years many state legislatures have put a "cap" on noneconomic damages in the amount of $250,000 to $500,000.

On rare occasions when the defendant's conduct has been grossly negligent, willfull, malicious, or with utter reckless disregard of the consequences of the acts, the courts allow *punitive damages*. These are in the nature of a criminal punishment or fine.

A basic concept of common law is to settle legal disputes peacefully within a period of time in a "civilized" manner. An alleged wrongdoer, whether he or she has committed a tort, a crime, or a breach of contract, should not be held in legal jeopardy in perpetuity. The plaintiff must bring the complaint against the defendant within a legislatively prescribed period of time, within the *statute of limitations*. Each jurisdiction sets its own statutes of limitations. If a lawsuit is not brought within the statutory period, the defendant may successfully have the lawsuit dismissed because the plaintiff failed to bring the suit in a timely fashion.

Frequently there is a question as to when the statute of limitations begins. Because many medical negligence injuries are latent and are not discoverable by the patient for a significant period of time that may be beyond the statutory period, almost all jurisdictions have adopted the "discovery" rule, which allows the statute of limitations to begin when they find out, or should have found out, about the alleged negligence.

Negligence

The law imposes certain specific responsibilities on the nurse with respect to both the duty and the standard of care to be given a patient. A nurse has a *fiduciary duty*, meaning a position of trust with the patient, and must exercise the degree of care and skill that a reasonably prudent nurse with similar training and experience practicing nursing would exhibit under similar circumstances (Annas, Glantz & Katz, 1981).

Negligence by the nurse can be defined as (1) the failure to do something that a reasonable nurse guided by those considerations that ordinarily regulate the conduct of nursing would do; (2) the doing of something that a prudent and reasonable nurse would not do; (3) the failure to exercise ordinary care under the circumstances; (4) conduct that a reasonably prudent nurse should realize involved an unreasonable risk of invading a patient's interest; and (5) a failure to do an act that is necessary for the protection or assistance of a patient.

To establish negligence on the part of a nurse, a patient must provide evidence that the nurse *owed a duty to the patient*, that the *duty was breached*, and that the *breach of duty has caused injury* to the patient *resulting in damages*. See Table 2-1 for a summary. The liability of nurses is reduced if they can show that the patient had *contributory negligence*, meaning conduct on the part of the patient that was a contributing cause to his or her own injuries. Another defense that may remove liability for nurses is if they can show that their act was in self-protection and a reasonable action or inaction in the face of danger (Walker, 1983).

In common law, patient's contributory negligence was an absolute and a

TABLE 2-1. REQUIREMENTS TO PROVE NEGLIGENCE IN A COURT SUIT

1. Nurse had a "fiduciary" duty to provide nursing care to the individual.
2. The duty was breached by violation of the standard of care.
3. The breach of duty was not reasonable self-protection by the nurse in fear of danger.
4. Injury occurred that led to calculable harm.
5. The injury was caused by the breach of duty.
6. Contributory negligence by the injured individual was not present (this reduces but does not remove nurse liability).
7. The statute of limitations for the injury has not been exceeded.

complete bar to any recovery for damages. Because this caused many harsh results, most states have adopted the doctrine of comparative negligence. Here, malpractice recovery places the economic loss on the parties in proportion to their fault. In a few states patients can still recover a percentage of their damages even where their own negligence exceeds that of the defendant.

Standard of Care. What does *standard of care* mean? Courts have generally expressed this by stating that in the performance of professional duties, nurses are required to exercise the same degree of care and skill that a reasonably prudent nurse with similar training and experience practicing nursing would exercise under similar circumstances. The degree of care required of nurses is relative, based on their qualifications, experience, and education. These are always taken into consideration in determining whether they acted with reasonable care in a given situation.

In the past, courts recognized a standard of care as applying to practices in the same or similar locality or community. Recently, national standards have been invoked for the health professions and hospitals. The more specialized a nurse becomes, the more likely the nurse is to be held to national standard. Thus, nurses need to be aware of both the community and national standards established by their professional organizations and organized specialty groups. Legally, "doing the best you can" is not a plausible defense (Bennett, 1983).

Where there is more than one recognized standard of care for a diagnosis or treatment alternative, and neither is used exclusively and uniformly by all practitioners in good standing, nurses are not negligent if, in exercising their best judgment they select one of the approved standard methods that later turns out poorly. In other words, choosing less than the best is not a legal liability.

Standardized Procedures. A standardized procedure is necessary when the function requires the nurse to perform procedures that require judgment based on medical knowledge beyond that usually possessed by a competent nurse in the area for which it is being considered.

Standardized procedures must be in writing and must be authorized by the health care institution. A written record of persons authorized to perform standardized procedures must be maintained by the institution. The standardized procedure must specify (1) the functions that the nurse may perform under specific circumstances; (2) any requirements that must be followed in performing that function; (3) the requisite education, experience, and training of the nurse performing the procedure; and (4) the methods for initial and continuing evaluation of the nurse's competence in performing the standardized procedure (Walker, 1980).

If a nurse without the necessary authority of a standardized procedure performs acts that result in injury to a patient, a presumption of negligence may result against the nurse. This has been called the *holding self out* doctrine; alleging that one can do something that in reality one is not qualified to do.

Protection of Patients and Public from Harm. Nurses are obligated to protect patients from injury by other patients as well as from injury by staff members and themselves. Therefore, nurses must record and report hostile patient behavior as indicative that the individual might become dangerously violent or assaultive toward others. Furthermore, the nurse manager also has a legal obligation to notify the institution's chief administrator when conditions of understaffing endanger patient welfare. Nurses must promptly and effectively communicate their observations. Furthermore, nurses are to observe patients more closely when their condition implies increased risk of hazard and document actions taken to protect these patients (Veatch & Fry, 1987).

Nurses also have a legal duty to protect the public from injury by dangerous patients. Nurse managers should ensure that the health institution in which they are employed has a clearly defined policy for dealing with violent patients. Managers must then ensure that nursing staff members follow the procedures to alert community members to the presence of a potentially dangerous patient in their midst.

Nurses must also protect the public from transmission of communicable diseases. All states require the reporting of certain health information concerning communicable diseases to specific government officials. Nurses need to know the statutes and protocols to fulfill them.

Equipment, Devices, and Material. Today, the professional nurse monitors complex physiologic data, operates sophisticated life-saving equipment, and coordinates the delivery of a myriad of health care services. To protect patients and employees from injury, the nurse must ensure that all equipment used in the course of patient care is safe and fully functional and that defective equipment is promptly reported, repaired, or replaced. Nurse managers must ensure that nursing staff members know how to operate and identify malfunctions of sophisticated equipment and provide necessary instruction in proper care and storage of the apparatus. They must also know their legal responsibilities to document and report defects and malfunctioning equipment even if others are designated as responsible for maintenance.

Medical Records

Legal Importance. Medical records are not only medically important, they are frequently legally crucial. There are recognized standards of record-keeping, which are accepted by professional organizations as well as by the courts. The courts will allow medical records to be introduced as evidence to impugn a health care provider's professional activities.

Good charting is a critical element of the nurse's duty to the patient. It documents the quantity and quality of care and contact given the patient. Nurses have a legal responsibility for accurate reporting and recording of patients' conditions, treatment, and responses to care. Entries must be timely, factual, relevant, pertinent, and material. To conform to the standard of care, nurses should record promptly as much and as often as they can, noting the date and the time (Greenlaw, 1982).

Changes, Corrections, Countersigning. A nurse is often asked to countersign entries in patient medical records for licensed pratical nurses, nurses aides, and student nurses. If the nurse's signature appears on the record in a capacity other than having personal knowledge of the particular events, he or she should explain that capacity and role clearly and note that he or she read and approved the entry; in the event of litigation his or her position will not be misconstrued.

Errors in nurses' charting must be corrected promptly in a manner that leaves no doubt as to the facts of the case. Every health institution should have a written policy and protocol, well publicized among all health care workers and students, that specifies that an erroneous chart entry is never to be erased or destroyed. Rather, it is to be crossed through, labeled as erroneous, signed by the individual correcting the error with date and time, and retained in the patient's record. Correct information is then entered. Tampering with medical records may result in large malpractice awards even when there has been no negligence. Nothing should ever be added, deleted, substituted, or removed.

Patient Access. Court decisions have held that because the patient's medical record is essential to proper administration, the medical record is the property of the hospital. In about 60 percent of the states, however, the patient or representative has a right to inspect the record while an inpatient and inspect and copy the record after being discharged from the facility. When supervising a patient's review of the record, nurses should explain only their entries in the record. Furthermore, the patient should be encouraged to go over the record with the physician. A physician who fails to cooperate should be reported to the administration.

Admissions, Discharges, and Transfers. There are a number of other legal responsibilities imposed on nurses including preparing nursing admission and discharge plans. This entire process has been revised with the legal establishment of the nurse as a health care provider and with the "corporate liability" concept, which establishes the nurse's role in quality of care.

The physician and the nurse are now mandated to have separate and complementary admission plans and orders concurrent with the admission of the patient. The more urgent the patient's problems the sooner these documents must be written. Discharge must now include a discharge plan. This should be done with the cooperation of the physician and other members of the health care team. It is the nurse, however, who has the ultimate responsibility of completing the discharge plan and recording it in the chart. All discharges must include documentation showing that the discharge is medically appropriate with plans for follow-up care and teaching of caregivers of the medical regimen after discharge. Premature discharge may result in legal actions against the physician, the hospital, and the nurse. Readiness for discharge is a responsibility of the entire health care team. Transfers must be documented in a similar manner.

Orders. A continuing mainstay of nursing practice is the carrying out of physician's orders. Nurses are now charged with knowing when an order is illegible, incomplete, ambiguous, or incorrect, and when not to implement it. This includes promptly informing the physician of a concern after confirming suspicions, so the physician can clarify or modify the order. Nurses are best served when they have a protocol to follow. Nurses have a duty to follow any order that is not patently erroneous (Katz, 1983).

When nurses are aware that execution of a physician's drug order is contrary to the manufacturer's recommendation or to the medical policy of the institution, they must defer execution of the order until conferring with the physician who wrote the order or with another physician who is authorized to act. If a particular physician regularly violates manufacturers' recommendations in ordering specific drugs, the nurse should report the problem in writing through the supervisor to the appropriate medical administrator.

Today, in many hospitals, ward secretaries or clerks transcribe orders. Ward secretaries or clerks should know that by law they are liable for their own errors and that they can be sued for negligence. Frequently, hospitals require that a transcribed order be countersigned by a professional registered nurse. Signing makes the nurse liable for any transcription errors.

A verbal order is legal but is a high risk legally. Verbal orders, oral or telephone, must be countersigned by the physician within 24 hours under a notation "read and approved" with date and time. Failure to countersign within the prescribed time should be followed by appropriate disciplinary action by the institution.

As to telephone orders, there is always the danger that the physician will misspeak or the nurse will mishear. Legal liability may be reduced if telephone orders are monitored by two health care professionals who are knowledgeable as to medications. This is one method for relieving a frequent source of patient injury and malpractice suits (Creighton, 1981).

Right to Refuse Treatment. A patient's refusal of treatment may involve an unwillingness to be resuscitated, a rejection of specific procedures, or an insistence on withdrawal of treatment. This is predicated on the right to privacy, which includes the rights to control one's own body and to consent to treatment. When contested, the courts have uniformly invoked the "benefit versus risk theory" in determining whether treatment should or should not be given. In addition, consideration has been given to the wishes of the patient and the family, as well as to those of the health care providers and the state.

Orders not to resuscitate (*DNR or no-code orders*) involving a patient who is in a hopeless condition have been termed valid by the courts, but these orders must be written. Furthermore the reasons for these orders should be documented, as well as the consent of a competent patient or the next-of-kin for an incompetent patient. *No-code* orders refer only to the decision not to resuscitate a patient after cardiac, pulmonary, or cardiopulmonary arrest arising from underlying pathological processes (Creighton, 1980).

Patients have a right to refuse treatment, says the law, even to the point of death when treatment will merely prolong inevitable death in the near future. *No treatment orders* are legal only at the patient's request and now generally include cardiopulmonary resusitation, nutrition, and hydration. They are not legal for withdrawing life support (i.e., respirator, intraveous fluids) from a patient who is unable to survive without them but not immediately facing death (Gargaro, 1984).

"Living wills" permit people to die as a natural course of a disease without the application of extraordinary means. These wills are filled out before the individual becomes incompetent and they direct the physician and the next of kin to take no artificial or heroic measures when there is no reasonable expectation of recovery. Courts generally have accepted those directions and enforced them when they have been challenged. A number of states have codified this right by statutes and have designated them as "natural death," "death with dignity," or "living will" statutes (Hershberger, 1982).

Informed Consent

The law in all states requires a physician to obtain informed consent of a patient before treatment. In the absence of that consent, the physician may be held liable in a civil lawsuit for battery, assault, and professional negligence. It has been held that an adult has the right, in the exercise of control over his or her own body, to decide whether or not to submit to lawful medical treatment (Bernstein, 1984a, 1984b).

To give informed consent to treatment, a patient should be told of the diagnosis, differential diagnosis, the nature of the diagnostic and therapeutic procedures to be performed, the *material* risks associated with that procedure, the prospect of success from the treatment, the prognosis or expectations, and the alternative courses of treatment that are available. Any special or unusual factors to be involved, such as the use of experimental drugs or techniques, the conducting of teaching or research, the use of cameras, must be revealed. *Material risks* include all risks that are reasonably forseeable as well as those that occur infrequently but are a threat to life or health. It is the physician's exclusive responsibility to convey the necessary information to the patient in language that the patient can understand at an appropriate time. The nurse is responsible to check that such consent has been obtained whenever possible, before treatment is begun (Cushing, 1984).

Recently the courts have mandated *informed refusal*, that is, when a patient refuses treatment, diagnostic or therapeutic, the physician has the duty to inform the patient of the perils and pitfalls of declining the care and management in a discreet, human, ethical, moral, professional manner.

Physicians may exercise professional, therapeutic discretion and not obtain informed consent if they believe it would be harmful, detrimental, injurious or hazardous to the patient to be told.

Durable Power of Attorney. Durable power of attorney is a document that gives the agent of the patient authority to consent or to withdraw consent to any care, treatment, service, or procedure to maintain, diagnose, or treat a physical or mental condition from that time on unless revoked by the patient orally or in writing. The agent also may examine medical records and consent to their disclosure. After death the agent may (1) authorize an autopsy, (2) donate the body or parts thereof, and (3) direct the disposition of the remains. This power is limited by any statement of the patient's desires or other limitations that are included in this document. In addition, no treatment may be given or withheld over the patient's objection at the time.

ADMINISTRATIVE LAW

History and Sources

Many of the legal doctrines applied by the U.S. courts are products of the common law that evolved over the centuries in England. This is a body of law based on judicial decisions that attempts to apply general principles to the specific situations that may arise. As society grew more complex, common laws became inadequate. Legislative bodies were then formed and their enactments became known as legislative or statutory law. These laws make up the bulk of U.S. laws as they exist today. Publications containing these statutes are known as codes.

Since the turn of the century another branch of law has become of great importance, that is, administrative or regulatory law. When the U.S. Congress or a state legislature desires to enact a program of regulation on businesses, or a program to confer benefits upon its citizens, it is difficult for the legislature to forsee the variations necessary for the proper execution of the law. To provide for these eventualities, the legislators have established administrative agencies clothed with power to promulgate the necessary rules and regulations, implement and monitor them, and enforce them.

Health regulations at the federal level are designed to carry out congressional intent as expressed in legislation. Examples of federal regulations affecting health facilities and programs include: Medicare, Medicaid, health planning, human experimentation, occupational health and safety, employment discrimination, food and drugs, medical devices, air and water pollution, reimbursement, radioactive wastes, controlled substances, peer review, collective bargaining, cost containment, and health education. At the state level, regulations implementing state legislation also cover a broad range of activity from facility licensure to preschool immunization.

Administrative rules and regulations are valid only to the extent that they are within the scope of the authority delegated by legislation. The legislature retains ultimate responsibility and authority by specifying what regulations the administrative body may make. Administrative rules and regulations are enforceable as law in the same way as statutes passed by legislatures or common law court decisions. Those involved with health care organizations should monitor proposed and final rules through these publications, their professional or agency associations, or other publications.

Quality Assurance

Quality assurance is concerned with identifying the specific elements of good patient care and seeing that those elements are present at each and every patient visit. Risk management begins whenever the quality assurance mechanism breaks down. The underlying basis of both programs is standards of care as determined by law, professional organizations, and the clinical expertise of members of the hospital medical, nursing, and other health care professional staff. The concepts of quality assurance and risk management overlap but are distinct entities (Orlikoff & Lanham, 1981).

Risk Management

Risk management focuses on the protection of the corporate assets by maintaining an acceptable level of care. The two major focuses of risk management are risk prevention and loss control. The risk manager works closely with the quality assurance coordinator to prevent incidents that may result in malpractice suits or general liability suits by patients, visitors, or employees (Monagle, 1985).

A number of states have mandated some form of risk management. The federal government is requiring it through rules and regulations controlling Medicare and Medicaid reimbursements. Insurance companies have made risk management a condition for coverage or for rate determination. Moreover, official hospital organizations, such as the American Hospital Association, are assisting in the development of risk management programs (Hirsh, 1979).

To reduce risk, any event or circumstance not consistent with the normal routine operations of the hospital, must be reported. *Incident reports* include two parts: part 1 is the documentation on the patient's chart of the facts by each health provider involved. Part 2 documents evaluations, assessments, conjectures, and opinions of health providers. Part 1 of the incident report can be subpoenaed by an attorney and used in a malpractice suit against the health care provider. Part 2 generally cannot be subpoenaed as it is not a classified "work product" (Creighton, 1983a, Orlikoff, Fifer & Greeley, 1981).

Supervision of Subordinates and Students in Nursing Practice

The nurse manager, as an agent for the health care institution, has a legal obligation to control the quality of nursing services to patients. This imposes the duty to observe, report, and correct the incompetence of subordinate personnel. The law is clear, a head or charge nurse is responsible for the quality of care given by all personnel assigned to the unit, whether or not these individuals have direct line reporting responsibility. To that end, the head nurse must also observe and evaluate the quality of care rendered by student nurses, clinical instructors, respiratory therapists, physiotherapists, laboratory technicians, and medical students, and, when these individuals render dangerous or inadequate care, report their failures to responsible individuals or remove the offender from the unit, or both. The head nurse also has a legal obligation to notify the chief administrator when understaffing endangers patient welfare (Greenlaw, 1981).

Nursing administrators have a legal duty not only to evaluate the quality of care given by a private duty nurse or nurse from a temporary agency, but also to check the identification and credentials of each nurse before allowing him or her to care for patients in the institution. This requirement is not removed when the agency claims responsibility for screening each nurse before employment.

Nurses as Instructor and Supervisor

Nurse administrators in hospitals with students should be aware of how the law regards students. Nursing students are responsible for their own actions and liable for their own negligence. When student nurses perform nursing services that are customarily performed only by registered nurses, they will be held to the standard of care of the registered nurse through the doctrine of "holding self out." Consequently, if nursing students know they are inadequately prepared for a particular assignment or duty or need additional supervision, they must inform the person responsible for their assignment and for supervision of the matter. The fact that they are students and may be a minor does not exempt them from liability or responsibility for their actions (Bernstein, 1982).

Instructors are responsible for the students' assignments and for their reasonable and prudent supervision. Accordingly, if they were to assign nursing students to perform duties for which the students were not fit or competent or had not been trained, or were to neglect or omit to supervise their performance to ensure professional competence, the instructors could be held liable if the student or patient suffered harm.

The inherent responsibility of nurses who supervise others—whether they be nursing students, registered professional nurses, practical nurses, aides, orderlies or attendants—is to determine which of the patient's needs can be safely entrusted to a particular person, and whether or not the delegated person is competent only if personally supervised (Creighton, 1982a).

Selection, Appointment, and Assignment of Personnel. Hospitals must exercise care in selecting their employees. The hospital should verify any required licenses and should check references and other information provided by the applicant to confirm that it is reasonable to believe the applicant is qualified for the position and free of medical conditions that may constitute a risk to patients or co-workers (Creighton, 1983c).

Nurse managers should be aware of the legal restrictions that affect the appointment and assignment of personnel. Any manager who ignores or departs from institutional hiring policies can be found negligent if an employee whom he or she appoints without appropriate screening later injures a patient. The nurse administrator is obliged either to relieve the nurse of a too difficult assignment or to provide needed preparation and coaching for the job. The more inexperienced and less skilled the work force, the more professional support and advice should be forthcoming from the nursing supervisor.

Because nurse administrators have responsibility to plan, staff, and supervise patient units to ensure safe and effective patient care, they have the right to temporarily reassign nursing personnel from one unit to another to compensate for emergency staff shortages. In shifting employees to compensate for personnel shortages, managers must take into consideration the capability of each nurse to discharge the anticipated duties in the temporarily assigned position (Creighton, 1982b).

Employees also have certain rights. They have a right to know the policies of the hospital and what is expected of them as employees, and the right to know what will happen if they fail to meet those expectations set out in the job description or in the policies and procedures of the hospital. Protocols spelled out in personnel policies should be followed conscientiously to reduce liability.

LABOR–MANAGEMENT LAWS

The National Labor–Management Relationship Act

Labor organizations have become a significant factor in hospital–employee relations. A number of different types of labor organizations are now recognized as collective bargaining representatives for groups of hospital employees. These include: (1) craft unions; (2) industrial and governmental employees' unions, and (3) professional associations. The professional associations, including the American Nurses Association, may be described as labor organizations to the extent that they seek goals directly concerned with wages, hours, and other employment conditions, and engage in bargaining activities on behalf of employees.

The National Labor–Management Relationship Act (NLRA) consists of the National Labor Relations Act of 1935, the Taft–Hartley amendments of 1947, and the 1974 nonprofit Health Care Institution amendments.

The 1974 amendments apply to "any hospital, convalescent hospital, health maintenance organization, health clinic, nursing home, extended care facility, or other institution devoted to the care of sick, infirm, or aged persons." Government hospitals are explicitly exempted by the NLRA. The courts have interpreted this to apply only to health care institutions that are *both* owned and operated by federal state or local governments (Miller, 1985).

The NLRA was enacted to eliminate industrial strife and establish the legal rights of employees, employers, and labor organizations. The act protects the rights of employees to join or refrain from joining a union and identifies their rights to bargain collectively through freely selected representatives. It also specifies the procedures for union selection that may include a secret ballot election supervised by the NLRB.

Section 7 of the Act ensures the right to "engage in other concerted activities for the purpose of collective bargaining or other mutual aid or protection." This phrase has a broad meaning and can be applied to groups of employees who come to administrators to complain about wages, hours, or working conditions. Section 7 includes rights to (a) engage in protected concerted activity, even though no union is on the scene; (b) join a union, even if that union is not officially acknowledged by the employer; (c) participate in organizing the employees in one's workplace or in other organizations; and (d) walk off the job to secure better working conditions.

National Labor Relations Board. The NLRA is administered by the National Labor Relations Board (NLRB), a quasijudicial agency. However, it cannot enforce its own decisions and must seek the assistance of the executive branch and court system to do so. The NLRB has two primary functions: to determine an employee's union representation status and to resolve any labor–management dispute. Thus, the NLRB investigates and adjudicates all complaints of unfair labor practices. It also conducts and oversees the secret ballot elections among employees to determine whether they wish to be represented by any labor union, and, if so, the choice of which organization (Health, 1983).

Legal Organizing Efforts: Process of Union Recognition. To become the collective bargaining unit for a group of health workers, a labor organization petitions the NLRB for an election as the collective bargaining unit. In the *petition,* a labor organization must demonstrate to the NLRB that there is a *showing of interest* by employees. The NLRB interprets this as 30 percent of the employees in the ultimate bargaining unit must have signed union authorization cards, or a list (Azoff & Friedman, 1982).

After a showing of interest, the NLRB has the authority to conduct *a hearing to determine appropriate bargaining units.* Congress felt that a multiplicity or "proliferation of bargaining units" would cause administrative problems including work stoppages and disruption of patient care. Thus, the NLRB limits the number of bargaining units in a hospital using the *community of interests* criterion. The NLRB's standard for community of interest has been: (1) similarity of skills, wages, hours, and working conditions; (2) collective bargaining history; and (3) desires of the employees. This usually results in one unit for registered nurses and another for nonprofessional nursing staff and other technicians such as x-ray or laboratory staff. The designation of a bargaining unit solely for registered nurses is still controversial because hospitals argue that it constitutes a proliferation of units that Section 9 of the 1974 laws sought to avoid. This controversy will be resolved if the NLRB moves to institute rules defining communities of interest.

A labor organization can become the *exclusive bargaining agent* for a bargaining unit four different ways. The most common is by winning the *secret ballot election* conducted by the NLRB. If a majority of employees vote for union representation, and more than one union is contending to represent employees, another election is held to select the union. Alternatively, an employer can *voluntarily recognize* a labor organization as the exclusive bargaining agent without an election. Recognition without an election can constitute an unfair labor practice when other labor organizations are also seeking to represent the employees. A third way that a labor organization can be recognized is by *order of the NLRB*. When the NLRB finds serious unfair labor practices, it has the authority to order the extraordinary remedy of recognition of a labor organization. A fourth way is termed *accretion*. If a labor organization has negotiated a contract for a bargaining unit at a hospital that subsequently acquires a new facility, under some circumstances the new unit employees are automatically covered by the preexisting contract. The entire process of union recognition is summarized in Table 2–2 (Swann, 1980).

Head Nurse: Union Member or Management? The NLRA defines *supervisor* as:

> Any individual having authority, in the interest of the employer, to hire, transfer, suspend, lay off, recall, promote, discharge, assign, reward, or discipline other employees, or responsibly to direct them, or to adjust their grievances, or

TABLE 2-2. PROCESS OF UNION RECOGNITION

Organizing efforts
    Solicitation
    Distribution
    Meetings
Showing of interest (30% of employees sign)
    Petition
    List
    Union authorization cards
Bargaining unit determination
    NLRB uses "Community of Interest"
    States which positions are included
Union certification as exclusive bargaining agent for unit
    Secret ballot elections for unionization and for selecting a union
    Voluntary employee recognition
    NLRB selection
    Accretion

effectively to recommend such action, if in connection with the foregoing, the exercise of such authority is not of a merely routine or clerical nature, but requires the use of independent judgment. (Sec 152 [11], 61 Stat. 138, 29 USC).

The wording of this section suggests several important conditions: (1) an individual need only satisfy one of the conditions to qualify as a supervisor; (2) independent judgment has been interpreted to require that a supervisor exercise his or her own discretion in directing, evaluating or selecting employees; (3) "effective" recommendations on personnel matters means they must be based on the supervisor's own investigation or assessment without the higher level supervisor's personal follow-up investigation or assessment; and (4) the mere title of supervisor does not confer supervisory status. Because supervisory status demands case-by-case analysis, the decisions in this area do not reflect a strictly uniform approach.

The determination of supervisory status is extremely important as supervisors are expressly excluded from the protections and rights of "employees" under the NLRA. Practical effects of this exclusion on supervisors include: (1) their votes will not be counted in Board elections; (2) exclusion from bargaining units; (3) no protection by the unfair labor provisions of the Act; (4) as legal agents of the employer, their actions may be judged to be unfair labor practices of the employer; and (5) possible requirement by higher management to assist in lawfully opposing union organizations.

The American Nurses' Association is a professional association, and qualifies as a labor organization under the NRLA. As a consequence, some hospitals have requested or even required all nursing supervisors and administrators to give up membership in the ANA. The U.S. Supreme Court has upheld the right of the health care agency to have such a policy. If no such policy exists, such nurses may belong to these associations but may not participate in resolving labor–management issues.

Labor Contracts

Good Faith Bargaining. Once a union is recognized, management must bargain "in good faith" with that union to establish a labor contract. For first contracts, the parties are legally bound to (1) meet at reasonable times to negotiate wages, hours, and other terms and conditions of employment in good faith, namely with an intent to reach an agreement and (2) to place into writing and execute a contract stipulating agreements when they are reached. Employers may not unilaterally change any terms or conditions once agreement is made; rather they must bargain with the union.

The NLRB looks at total conduct in the context of the bargaining relationship to justify bad faith bargaining charges. Although no set number of meetings is required, the NLRB carefully considers the number of meetings, the substantive nature of the meetings, the initiative of the employer in scheduling meetings, and the delays or cancellations of meetings. In making arrangements or sending documents and minutes, a hospital should ensure that everything is sent by certified mail. Such documentation may be essential for defending management against a charge of refusal to bargain.

Unfair Labor Practices. The term *unfair labor practice* relates to any activity carried out directly or indirectly by either the employer or by the union that violates the NLRA. Employer and union activities that are unlawful are set forth in Section 8 of the Act. Employer unfair labor practices may be outlined as follows:

1. Interference, restraint, or coercion of employees in the exercise of their rights to join or form unions or not as they desire and to engage in collective bargaining and corrected activities.
2. Employer domination of or assistance to a labor organization. It is unlawful assistance for an employer to favor one union over another.
3. Encouragement or discouragement of membership in labor unions by discrimination in hire or in tenure, terms, or conditions of employment.
4. Discrimination against employees for filing charges or giving testimony under the Act.
5. Refusal to bargain collectively with the representative of the majority of the employees or the designated exclusive bargaining agent (union).
6. Refusal to bargain collectively concerning wages, hours, or terms and conditions of employment.
7. An employer may not refuse to provide statistical data to a union for collective bargaining that does not invade the employees' right to privacy. This includes financial statements of its health and welfare, retirement and pension funds. (Regan, 1982).

Subject of Bargaining. The NLRB mandates that the labor contract include wages, hours, and terms and conditions of employment. It is forbidden to contract for illegal employment practices or that employees join a union before they have been employed 30 days. Any other subject that both parties agree to bargain about is permissible including quality of work life issues. Once signed, a labor contract must be in effect for 12 months.

An important point of negotiation in any new collective bargaining agreement is the *union security clause.* This clause describes who will be required to join the union. Unions generally prefer a closed shop, meaning all employees must join and that union dues, fees, and assessments will be subtracted from the employee's salary and forwarded to the union. Other arrangements vary from no requirement to certain groups of employees required to join or a service fee imposed on all employees with optional membership. Twenty-one states have made union security clauses unlawful. Statutes forbidding such agreements are generally called *right to work* laws on the theory that they protect employees' right to work if they refuse to join the union (Rutkowski & Rutkowski, 1984).

Administering the Contract. After negotiating a labor contract, the hospital should spend no less care on its administration. Managerial rights that have been established at the bargaining table, sometimes at a high price, can be eroded or entirely lost through inattention. The entire managerial team, especially first-line and second-line supervisors, should know the aspects of the contract applicable to their responsibilities. Of particular importance is the problem of discipline. Managers must be trained to administer discipline by the appropriate procedures under the contract. Grievances are formal written complaints alleging a violation of the labor contract and must follow agreed procedures or may be prosecuted as an unfair labor practice.

Strikes

There are six types of strikes. Only two, economic strikes and unfair labor practice strikes are legal. The *economic strike* is called by the union in support of an unrequested demand. A striker cannot be discharged for participating in an economic strike, only replaced. An *unfair labor practice strike* is over the employer's unilateral actions on mandatory subjects of bargaining or the infrequency of the meetings. When the strike is over, the hospital may be required to reinstate striking employees with their full rights and privileges if the hospital is found to have committed the alleged unfair labor practices.

A union may call an illegal *organizational strike* when the employer refuses to recognize the union without an election. Strikes or partial strikes planned and staged by employees without the approval of their union are *wildcat strikes*. Such strikes typically occur when there is a no-strike and no-lockout clause in the contract and union members believe that they have suffered because the employer has committed serious NLRA violations that undermine the union. Employees may also spontaneously call a *surprise strike* without the knowledge or consent of the union. A *sympathy strike* may be called by an employee or another group of employees in support of a legal strike by another union group. The NLRB may seek legal recourse to fine unions for illegal strikes called by themselves or employees.

The 1974 amendment to the Taft–Hartley Act specifies that a union must give a ten-day notice before striking or picketing a health agency. Conversely, an employer must give similar notice before locking employees out. There is no notice requirement for an unfair labor practices strike.

The courts have ruled that *actions* such as working by the book, reporting sick, refusal to perform any task not in the job description, and mass resignations are not the equivalent of strikes and, therefore, are not governed by strike rules.

Deunionization

Petitions. When a union receives NLRB certification, the majority status of the union must be recognized for one year. Decertification petitions may not be filed until 60 days before the first anniversary of the contract. There must also be evidence that 30 percent or more of the employees desire a change. The NRLB will conduct an election if satisfied that reasonable doubt of majority support is present.

Another way to decertify a union is if a rival union petitions the NLRB for an election to determine if employees wish to change unions. The same rules of timing and 30 percent or more employees showing interest in change must be met. The NLRB response is to hold elections (1) if the employees desire to be represented by any union and (2) to decide which union.

Mediation and Binding Arbitration. The 1974 Health Care amendments to the National Labor Relations Act established special provisions for strikes in health care institutions when the parties report to the NLRB they are unable to resolve their problems. They must also report this to the Federal Mediation and Conciliation Service (FMCS), which *may* require *mediation* before any strike may be legal. If so, the FMCS will then appoint a Board of Inquiry to investigate the dispute, stipulate the facts discovered, and write recommendations that are advisory, not binding, to the involved parties. If no settlement is reached after the parties consider the recommendations and the mandatory time periods have lapsed, the union may strike after it has provided the FMCS and the employer with a ten-day notice.

Like mediation, *binding arbitration* involves third-party intervention on unsettled issues in collective bargaining. The invocation of binding arbitration may be included in the contract or may be a mutual decision of the parties at the time of the dispute. An arbitrator holds a hearing on the issues in dispute between the hospital and the union and makes a decision that is binding to both parties. Binding arbitration decisions are obligatory on the parties and disagreement by management or the union may not result in a lock-out or strike.

HEALTH CARE EMPLOYMENT LAWS

The federal and state governments have enacted a variety of laws regulating compensation and benefits of employees. Nurse administrators should be aware that these laws exist and govern health care institutions.

Workers Compensation

Every state has some form of workers' compensation legislation that is designed to assure that employees will be compensated for losses due to accidental on-the-job injuries or employment-related illness. When the workers' compensation law applies, the employee is barred from suing the employer for the injury. The only way courts become involved is if there is an appeal concerning the decisions of the state official or agency administering the law (Larson, 1983).

In cases not routinely paid by the insurance carrier, the matter goes to a hearing before a state commission to determine questions of liability. Any injury caused by the job is covered. The key question is whether the condition arose out of or occurred in the course of employment. This definition is broad enough to cover the more common workplace injuries (occupational diseases, the cumulative effect of a working lifetime, even accidents that happen away from the normal workplace). Thus, almost everything that happens to an employee during the workday is covered by workers' compensation, and in some jurisdictions on the way to and from work, particularly if the employee is on call and in residences supplied to such employees. Under workers' compensation laws, nurses have been compensated for disabilities arising from falls, assaults, pranks, heavy lifting, and infections contracted from patients (Creighton, 1984a, Sosin, 1984).

Occupational Safety and Health Act

The Occupational Safety and Health Act of 1970 was enacted to "assure safe and healthful working conditions for working men and women." Among other provisions, the law requires the isolation and placarding of patients with serious infectious diseases; the placarding of areas containing ionizing radiation; the proper grounding of electrical equipment; controlling the atmospheric concentration of alcohol, formalin, and ether vapor; and the protective storage of flammable and combustible liquids. The statute provides that when no federal standard has been established, state safety rules remain in effect. Hospitals can be sanctioned for not providing a safe working environment for employees. Space prohibits a detailed discussion of the law, the administrative and court decisions. Nurse managers concerned with this problem should familiarize themselves with this information.

Equal Employment Opportunity Law

The federal government has enacted several laws to expand equal employment opportunities by prohibiting discrimination on various grounds, including sex, age, race, religion, handicap, pregnancy, or national origin. These are enforced by the Equal Employment Opportunity Commission (EEOC). There are also numerous state laws addressing equal employment opportunities. In hiring and assigning nursing personnel, the manager should abide by those federal and state laws that protect employees' civil rights.

One of the few exemptions permits religious institutions to consider religion as a criterion in their employment practices. Other institutions need not employ an individual whose religion interferes with the normal operation of the hospital (Regan, 1980).

The Age Discrimination Employment Act extends civil rights to include nondiscrimination of persons from 40 to 70 years of age for all employment-related purposes. Mandatory retirement is prohibited for persons under 70, except for certain exempted executives. The Act applies to governmental and private employers of 20 or more persons. There are exceptions for bona fide occupational qualifications, bona fide seniority systems, and reasonable factors other than age, such as physical fitness (Age, 1984).

In 1978, Title VII of the Federal Civil Rights Act of 1964 was amended to prohibit discriminatory treatment of pregnant women for all employment-related purposes. No special considerations are required. If leaves are offered for disabilities, similar leaves must be offered for maternity. Mandatory maternity leaves that are not based on inability to work violate Title VII. Some states require employers to offer a leave of absence for pregnancy. Thus, it is important for the nurse manager to be familiar with the details of federal and state laws, and the decisions incident to these laws.

The Equal Pay Act is designed to prohibit discriminatory compensation policies based on sex. Equal work is defined as work requiring the same skill, effort, and responsibility that is performed under similar working conditions. In general, the courts have required equal pay except when the hospital has been able to prove actual differences in the work performed during a substantial portion of work time (Alessi, 1983). The courts have adopted a case-by-case approach to the determination of whether work is equal.

There are three legal bases for establishing employment discrimination: (1) when work rules or employment practices are not applied in a consistent fashion; (2) when an employment practice, such as a written employment test, has an adverse impact on minorities and cannot be justified as job-related; and (3) when minorities are in a disadvantageous position because of prior discriminatory practices (Creighton, 1983b).

Fair Labor Standards Act

The Fair Labor Standards Act establishes minimum wages and maximum hours of employment. The employees of all nonprofit and proprietary hospitals are covered by this act. However, bona fide salaried executive, administrative, and professional employees are exempted.

Most employers are required to pay overtime rates for work that exceeds 40 hours in seven days. However, the law permits hospitals to enter into agreements with employees, establishing an alternative work period of 14 consecutive days, rather than the usual seven-day week. However, the hospital is not relieved from paying overtime rates for hours worked in excess of eight hours in any one day, even if no more than 80 hours are worked during such a period.

Sexual Harassment

The Equal Employment Opportunity Commission (EEOC) published final guidelines on November 10, 1980 affirming that sexual harassment in the workplace violates Title VII of the 1964 Federal Civil Rights Act. Under these new guidelines, the employer can be liable for sexual harassment by co-workers and nonemployees, as well as supervisory and managerial staff. Employers will be considered absolutely responsible for the sexually harassing acts against employees regardless of whether the specific acts complained of were authorized, sanctioned, or even forbidden by the employer and regardless of whether the employer knew or should have known of their occurrence. Employer liability for acts against workers may be minimized by the employer taking immediate and appropriate corrective action in instances of sexual harassment. The EEOC will consider the extent of the employer's control and any other legal responsibility in determining employer liability for acts of nonemployees.

BIOGRAPHICAL SKETCH

Dr Hirsh received his medical degree, from the Georgetown University School of Medicine, and his law degree from the American University Washington College of Law. He practiced internal medicine for over 30 years and has been teaching legal medicine for the past 16 years. He is board certified in Internal Medicine and Legal Medicine.

Dr Hirsh is President and a Fellow of the American College of Legal Medicine. He serves as a Member of the Board of Trustees of the American Board of Legal Medicine. He has been a member of various medical and legal societies.

At present Dr Hirsh is Editor-in-Chief of *Trauma* and is an Editor of *Medicine and Law* and *Medical Trial Technique Quarterly.* He serves on the Editorial Board of *Legal Aspects of Medical Practice* and has been Editor of several medicolegal publications. He has published over 300 articles in medical, scientific, legal, and medicolegal journals and has authored or co-authored 15 books.

At various times Dr Hirsh has been a consultant to governmental agencies and also pharmaceutical and consultant firms. He has been a guest lecturer in over 275 programs involving medical, legal, and medicolegal organizations, locally and nationally. He is a Distinguished Visiting Professor at George Washington University in the Department of Health Services Administration. He has held professional rank in several of the local universities.

SUGGESTED READINGS

Nursing Practice

Helen Creighton's monthly column on law in *Nursing Management*
Northrup, C.E. (1987). *Legal issues in nursing.* St Louis: CV Mosby Co.

Labor Law

Rutkowski, A.D., Rutkowski, B.L. (1984). *Labor relations for hospitals.* Germantown MD: Aspen Systems.

Administrative Law

Miller, R.D. (1985). *Problems in hospital law* (2nd ed.). Germantown, MD: Aspen Systems Corp.
The journal: *Law, Medicine and Health Care*

Employment Law

Jernigan, D. (1988). *Human resource management in nursing.* Norwalk, CT: Appleton & Lange.

Larson, A. (1983). *Workmen's compensation for occupational injuries and death.* New York: Matthew Bender & Co.

REFERENCES

Age Discrimination & Nurses. (1984, January). Pamphlet No. 4, *Texas Nursing,* *58*(1), 28–29.

Alessi, D.J. (1983). *Proving sex-based wage discrimination under federal law.* Kansas City: American Nurses' Association.

Annas, G.J., Glantz, L.H., Katz, B.F. (1981). *The rights of doctors, nurses and allied health professionals.* New York: Avon Books, pp. 159–161.

Azoff, E.S., & Friedman, P.L. (1982). Solicitation-distribution rules: A developing doctrine. *Hospital Progress, 63*(2), 44.

Bennett, H.M. (1983) The legal liabilities of critical care: The good samaritan act. *Critical Care Nurse, 3*(3) 24.

Bernstein, A.H. (1982). Medical and nursing students v. their schools. *Hospitals, 56,* 98–102.

Bernstein, A.H. (1984). Informed consent, Part 1. *Hospital Medical Staff, 13*(11), 2–6.

Bernstein, A.H. (1984). Informed consent, Part 2. *Hospital Medical Staff, 13,* 4–8.

Cohn, S.D. (1984, April). Prescriptive authority for nurses. *Law, Medicine & Health Care,* 72–76.

Creighton, H. (1980). Withdrawal of life support systems. *Superv. Nurse, 11,* 52–54.

Creighton, H. (1981). Telephone orders. *Superv. Nurse, 12*(3), 48–52.

Creighton, H. (1982a). Students' unsatisfactory clinical performance. *Nursing Management, 13*(2), 47–49.

Creighton, H. (1982b). Liability of nurse floated to another unit. *Nursing Management, 13*(3), 54–55.

Creighton, H. (1983a). Incident reports subject to discovery? *Nursing Management, 14*(2), 55–57.

Creighton, H. (1983b). Hospital guilty of racial discrimination. *Nursing Management, 14*(3), 20–21.

Creighton, H. (1983c). Value of careful personnel records. *Nursing Management, 14*(6), 38–40.

Creighton, H. (1984a). Recovery for on-the-job injuries or illness. *Nursing Management, 15*(3), 70–71.

Creighton, H. (1984b). Nursing judgment. *Nursing Management, 15*(5), 60–63.

Creighton, H. (1986). *Law every nurse should know* (5th ed.). Philadelphia: W.B. Saunders.

Cushing, M. (1984). Informed consent and M.D. responsibility. *Am. J. Nursing, 84*(4), 437–440.

Fiesta, J. (1983). The law & liability: A guide for nurses. New York: John Wiley and Sons.

Gargaro, W.J., Jr. (1984). Criminal prosecution for discontinuance of life support, Part 4. *Cancer Nursing, 7*(2), 57–58.

Greenlaw, J. (1981). Understaffing: Living with reality. *Law, Med. & Health Care, 9*(9), 23–24.

Greenlaw, J. (1982). Documentation of patient care: An often underestimated responsibility. *Law, Med. & Health Care, 10*(9), 172–174.

Greenlaw, J. (1980). Ethical dilemmas: Reporting incompetent colleagues II: Will I be sued for defamation? *Nursing Law and Ethics, 1*(5), 5–6.

Guarriello, D.L. (1982, October). Nursing malpractice litigation: Toward better patient care. *Trial*, 77–80.

Hershberger, W.S. (1982). Ins and outs of wills require expert advice. *Nephrology Nurse, 4*(1), 43–44.

Hirsh, H.L. (1979, November). Hospital risk management. *Urban Health*, 24.

Hirsh, H.L. (1981). On law and medicine: The courts have a new view of nursing. *American College of Physicians Observer, 1*(8), 2, 10.

Katz, B.F. (1983, April). Reporting and review of patient care: The nurse's responsibility. *Law, Medicine & Health Care*, 76–79.

Larson, A. (1983). *Workmen's compensation for occupational injuries and death.* New York: Matthew Bender & Co.

Miller, R.D. (1985). *Problems in hospital law* (5th ed.). Germantown, MD: Aspen Systems Corp.

Monagle, J.F. (1985). *Risk management, A guide for health care professionals.* Germantown, MD: Aspen Systems Corp.

Northrop, E.E. (1987). *Legal issues in nursing.* St Louis, MO: C.V. Mosby.

Orlikoff, J.E., & Lanham, G.B. (1981). Why risk management and quality assurance should be integrated. *Hospitals, 55*(11), 54–55.

Orlikoff, J., Fifer, W., & Greeley, J. (1981). *Malpractice prevention liability control for hospitals.* Chicago: American Hospital Publishing, Inc.

Philpott, M. (1985). *Legal liability and the nursing process.* Toronto: W.B. Saunders Company Canada Ltd.

Pozgar, D. (1983). *Legal aspects of health care administration* (2nd ed.). Germantown, MD: Aspen Systems Corporation.

RNs and criminal assault: Legal rights. (1982). *Regan Rep. Nurs. Law, 23*, 2.

Regan, W. A. (1980). Hospital employees, religious rights. *Regan Rep. Nurs. Law, 20*(9), 2.

Regan, W.A. (1982). Nurses' rights in collective bargaining, solicitation. *Regan Rep. Nurs. Law, 22*, 2.

Rhodes, W.B., & Miller, R.J. (1986). *Nursing and the law* (4 ed.). Germantown, MD: Aspen Systems Corporation.

Rowland, H., & Rowland, B. (1984). *Nursing administration handbook.* Germantown, MD: Aspen Systems Corporation.

Rutkowski, A.D., & Rutkowski, B.L. (1984). *Labor relations for hospitals*. Germantown, MD: Aspen.

Sosin, J.S. (1984). What to do if you're hurt on the job. *RN, 47*, 13–15.

Swann, J.P. Jr. (1980). *NLRB elections: A guidebook for employees*. Washington, D.C.: Bureau of National Affairs, Inc.

Veatch, R.M., & Fry, S.T. (1987). *Case studies in nursing ethics*. Philadelphia: J.B. Lippincott Co.

Walker, L.J., (1980). Nursing 1980: New responsibilities, new liabilities. *Trial, 16*(12), 42–47.

Walker, D.J. (1983). Legal rights and responsibilities of the nurse. In N. Chaska (ed.), *The Nursing Profession: A time to speak*. New York: McGraw-Hill, pp. 49–59.

Wiemerslage, D. (1983). Torts: Doctrine of precedent. *Crit. Care Update, 9*, 27–37.

APPLICATION 2–1

Managing Unionized Nurses

Mary Suzanne Hudec
Mary Dowling Willigan

ORGANIZING A UNION

Scenario

As the Director of Nursing of a 500-bed hospital, you have been made aware by your management staff that the State Nurses' Association (SNA) is campaigning to represent all the registered nurses as their collective bargaining agent. The SNA is distributing literature on the benefits and advantages of union representation. In addition, the SNA is attempting to obtain signatures for eligibility of a National Labor Relations Board (NLRB)-conducted election. Hospital administration and nursing management are concerned about their roles. A meeting has been called to discuss management's responsibilities and to plan a course of action.

Discussion

Management must recognize that employees have the right to organize, as stated by the National Labor Relations Act (NLRA). Management must not obstruct organizing activities or exercise reprisal against employees involved. The following are recommendations for management during the campaign.

This article was prepared on the author's personal time and was not part of their official responsibilities with nor should it be attributed to either the Veterans' Administration or the National Institutes of Health.

Recommendations

- Remember that the union is seeking to become the spokesperson for your employees, not an outside organization, a co-manager, or a threat to management.
- Dispel any personal biases toward unions in responding to organizing activities.
- Permit employees to campaign for a union as long as the activities do not interfere with the work of the organization. Solicitation is permissible in nonwork areas during nonwork times, including lunch hours and scheduled breaks. Prounion propaganda, such as buttons and badges, is generally permissible unless it interferes with the agency's mission.
- Investigate the past history of the union and its prior activities and practices.
- During the campaign and the election, management should maintain a fair and reasonable posture in dealing with issues of concern to employees.
- Give factual information if questioned by employees regarding the union.

NEGOTIATING A CONTRACT

Scenario

After the NLRB-conducted election, the SNA achieved certification and is recognized by management as the exclusive representative of the nursing employees. The union has presented management with a package of proposals for negotiation of a contract. As the Director of Nursing, you must plan a course of action.

Discussion

Management is obligated to negotiate. Because this is the initial contract being negotiated, management should recognize its responsibility to secure an agreement that permits management to manage. The following are recommendations for management before and during negotiation.

Recommendations

- Review the NLRB union certification and become knowledgeable of basic NLRB tenets.
- Meet with the hospital's labor attorney to review all proposals. Use consultants as appropriate.
- Develop a negotiating team and team behaviors.
- Prepare for formal negotiations; Do your homework.
- Obtain input from the grassroots of the organization, so that management is aware of the issues. Be sensitive to all proposals.
- Analyze proposals beyond their language. What is the underlying issue

the proposal deals with? Are there more acceptable commitments that may satisfy the union?

- Anticipate demands that will be made. Review all past grievances and problems, especially problems or issues that have arisen in the last year.
- Establish priorities. What items could management make concessions on and which ones is it necessary to hold the line on?
- When developing management proposals, establish original proposals, and have fall-back positions.
- Bargain in good faith. Demonstrate a sincere intent to reach an agreement regardless of whether an impasse eventually develops.
- Maintain mutual respect between negotiating parties.
- Listen attentively and do not be intimidated.
- Objectivity is the most essential quality of a negotiator. The negotiator must not use resentment or anger.
- Avoid flat rejections of union proposals when possible. Do not make commitments you cannot keep.
- Do not report specific details of the negotiation process outside of the proceedings. Relate only general information, otherwise, negotiations may be jeopardized.

CONTRACT ADMINISTRATION

Scenario
A nurse requests three weeks vacation during the peak summer vacation period. The head nurse denies the request, explaining that because of the number of requests for leave, only two weeks can be approved. The employee and the union steward meet with the head nurse alleging that the disapproval is in violation of a provision of the negotiated contract and past management practice. The employee threatens to file a grievance if the head nurse does not approve the leave.

Discussion
Administering the contract is a responsibility of all levels of management. It is the middle manager and the first-line supervisor who interpret and apply the contract on a daily basis.

After the contract is signed, differences will exist on the content, meaning, and application of certain contract language. Contract administration is a dynamic activity, not a static body of cut-and-dried knowledge. Controversy is unavoidable.

Recommendations

- *Know* your contract, this includes all levels of management.
- Train the management staff in the contract, especially on the intent of contract language, which may be deliberately ambiguous.

- Apply the contract fairly and consistently. A supervisor's actions or behaviors can establish contract interpretation or change the intent of the contract.
- Examine management's past practices before taking action.
- Review with managers what they can and cannot say or do. It is illegal to spy on union activities, make promises contingent on nonunion participation, interrogate or threaten employees about union involvement.
- Read and interpret the contract fairly. Apply the contract in a firm and consistent manner.

UNFAIR LABOR PRACTICE

Scenario

The community has been suffering from a severe nursing shortage and your hospital has not remained immune. As the Director of Nursing, you have used all available resources. Bed census has been decreased by 20 percent and most recently, you have reassigned a proportion of the specialty staffs (OR, dialysis, etc.) to the general medical–surgical units. Management did not consult the union before the changes in assignments and work functions. Due to the failure of management to bargain the above changes, the union filed an unfair labor practice.

Discussion

Management has the right to decide employee workload, but if changes are made in organizational policy regarding the workload or working conditions, the union has the right to be informed in advance and to negotiate these changes. Management, however, is ultimately responsible for the delivery of patient care. In this scenario, management directly violated a right of the union by failing to discuss the issue with the union. This is in direct violation of one party's rights granted by the labor relations law. Either party may be found culpable for failing to live up to its obligation.

Recommendations

- Immediately investigate once an unfair labor practice has been filed.
- Examine the possibility of resolving an unfair labor practice charge informally.
- Admit the mistake at the onset, if management is wrong. If management is in the right, however, do not be intimidated.
- Be willing to compromise, in many cases it is not important to prove who is wrong.
- Allowing the union an opportunity to "save face" may have long-range benefits in some instances.
- Work with the Director of Personnel as a team.

GRIEVANCES

Scenario

On the night shift of a medical–surgical unit, there are two registered nurses and one nursing assistant on duty. The unit is very quiet and one of the registered nurses locks himself in the treatment room to sleep. The other RN, the charge nurse, is unaware of the nurse's actions. During the night, a patient develops respiratory distress and subsequently cardiac arrests and expires. A code has been called. The charge nurse, unable to locate the other RN, notifies the night supervisor of the incident. After a thorough investigation of the incident by management, the sleeping employee is fired. The union files a grievance on behalf of the employee. The union's position is that the nurse had been employed at the hospital for over ten years and the employee was denied the right to counseling concerning the sleeping.

Discussion

Most contracts specify that if both parties are unable to satisfactorily resolve a grievance, through the grievance procedure, the process ends in binding arbitration. Management should examine each grievance very carefully at every step to determine whether settlement or resolution is more advisable than rejection of the grievance. A grievance should not automatically be considered as a threat to management's authority.

Winning or losing is not always the most important issue. The cost of personnel time to prepare for testimony, its effect on staff and patients, the potential long-term adverse effects on labor–management relationships, legal fees incurred, and the realization that the arbitrator's decision is binding should be examined and weighed by management. If management, however, is committed and confident of its position, they should proceed through arbitration.

Recommendations

- Place a high priority on resolving dissatisfactions of employees consistent with accomplishment of overall goals.
- Carry out the provisions of the contract and personnel policies consistently.
- All levels of management must know the labor contract and other personnel policies.
- Act with deliberation, investigate carefully, and get all the facts. Be available and encourage a full discussion of the incident.
- Make a strong effort at the first-line management level to resolve grievances at the first step of the grievance procedure.
- Follow the steps of the grievance procedure exactly as outlined in the contract. Adhere to all time requirements, otherwise the outcome of the grievance may be jeopardized.

- Treat the union official as a professional. In preparing and presenting the grievance, the union offical has equal status with the management official.
- Consider resolving the grievance before arbitration. If the grievance does go to arbitration, solidify management's position remembering that the arbitrator's decision is binding.

ATTITUDES AND RELATIONSHIPS

Scenario
As Director of Nursing, you have formulated the following goals and objectives:

- To promote shared responsibility for planned change.
- To identify recurrent problems in patient care.
- To formulate/revise standards of care.
- To implement nursing service goals addressing clinical practice issues.

The goals are not being realized. You are considering approaches to attain these goals, but you are unsure of how to get union input.

Discussion
Management does not need to ask the union's approval for every administrative decision, however, informing union leaders of planned change before implementation provides constructive suggestions to management and increases cooperation with employees. It is imperative that union leaders acknowledge management's need for efficient and effective delivery of nursing services, otherwise, patient care ultimately suffers.

Recommendations

- Use the union as a vehicle for nurses concerns.
- Allow the union input on issues other than benefits and economic matters.
- Adopt a cooperative versus an adversarial role in allowing the union input into nursing practice issues and standards.

BIOGRAPHICAL SKETCHES

Mary Suzanne Hudec is the Chief, Nursing Service at the Washington, D.C. Veterans Administration Medical Center. She began her VA career as a staff nurse, holding progressively responsible positions in nursing administration at various VA Medical Centers before being selected as Chief, Nursing Service at the Dayton, Ohio VAMC. Ms. Hudec also served in active duty status with the U.S. Navy during the Viet Nam War and was assigned to the hospital ship USS Sanctuary. Ms. Hudec has a BS in Nursing from the College of Mount St.

Joseph, a MSN from the University of California at San Francisco and is past President of the National Capital Area Chapter of American Organization of Nurse Executives.

Mary Dowling Willigan was completing her graduate studies in Nursing Administration at George Mason University at the time of this writing. Her clinical expertise is critical-care nursing. She received her BA in nursing from Niagara University and is a certified critical-care registered nurse. She is currently a nurse administrator at the Memorial Sloan-Kettering Cancer Center in New York City.

APPLICATION 2-2

Designing a Nursing Risk Management System
Leigh Wintz

THE ENVIRONMENT

The field of risk management is relatively new. Interest in such programs has been triggered by a variety of factors: an emphasis on quality assurance, the crisis in insurance, asbestos, AIDS, chemotherapy agents, and radiation. Boards of directors are demanding programs that will protect the resources and assets of the corporation (Stock, 1986).

Health care providers are committed to providing the highest possible quality of care in a setting that poses the least risk to patients, visitors, and staff. Strong quality assurance and risk management programs are essential to achieving this goal. Quality assurance means making sure that each patient receives the best possible care, while risk management means making the environment as safe as possible for everyone—patients, visitors, and staff. The main objective of a risk management program is to protect an institution's resources and assets.

INCREASING ACCOUNTABILITY

Nursing is a vital component of any effective risk management program. Nurses are expected to provide quality care, even in an environment with restricted resources. Although nurses can, and are now more frequently being held individually liable for negligent acts, employing institutions also bear the financial burden of malpractice and negligence suits involving the quality of nursing care rendered. Identifying and correcting deficiencies in nursing practice can significantly reduce the potential harm for patients, visitors, and staff and prevent financial loss.

A recent study by the Virginia Insurance Reciprocal ("A Closer Look", 1986) showed that 18 percent of the total number of new claims was based on nursing errors. In addition, 23 percent of the total claim dollars were based on nursing error. The vast majority of these claims were based on the failure to monitor or assess adequately a patient's nursing needs. One of the critical situations that contribute to hospital liability is nurses who are placed in charge of a unit without ever having been given the management training to perform this responsibility.

The majority of successful suits against nurses falls into one of eight risk categories: (1) administration of medications, (2) assisting in the surgical suite, (3) falls, (4) burns, (5) electrical shock, (6) nosocomial infections, (7) mistaken identity, and (8) misinterpretation of signs and symptoms. Therefore, it is logical and prudent initially to design a program that concentrates on risk reduction in these areas.

THE RISK MANAGEMENT PROGRAM

The Risk Management Plan

A risk management program specific to nursing service in an institution must interface with the existing institutional program. Nurse administrators should be familiar with the institution's plan and work with the risk manager to ensure that all systems are working together to accomplish the same objectives.

The institution's risk management plan itself should include:

1. Statements of purpose, authority and objectives.
2. Relevant board and committee structure.
3. The relationship of risk management to quality assurance, in-service education, the patient advocacy and guest relations programs, occupational health and safety, fire safety, and security programs.
4. Incident reporting and other risk detection policies, procedures, trending, and analysis.
5. Risk prevention and loss control programs.
6. Risk financing plans, including recommendations for types and levels of insurance coverage.
7. Claims management program.
8. A mechanism for program evaluation on a yearly basis.

In addition to the risk management plan, nurse administrators will also want to obtain a copy of the risk manager's job description to fully understand the unique and important role of this individual in the institution. This individual may already be familiar to you as many risk managers are registered nurses with experience in quality assurance or nurse attorneys. This person is a valuable resource in the design of a program specific for nursing.

There are two major components of a well-designed risk management program: risk identification and risk control.

Risk Identification

The risk identification aspect of risk management very closely resembles quality assurance. It is imperative that the programs be integrated or there can be a great deal of duplicated effort.

Risk identification is accomplished by the routine collection of incidents and adverse patient occurrences (APOs). Nurses must be educated about what to report as an APO. They are indicators of possibly less than optimal patient care, such as infant birth injury, unexpected return to the operating room, or unexpected transfer to intensive care. It is important that nursing personnel reporting such events feel absolutely free of reprisal. They should not attempt to evaluate the incident, but merely report its occurrence in a timely manner. This, too, helps ensure that reporting is just a routine part of procedure. Even where no patient injury is apparent or likely, the frequency and location of such events and the trending of this information is important for the risk control aspects of the overall program.

Nursing Specific Indicators. The nursing service may want to collect and trend their own adverse patient occurrences through the routine reporting and collection of those events that may lead to nursing liability and for which the responsibility of risk minimization lies clearly within the nursing service. Results of such activities would then be reported and integrated into the overall risk management program.

Reporting of such events is most easily accomplished through the use of a standard form available on each unit.

Table 2-3 includes a list of the type of indicators that provide a basis for routine monitors of nursing practice. Such a list needs to be adapted to be specific to the institution. The list provides feedback on nursing situations likely to result in patient dissatisfaction with care and, therefore, possible law suits.

The collection of such data gives a wealth of topics for quality assurance studies. The appropriate policy or procedure should contain statements specific enough to become criteria for either retrospective or concurrent studies. Results of the study can direct educational efforts for specific nursing units or for the nursing service in general.

After identification of those areas that are to be monitored continuously, it is necessary to determine what is to be done with the information once it is collected.

Case By Case Analysis. A case by case analysis is an important aspect of risk identification. Each case must be evaluated to determine if the event is serious

TABLE 2-3. RISK MANAGEMENT INDICATORS: NURSING SERVICE

Please check any applicable indicators. Send the completed form to the Nursing Quality Assurance Coordinator.

[ ]   Patient left against medical advise
[ ]   Medication error
[ ]   Skin breakdown during hospitalization
[ ]   Unsuccessful cardiopulmonary resuscitation
[ ]   Patient fall
[ ]   IV infiltration or complication from a peripheral or central IV line or heparin lock device
[ ]   Transfusion reaction
[ ]   Nosocomial infection
[ ]   IV, Foley, or nasogastric catheter not changed according to policy
[ ]   Postoperative atelectasis or pneumonia
[ ]   Hemorrhage or hematoma after an invasive procedure
[ ]   Fecal impaction
[ ]   Aspiration of food or foreign body
[ ]   Lumbar puncture headache (includes postmyelogram/postspinal anesthesia)
[ ]   Repeated patient complaint (for more than 24 hours) of ineffective pain management
[ ]   Missed or untimely transcription of order
[ ]   Incorrect or inappropriate isolation
[ ]   Missing intake and output entry noted
[ ]   Disposable item being reused
[ ]   Failure of a physician to respond in an emergency

Date of occurrence _____ Time of occurrence _____
Date reported _____ by _____

Nursing QA use only (attach and complete data abstract):

                                                    addressograph

_____ Date received
_____ Date analysis completed
_____ Date abstracted

enough to pose potential liability. The nurse administrator evaluating the case should be clinically competent, intimately familiar with policy and procedure, and have enough authority to take corrective action immediately if necessary. In some instances, it will be determined that every possible, prudent precaution was taken to prevent a situation but that it occurred anyway. In this case "the standard" was met.

When analyzing a case, it will be necessary to review the medical record. Depending on the timing of the referral and the nature of the reported event, this may happen while the patient is still under care or after discharge. To analyze all cases in the same manner and cover all aspects of analysis, the use of a standardized form, such as the one in Table 2-4, is recommended.

Work closely with the risk manager to determine the type of case that should

TABLE 2–4. DATA ABSTRACT FOR ANALYSIS OF RISK MANAGEMENT INDICATORS: NURSING SERVICE

1. Describe the extent of patient injury:

   Severity score:
   [ ] 0 – No injury or ill effects
   [ ] 1 – Emotional injury or upset
   [ ] 2 – Physical discomfort
   [ ] 3 – Injury or damage requiring additional nursing measures
   [ ] 4 – Injury or damage requiring additional hospitalization and/or treatment by MD
   [ ] 5 – Potential permanent damage or death

   (Cases with severity scores of 3, 4, or 5 should be referred to the Hospital Risk Manager immediately.)

2. Describe staff actions that contributed to the event/injury:

   Presence of staff actions: [ ] yes [ ] no

3. Describe patient actions that contributed to the event/injury:

   Presence of patient actions: [ ] yes [ ] no

4. Were any policies, procedures, or protocols violated by the nursing staff?
   [ ] yes [ ] no

5. Was the standard of care met by the nursing staff? [ ] yes [ ] no

6. How frequent is this type of event on this unit?

7. Attributable cause (check all that apply):
   [ ]   Failure to follow established policy, procedure, protocol
   [ ]   Failure to make an adequate assessment
   [ ]   Failure to take the appropriate action after an assessment
   [ ]   Failure to communicate adequately with other health team members
   [ ]   Failure to communicate adequately with patient/family
   [ ]   Failure to implement a physician or nursing order
   [ ]   Equipment failure
   [ ]   Patient caused event/injury
   [ ]   Other _____

8. Cause to be attributed to the following unit and/or nurse: _____
   (unit code #) _____ (RN code #)

9. Actions taken:
   [ ]   Referred to hospital administration _____
                                              date
   [ ]   Referred to hospital risk manager _____
                                            date
   [ ]   Trend only

10. List immediate actions taken to prevent recurrence:

11. State any recommendations to change policies or procedures that would prevent recurrence.

Analysis by _____ date _____

be referred right away and those that may be deferred. Remember, for there to be liability, there has to be a breach of duty and some injury must result as a breach of that duty.

Next, use the appropriate nursing policy to make a determination about whether the standard of care was met or not met. Did the nurse do everything the way it was supposed to be done? If not, was there a reasonable exception that is clearly documented in the medical record?

It is also necessary to determine the attributable cause. Sometimes it is difficult to determine what caused an event. If reasonable care has been taken by staff to deliver quality care by acceptable standards, it would be hard for a jury to determine against the hospital and staff. It is not necessary to spend hours and hours on this aspect of analysis. Let the risk manager do this.

Trend Analysis. Trending involves the regular recording of certain items for each event referred. Although manual pattern analysis is certainly an option, the use of a personal computer spread sheet program allows for the generation of more accurate and extensive data reports in a much more rapid manner.

Quarterly and yearly summary reports are recommended, however, the database is continually built on and added to. Be certain to allow for the addition of indicators and easy modification of reports once experience has demonstrated what is meaningful and useful within nursing service, administration, and the overall risk management program.

Reports should include the number of risk management indicators that occurred in a given time frame, where they occurred, on what types of patients, during what shifts, and to what practitioners. Using this method, actions to reduce the risks can be targeted to the necessary groups. Remember that the numbers are dependent on self-reporting. In the beginning of a program, numbers may increase as reporting becomes more complete and occurs closer to 100 percent of the time.

Stagger monthly reporting so that one-fourth of the list of indicators is reported each quarter. The numbers will probably not warrant reporting more frequently than this and staggered reporting prevents the nursing committee with oversight responsibilities from becoming overwhelmed by the data and unable to make the appropriate recommendations for problem resolution. For such committees not to be influenced by past behavior or bias toward individuals, it is customary for nursing units and individual practitioners (if appropriate to the data) to be presented in a coded form.

Risk Control

The second aspect of a risk management program is risk control, which entails risk avoidance, loss prevention, and risk reduction.

Risk avoidance requires a very proactive risk management system in which actions are taken to correct identified problems. Policies are changed as indicated by data and trend analysis. Active in-service programs are offered to employees as indicated by their individual needs and salaries are based on specific performance standards being met or exceeded. Through such measures, the environment is made as safe as possible and all employees are aware of their role in the risk management program.

When a patient, visitor, or staff member is involved in a potentially litigious situation, the hospital-wide risk management system is activated immediately to prevent or reduce losses through legal action. It is important to remember that most patients sue not just because an error has been made in the delivery of care, but because they are angry. Informing people that you are aware that something has not gone the way it was supposed to and taking all the necessary

TABLE 2-5. MEDICATION ERROR ANALYSIS: NURSING SERVICE

Patient name _____ MR# _____
Room # _____ Attending MD _____
Primary RN _____ RN who made error _____
Date of error _____ Time of error _____

1. Describe the error:

2. Type of error (check all that apply):
   [ ] Charting
   [ ] Omission
   [ ] Extra dose
   [ ] Unordered drug (wrong patient or wrong drug)
   [ ] Wrong dose
   [ ] Wrong route
   [ ] Wrong time
   [ ] Other _____

3. Contributing cause (check all that apply):
   [ ] Unclear order not reviewed with physician
   [ ] Nurse selected and administered wrong drug
   [ ] Nurse misinterpreted Kardex
   [ ] Nurse miscalculated or mismeasured
   [ ] Verbal order misunderstood
   [ ] Nurse gave medicine to wrong patient
   [ ] Nurse did not read drug label
   [ ] Transcription error
   [ ] Nurse misread dosage ordered
   [ ] Nurse failed to use Kardex
   [ ] Pharmacy error
   [ ] Nurse used poor judgment
   [ ] Uncommon dosage schedule ordered
   [ ] Nurse administered drug prepared by others
   [ ] Other

Analysis by _____ Date _____

TABLE 2-6. PATIENT FALL ANALYSIS: NURSING SERVICE

Patient name _____ MR# _____
Room # _____ age _____ Attending MD _____
Primary nurse _____ RN assigned _____
Date of fall _____ Time of fall _____
Activity orders in effect at time of fall:

MD _____

RN _____

1. Has patient fallen before? [ ]   yes   [ ]   no
2. Was patient identified in care plan as being at risk for a fall? [ ]   yes   [ ]   no
   If yes, was the fall protocol followed? [ ]   yes   [ ]   no
   If no, was the prefall assessment adequate? [ ]   yes   [ ]no
3. Type of fall (check all that apply):
   a. General:
      [ ]   Observed
      [ ]   Unobserved
      [ ]   Call light on
      [ ]   Patient attended by staff at time of fall
      [ ]   Staff not in attendance at time of fall
   b. If from bed to floor:
      [ ]   Bed rails down/no restraints
      [ ]   Bed rails down/restrained (type _____)
      [ ]   Bed rails up (# _____)/no restraints
      [ ]   Bed rails up (# _____)/restrained (type _____)
   c. If from chair or equipment to floor:
      (type of chair or equipment _____)
      [ ]   No restraints
      [ ]   Restraints (type _____)
   d. If fall occurred while ambulating:
      [ ]   Occurred in hall
      [ ]   Occurred in bathroom
      [ ]   Occurred in patient room
      [ ]   Occurred elsewhere (_____)
4. Cause of fall (check all that apply):
   [ ]   Equipment failure
   [ ]   Patient incontinent
   [ ]   Patient refused siderails
   [ ]   Patient refused restraints
   [ ]   Patient violated activity orders
   [ ]   Patient unable to follow instructions
   [ ]   Patient removed restraints
   [ ]   Patient lost balance/became dizzy/fainted
   [ ]   Visitor assisted patient in ambulating without assistance
   [ ]   Staff member did not/could not respond to call light in a timely manner
   [ ]   Restraints applied improperly
   [ ]   Wet/slippery floor
   [ ]   Wheelchair brakes not locked
5. Comments:

Analysis by _____ Date _____

steps to correct the matter to the extent possible, will go a long way toward reducing losses.

Potential problems and threats of legal action are to be reported to the hospital risk manager immediately. The risk manager will triage the situation and call in the appropriate parties, such as members of the administrative staff, legal counsel, or the insurance company, as necessary. Usually the patient or family members will be visited and a full explanation of the events will take place. Frequently, parts or all of a hospital bill that may be incurred as a result of an adverse patient occurrence are waived. This helps to establish the care and concern necessary to maintain good communication with an aggrieved party. In cases where there is no question of negligence, hospital and insurance company personnel will seek out-of-court resolution to avoid additional financial losses.

TWO CLASSIC RISK MANAGEMENT TOPICS FOR NURSING

There are two areas of risk management that are most familiar to the nursing service: medication errors and patient falls. Let us reexamine these familiar topics in light of a proactive risk management system.

Nurses have been trying to deal with medication errors for years. By creating subcategories of medication errors that clearly describe how the error occurred, strategies to reduce errors can be targeted. A standardized form for consistent and easy trending, such as the one in Table 2-5, is recommended for analyzing medication errors. A copy of the form should be sent to the hospital risk manager as well as retained in nursing service.

Nursing has also been studying patient falls and profiling the type of patient who is most apt to fall. Profiles have been used for quite sometime with little success in reducing incidence. Information may be used more fruitfully for trending by establishing categories of types of falls and reasons for the fall, rather than only patient characteristics, to assist in defining specific strategies for risk reduction. A sample form for analysis is shown in Table 2–6.

BIOGRAPHICAL SKETCH

Leigh Wintz was Administrative Director of Patient Services at Prince George's Hospital Center, a 555-bed acute care facility in Cheverly, Maryland when she wrote this application. In that capacity, she had responsibility for the hospital's quality assurance, utilization review, and risk management systems, as well as the departments of Social Work, Discharge Planning, Infection Control and Patient Transport Services. Her unique background as a nurse in quality assurance gave her the ability to understand the points of view of both nursing and administration and made her a valuable member of the senior management team. She is now the President of the General Federation of Womens Clubs in Washington D.C., which is a large non-profit volunteer community service organization.

REFERENCES

A closer look-Nursing error and litigation. (1986, January/February). *Reciprocal News, 9*(1), 1.

Stock, R. (1986). Risk management: Minimizing errors and liability. *Dimensions, 63*(1), 22.

3

Health Policy

James D. Vail

Health care policy and its formation is relevant knowledge for all nurses. This policy is reflected in the guidelines for action by each of the major professional nursing organizations. For example, the American Nurses' Association has published a Social Policy Statement and distributes a video tape that provides basic information for nurses who wish to participate in the health policy process. Participation in health policy formation and knowledge of current laws, regulations, and accrediting standards is one responsibility of any nurse administrator.

What is public policy? Policy, in general, is "a course of action (or inaction), either explicit or implicit, that is consciously or purposely chosen in the interest of addressing concerns or resolving some problem in a particular or specific way" (Moccia, 1984, p. 481). Public policy is, "whatever governments choose to do or not to do" (Dye, 1984, p. 2). MacPherson (1987) finds this definition useful because it focuses not only on government action but also on government inaction.

What is the relationship between public policy and politics? Politics is the science and art of government. Diers (1985) relates the two saying "policy deals with *shoulds* and *oughts,* while politics is the use of power to persuade or otherwise change." She also states, "politics is reactive; policy is proactive" (p. 422). MacPherson (1987) takes issue with this statement saying, "health care policy as a form of public policy can, on the contrary, be reactive or proactive, and instead of being separate from politics is created and maintained through complex political–economic alliances" (p. 7). This author concurs with MacPherson that the separation is only analytical.

Health policy may be best described by the example of the 1965 Medicare and Medicaid legislation. Because this major piece of federal legislation addresses the medical assistance needs of those citizens over 65 years of age, it also touches on who is responsible for the welfare of this social group—which is, in fact, social policy. Social policy addresses the intrasocietal relationships among individuals, groups, and society as a whole. Health policy is a subset of social policy that addresses how and by whom health care is delivered and financed and environmental influences on the nation's health. Social issues are only considered insofar as they influence people's health.

This chapter is organized to first give a brief historical review of American health policy and the role politics plays; then describes forces shaping health policy and the reorganization of health policy; and finally discusses the future of health care delivery and health policy.

HISTORICAL REVIEW

Health care statutes and health policy are made on at least three governmental levels: federal, state, and local county or city. There are no distinct lines between responsibility of one level of government and another.

Historically, health care was perceived as a *local* problem and various methods were developed to manage the health needs of local areas. Some of those methods included the establishment of almshouses and poorhouses, which later became the nation's first hospitals. Epidemics made it necessary for local authorities to generate health policy to protect the public. Early policies mandated health examinations and quarantine. Those early efforts at protecting the public have evolved into the present local (city, town, county) and state health departments, which promote the health of its residents through monitoring sanitation, immunization programs, and providing other health services.

Although early health policy was primarily determined by local jurisdictions, in the last two decades there has been a great increase in the federal government's determination of a national health policy. Even so, in every state some responsibility for determining health policy is delegated to local authorities. In many instances health policy is determined at a higher level of government, but interpreted and implemented at the state or county level.

The earliest involvement of the federal government in health care is thought to have been around 1798 through the establishment of a Marine health service for sick and disabled seamen (Cray, 1970). Although these services were established by Congress, they were supported by a tax levied against the seamen's wages. It was not until 107 years later that the federal government supported these services out of general tax revenues.

Over the years the federal government has become more and more involved in health policy. Today, all three branches of government are involved: statutes from the legislature, court decisions from the judiciary branch, and administrative regulations and actions from the executive branch. Hawkins and Higgins (1982) summarize the general function of the federal government in health care as: "providing direct care for certain groups such as Native Americans, the military, and veterans; safeguarding the public's health by regulating quarantine and immigration and the marketing of food, drugs, and biologicals; preventing environmental hazards; giving grants in aid for health care delivery to states, local areas, and individuals; and conducting and supporting research" (p. 24).

Even though the Constitution does not define a role for the federal government in health care either as a provider of service or as a payer for services rendered by others, over the years the federal government has assumed a major role in health related issues primarily in policy setting and economic controls (Cray, 1970).

There are no less than 13 cabinet-level departments that exercise health care policy. These are: Department of Agriculture, Department of Defense, Department of Housing and Urban Development (HUD), Department of the Interior, Department of Labor, Department of Justice, Department of State, Department of Commerce, Department of Energy, Department of Transportation, Department of the Treasury, Department of Education, and the Department of Health and Human Services (DHHS). The health policy agencies, which operate directly under the authority of DHHS, include: Health Care Financing Administration (HCFA), the Social Security Administration, the Office of Human Development Services, and the Public Health Service (USPHS) (U.S. Dept. of Labor, 1979). Additionally, there are no less than 17 independent federal agencies concerned with the health of the nation. To name a few: ACTION, The Consumer Product Safety Commission, The Federal Trade Commission, and the Veterans Administration. There are also several "quasi-official" agencies concerned with health and health policy, such as the Smithsonian Institution, which is an independent trust and sponsors research on such topics as human nutrition, preservation of the environment, and disease prevention (U.S. Dept. of Health, Education and Welfare, 1978).

Although the Constitution does not define a role for the federal government in health care matters, it does define a role for the states. The states are delegated police powers to enact and enforce laws to protect their citizens (Jonas, Banta, & Enright, 1977). Burton and Smith (1970) have identified four major roles of the states in health care policy.

- Quality control over licensure, vital statistics, health care delivery distribution, medical laboratories, fire and sanitation through legislation, regulations and enforcement.
- Administration of federal reimbursement programs, especially Medicaid.
- Policy influence on communicable disease control, data collection, and assessment.
- Delivery of service: maternal child health care, public health nursing, keeping vital records, clinic services, laboratory services, health education, mental health care, state hospital care, local health screening.

States have also begun enacting statutes and developing policy supporting living wills and death with dignity issues.

When examining the roles played by the various actors in health policy making the private sector must not be overlooked. According to Duval (1977) the traditions of American health care are rooted in the private enterprise system. Private independent providers, hospitals, nursing homes, insurance companies, voluntary charitable agencies, and professional associations all influence health care delivery and policy.

It is interesting to note that throughout this century two of the nation's largest and most influential professional organizations, the American Nurses' Association (ANA) and the American Medical Association (AMA), have regularly taken opposing positions regarding major health care legislation. The most noted example of position difference between the ANA and the AMA related to legislation centered around national health insurance.

As far back as 1920 the AMA House of Delegates announced, "opposition to the institution of any plan embodying the system of compulsory contributory insurance against illness, or any other plan of compulsory insurance which provides for medical service to be rendered contributors or their departments, provided, controlled or regulated by any state or federal government" (Feingold, 1966, p. 85). From that time forward the AMA has fought almost all proposed legislation that would create a national insurance plan or national health care services. Congressional Hearings (Marmor, 1970), in 1961, recorded the position of various organizations *for* and *against* health insurance for the aged (Medicare). Leading the list *against* such legislation were the AMA, the American Hospital Association, the Life Insurance Association of America, and the National Association of Blue Shield Plans.

Marmor (1970) wrote that the AMA is an organization with conflicting roles. "As a type of professional trade union, it is committed to improving the status of physicians. As a scientific organization, the AMA sponsors research and regulates medical practice. As a political pressure group, it has fused these roles, linking, and to some extent, confusing the issues on which physicians speak as scientific authorities and as self-interested professionals. Its broad lobbying aim has been to convince the American public that physicians are the sole authority that can properly decide on the organization, financing, and regulation of medical care practice" (p. 27).

Organizations *supporting* health insurance for the aged were: the ANA, the AFL–CIO, the American Association of Retired Workers, the National Association of Social Workers, and the American Geriatric Society. The ANA not only supported the proposed Medicare legislation, it has always supported comprehensive health care services for all Americans. The National League for Nursing (NLN) also has a policy statement supporting eventual establishment of a comprehensive national health insurance program (NLN, 1979).

In the 1850s Florence Nightingale wrote many letters to the British Parliament in an effort to improve health conditions for soldiers fighting in the Crimean War, as well as for those committed to hospitals. In 1858 she wrote a study entitled *Notes on Matters Affecting the Health, Efficiency, and Hospital Administration of the British Army*, which was "respectfully received by Her Majesty's Government" (Kalisch & Kalisch, 1986). This action by Nightingale was probably the earliest recorded effort of nursing's influence on national health policy through the direct "lobbying" of the government.

What worked then works today—bringing issues to the attention of federal lawmakers through letter writing, congressional testimony, lobbying, and other political activities. Jordan (1983) writes, "nurses' beliefs and standards for health care will not survive in the future if exercised *only* at the bedside of patients and clients" (p. 83). Today, nursing is represented by both professional lobbyists from the Council of ANA, NLN, American Association of Colleges of Nursing, and American Organization of Nurse Executives, specialty nursing organizations, and by grass roots political action by nurses organized in Political Action Committees (PACs). Over 40 states have registered PACs, and nursing's ability to make sizable contributions and endorsements is growing. Skaggs (1985) reports that campaign contributions have soared over the past couple of years, mainly through the efforts of state PACs. At the conclusion of the 1985 election cycle, one state PAC saw 90 percent of its endorsed candidates selected. Today, many candidates seek nursing's endorsement.

Policy is slow at being formulated and even slower at being disseminated, implemented, enforced, and evaluated. From the time health legislation (which would result in health policy) is introduced until it is implemented can be as long as 10 to 12 years or even longer. The Medicare–Medicaid legislation is just one example of this prolonged process. Although the first Medicare bill was introduced as early as 1952, with years of preliminary debate before that, the bill did not actually pass and become law until 1965, some 13 years later. Marmor (1970) writes, "serious congressional interest in special health insurance programs for the aged developed in 1958, six years after the initial Medicare proposal. From 1958 to 1965, the Committee on Ways and Means held annual hearings which became a battleground for hundreds of pressure groups" (p. 25).

Plans for National Health Insurance have been in the making since 1912 when President Theodore Roosevelt's Progressive Party included a plan as a plank of the party platform. Since that time, through every administration, and through every Congress there has been some effort to create a National Health Insurance Plan, but to no avail. Refer to Table 3-1 for a list of the most common proposals that have been introduced, none of which have passed and become law. Nursing must continue to evaluate critically proposals that would provide more comprehensive health care to all citizens.

FORCES SHAPING HEALTH POLICY

The forces shaping health policy can basically be sorted into two groups: political and social. Each, however, is not a distinct entity. Whatever happens in the political arena directly impacts on social relationships and vice versa. The two groups are different, but not separate; simple appearing, but not simplistic. Both groups are also affected by world events such as economic changes.

The issues that shape health policy today are the same as in the past—natural events, discoveries, and upheavals. Current examples are increased ease of mobility around the world; the AIDS virus; the development of birth control measures; and the rapid growth of new technology.

To identify major forces driving the various social trends and political issues

TABLE 3-1. PROPOSALS FOR NATIONAL HEALTH INSURANCE

Health Security Act H.R. 21; S. 3 (AFL–CIO support)	National Health Care Services Reorganization and Financing Act H.R. 1 (AHA support)
National Health Care Act of 1976, H.R. 5990; S. 1438	National Health Insurance Standards Program Family Health Insurance Plan. (Nixon Administration) S. 1623; H.R. 7741
Griffiths AFL–CIO Plan of 1970, H.R. 22	National Health Insurance Act, H.R. 94
Pettengill Proposal 1969	Comprehensive National Health Care Act of 1975, H.R. 8887
Kennedy/Waxman Labor Coalition	Carter Administration Proposal
Comprehensive Health Insurance Act of 1974, H.R. 4747	Comprehensive Health Care Insurance Act of 1975, H.R. 6222 (AMA support)
Catastrophic Health Insurance and Medical Assist. Reform. H.R. 10028; s. 2470	National Health Insurance and Health Services Improvement Program, S. 836
National Voluntary Medical and Hospital Services Insurance	National Family Health Protection Act, H.R. 3672
National Health Standards Act, S. 2644	Medical Expense Tax Credit Act, S. 600
Long Catastrophic Plan	

pertinent to health policy is difficult because their interactions are so complex. Some of the major forces are:

- Political forces
    Economics
    Health systems
    Professional organizations
    Health care rights
    Legal and ethical decisions
    Consumer special interest organizations
- Social forces
    Demographics
    Types of services
    Technology
    Scope of practice
    Education
    Epidemics

Political Forces

Health care is now the nation's second largest industry (Hawkins & Higgins, 1982). With health care costs continuing to spiral it is no accident that whereas the primary U.S. health political issue of the 1950s and 1960s was *guaranteed access*, it has shifted in the 1980s to *cost containment*. In 1950, total expenditures for health services were $12.7 billion—approximately $82 per person. By 1983, health care expenditures were $355 billion, an average of $1,459 per person (Gibson & Waldo, 1984). In 1986 those expenditures jumped to $458 billion, an amount equal to 10.9 percent of the gross national product (GNP). An increase of 22 percent in just three years. It is predicted that by the year 2000, American health care costs will consume more than 12 percent of the GNP. Thus not only has the percentage increased over time, the rate of increase has also accelerated. In 1986 spending for health amounted to an allocation of resources equal to $1,837 per person. For a graphic view of the nation's health dollar: where it came from and where it went, refer to Figure 3–1.

Some of the factors contributing to increased costs are:

- An older and more chronically ill population.
- Increased use of Medicare and Medicaid.
- Increased number of diagnostic procedures and overutilization of other medical services.
- Increased use of technology.
- Overutilization of hospital beds, and particularly expensive intensive care beds.

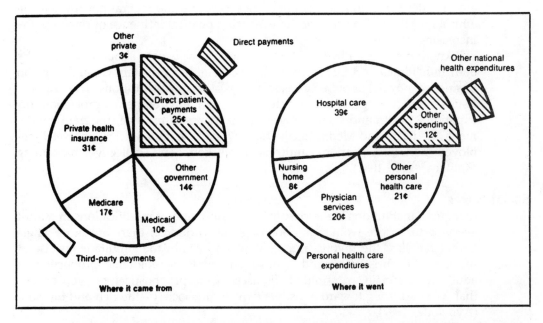

Figure 3-1. The nation's health dollar: 1986. Almost three-quarters of national health expenditures were channeled through third parties. Nearly two-thirds were channeled through private hands. The bulk of that expenditure was for patient care, and the remaining 12 percent was spent on research, construction, administration, and government public health activity. *(Source: Health Care Financing Administration, Office of the Actuary. Data from the Division of National Cost Estimates.)*

- Increase in malpractice suits with a subsequent increase in malpractice insurance and the practice of "protective" medicine.
- Limited supply of nurses.
- Long hospital stays.
- Health policies developed and implemented according to a "sickness" model, rather than as "health" model.

The political forces impacting on the economics of health care are varied and interconnected. For example, the types of health systems available to the consumer is largely determined by other forces such as professional organizations, laws and regulations, payment mechanisms, and the ethics of health care delivery.

Ethical decisions reflect the economic and political values of society. One could argue that values and ethics should not be legislated. This may be true, but it is also true that laws and regulations about health often legislate moral reasoning. The laws concerning ethical questions related to death, such as honoring living wills, the right to die, organ donations, and paying for abortions with federal funds, are based on moral choices that have great political and economic impact on society. Ethically, there are no right and wrong answers, but there are legal and illegal answers. One arena where ethical issues are debated are Presidential Commissions appointed to advise the federal government on ethical questions. One sign of the increasing political influence of nurses is the increasing membership on such panels.

Another political force is the increasing consciousness about legal rights by both individuals and institutions. Rights are either privately created (e.g., in business contracts) or publicly based in legislation or constitutions. The "rights" issues in the health care arena include: abortion, environmental protection, occupational health and safety, physician standards of practice, program entitlement (Medicare and Medicaid coverage; workers' compensation), hospital employee nondiscrimination, antitrust protection, and collective bargaining (Kaluzny et al., 1982).

Social Forces

Our social institutions are currently undergoing radical modifications in almost every sector. More women are entering the workforce; there are more single parent families; the divorce rate continues to climb; the simultaneous rise of fundamental christianity and agnosticism; and the epidemic proportion of adults with socially transmitted diseases. Some prognosticators even believe that we are drifting toward a distinct two-culture society—the rich and the poor (Aydelotte, 1987).

Should this occur, an even greater portion of the nation's health care cost may be borne by the federal government. The health care policy of the last four administrations (Nixon, Ford, Carter, and Reagan) has been one of cost control (Lewis, 1983). The Reagan Administration attempted to redirect public responsibility by *reducing controls and regulations* on the health care market, and encouraging *competition* and *private enterprise* (Davis, 1983a, b). According to Aydelotte (1987) the forces that are driving costs upward are of two types: the *cost* of providing the service and the *demand* or use factors, such as requirements of the aging population. Increased competition may increase productivity and be an incentive to improved business practices in health care delivery, but the greatest increases in costs are currently due to new medical–technological devices, new surgical procedures, increased medical litigation, and increased charges for pharmaceuticals. Reduction in these costs is tied to increased governmental regulation.

Demand is an even more complex issue. In 1985 one-fourth of the total cost spent on health care was the result of intensity of care and the length of stay of those over 65 years of age (Aydelotte, 1987). As technology effectively increases the median age of the American population, demand will continue to rise. This leads to an examination of the social policy of health care, that is, health as a social good.

An issue basic to any health care policy is what amount of the GNP should be given to health care and how it should be rationed. Deeply rooted in this issue are social forces such as: (1) Education—How will health care providers be educated? And, how will this education be financed? (2) Types and availability of services—Should cost be considered? (3) Technology—What technology should be available and how should it be used? (4) Resources—What economic and manpower resources should be used to secure a healthy nation? (5) Scope of practice—Who should do what at what price? (6) Ethics—What is the government's moral responsibility for access to what health care?

With an ever increasingly large number of uninsured Americans (35 million) and with the increasing AIDS epidemic, the issue of national health insurance may be reexamined. AIDS is an expensive chronic terminal illness that can cost up to $150,000 to treat. This epidemic has revealed many shortcomings in both private and public insurance plans as well as government disability coverage. The Health Insurance Association estimates the total bill for AIDS, not including the cost of the new drug AZT, and other related illnesses will reach $40.5 billion between 1987 and 1991, straining the capacity of hospitals, nurses, doctors, and social workers to care for an increasing number of patients (Trofford, 1987). Howard H. Hiatt of Harvard Medical School and author of *America's Health in Balance*, writes, ''The growing burden of AIDS may be what forces us to look at some type of national health insurance plan. We are the only industrialized country except for South Africa that does not have universal coverage'' (Trafford, 1987 p. 15). The health political issue of the 1990s may be national health insurance.

REORGANIZATION OF HEALTH CARE DELIVERY

Paying for health care, whether it is paying the doctor, the hospital, or the nursing home has become a perennial health policy issue. Every administration post-

World War II has been faced with what to do about rising health care costs. Ironically, each administration has failed and costs have continued to rise through each administration, no matter what has been done. This observation of failure is based on social, economic, and political indicators. From the social standpoint none of the social reforms of the Johnson administration produced their desired changes and, almost all have been dismantled by the end of the Reagan Administration. Although the Carter Administration seemed to recognize the link between social and health issues, the Reagan Administration seemed to treat them as two separate issues. Neither approach was able to reduce rising costs, improve infant mortality, or otherwise show significant improvement in the nation's health or cost effective health care delivery. Regardless, dramatic changes in the organization of health care delivery have occurred in the last 10 years.

Historically, doctors and hospitals have received reimbursement under two completely different systems. Hospitals evolved as charity organizations usually sponsored by churches and voluntary associations depending on charitable gifts and public grants. It has only been during the twentieth century that hospitals have charged their patients. Hospital's missions have always focused on public service. Their Boards of Trustees were prominent citizens able to generate philanthropic donations. The business aspects of a hospital were seen as less important than community service. Profit-making or proprietary hospitals were disdained and widely believed to give inferior care.

On the other hand, doctors have always charged their patients as self-employed businessmen. They set fees covering both their personal income and their operating costs. As their social prestige has grown since the early 1900s, so have their incomes. Glaser (1986) notes that the trend in the United States has been away from self-employed solo practice while preserving traditional payment methods. More than one-half of American office doctors now are organized in partnerships, and in single or multispecialty groups. In contrast, European doctors have preserved the model of solo practice, having been guaranteed their costs and income by the official fee schedules of national health insurance.

The entire American health care system, since the early 1900s has been dominated by physician groups. Krause (1977) delineated five types of health worker groups, classified in a hierarchical relationship to physicians. The first direct competitors: osteopaths and chiropractors. The second type includes independent nonphysician specialists: dentists, podiatrists, opticians, optometrists, and pharmacists. Subservients, such as nurses and allied health workers, form the third type. The fourth type is comprised of deviants such as quacks and imposters, and the fifth consists of nonmedical health care administrators. The domination of physicians seems to be lessening since 1965 as shown by the passage of Medicare, the rise in consumer political action and self-help groups, and the increased autonomy of other health care providers.

The nursing shortage and the effort to identify innovative ways to deliver safe, effective care is not new to nursing. After World War II there was such a shortage of nurses that large numbers of unskilled workers were introduced into the system for minimal pay. These included: licensed practical nurses (LPN), nurses' aides, and orderlies. With the introduction of these workers, "functional nursing" was born. Functions, not patients, were assigned to the nursing assistants and thus the patient's care became fragmented and no *one* person could claim full responsibility and accountability for the patient's nursing services.

In an effort to try to "correct" this approach, team nursing was introduced. Marram, Schlegel, and Bevis wrote, "there were not enough nurses to do the job and not enough supervisors and head nurses to provide adequate supervision to poorly trained personnel. Team nursing seemed an answer to a profession in a care delivery crisis" (p. 15). Although team nursing may have provided a more organized appearance, it lacked theoretical soundness and, in fact, yielded no real change in the delivery care methods.

Several other attempts to address the staffing shortage followed in rapid succession. In an attempt to address the "professionalism" aspect of nursing, the concepts of *clinical nurse specialist* and *practitioner* were introduced. Although they are both very popular nursing specialties today and are well grounded in graduate education, they did not alleviate the problems caused by staffing shortages.

Still in quest for the best solution, yet another modality of care delivery was spawned—the concept of primary nursing. Many nursing administrators interpreted this concept to mean an all-RN staff and promptly set about trying to establish all-RN staffs by eliminating the LPNs, aides, and other nursing helpers. While primary nursing has been demonstrated to be a cost-effective method of delivering nursing care, there simply were not enough nurses available for this approach to withstand the demand created by an ever-increasing older, sicker population and the introduction of diagnostic-related groups (DRGs) and other prospective payment systems. Thus, as we leave the 1980s and enter the 1990s, we have come full circle. The profession is still experiencing a nursing shortage, and again, the concept of using paraprofessionals and team nursing is coming back into vogue under the labels of differentiated staffing or case management.

As the nursing shortage crisis continues, nursing administrators across the country are exploring ways of delivering safe, effective care with limited personnel resources. Many of the previously used methods of care delivery, such as, functional nursing and team nursing, as well as the reintroduction of nurses' helpers—nursing assistants, aides, and nursing technicians—are again being tried in the workplace. Hopefully, this time around these paraprofessionals will serve to *extend* professional nursing care and not replace it. David A. Reed, President of SamCor Inc., Phoenix, and Chairman-Elect-Designate of the American Hospital Association, wrote, "whatever and whenever possible the institution has to free the nurse to nurse. You have to supplement support services that maximize the productivity of the nurse" (1988, p. 44). Reed is advocating what was advocated after World War II—use support staff and services to permit the nurse to do what he or she is prepared to do, nurse.

New Primary Provider

Emergence of the so-called "new professionals" in the early 1970s was a forerunner to the reorganization of health care delivery. The professionals consisted of nurse practitioners (NPs) and physician assistants (PAs). Eastaugh (1981) refers to these new health workers as physician extenders (PEs) and portends that the rapid growth in PE training programs in the 1970s was a by-product of the unmet consumer demand for primary care and the perceived neglect of the human side of medicine. He goes on to say that "the promise of PEs is best described in terms of improved access to care, improved practice, productivity, health education counseling, comprehensive planning in patient management, and lower unit costs" (p. 119). Nurses contend that NPs are doing nursing and not medicine, but they do agree that they are primary health care providers.

The struggles of NPs and PAs to provide independent primary care has increased public awareness of the resistance of organized medicine to any form of competition. The report of the Macy Commission (1976) suggests that the continued success of NPs and PAs will not only have a positive impact on the quality of health care, but will also encourage the development of other nonphysician competitors.

In 1981 the Public Citizen Health Research Group issued a policy statement calling on the federal government to assist consumers and in particular Medicare beneficiaries in avoiding high-priced physicians. Consumerism has extended its interests beyond simple price disclosure activities to include expanded information on quality and availability of care. Access to information is a necessary condition for stimulating competitive markets. Organized medicine, however, has resisted efforts to supply consumers with more information concerning cost, quality, and access (Eastaugh, 1981).

Traditional Delivery System

In recent years the health care delivery system has undergone numerous changes. The traditional system consisted primarily of (1) physicians, giving all primary care as the only provider authorized for insurance payment. (2) The focus of medical intervention was "cure of acute conditions" because prevention was not covered by health insurance. (3) Physician referral to hospitals for all types of secondary care as outpatient care was usually not covered by employer health insurance. (4) Hospital discharge only when patients were well enough to care for themselves at home and medically stable; again because home care was not covered by health insurance. With hindsight we can see that all four items are costly alternatives driven by financial incentives.

Medicare–Medicaid

It was Public Law 89-97, Titles 18 and 19, of the Social Security Act and Public Law 98-21, the Social Security Amendments of 1982 that served to change the "traditional" way of health care delivery in the United States. Public Law 89-97 Title 18, known as Medicare, provided for medical health insurance for citizens over the age of 65, and Title 19, known as Medicaid, provided for medical assistance for the indigent, financed by state and federal funds, and implemented at the state level. These laws have led the federal government to have a major interest in both the quality and cost of health care services. Implementation also created unprecedented demand for health care services and a reexamination of health care as a civil right.

Although PL 89-97 was a major step forward in addressing some of the major issues of health care, the Medicare and Medicaid programs using the traditional retrospective payment system have been extremely costly to operate, and their oversight has brought to light the fragmentation and lack of economic controls on the delivery system. The ease of abuse of the Medicaid and Medicare programs by some physicians and hospitals has not helped the financial stability of the system.

Many attempts have been made by every administration since 1965 to control the cost of Medicare and Medicaid. These attempts have increased public awareness of the "runaway" nature of health care spending in the United States. Despite caps, peer review organizations, reporting systems, and investigations, costs continue to rise. Some experts forecast that health care expenditures will exceed $1 trillion in the 1990s.

Prospective Payment

On April 20, 1982 President Reagan signed Public Law 98-21, the Social Security Amendments of 1982, which established the prospective payment system (PPS) for Medicare and Medicaid. The passage of the Tax Equity and Fiscal Responsibility Act (TEFRA) has significantly influenced the health care payment system by changing the amount and type of reimbursement hospitals receive for inpatient services. Shaffer (1984) writes, "this legislation will revolutionize the American Health Care delivery system and its impact will be felt in every sector." He goes on to say that, "PL 98-21 is a milestone in the history of health care and is the most dramatic health care legislation since the passage of Medicare in 1965" (p. 33). This law focuses on prospective reimbursement policies for hospitals based on DRGs. The purpose for this law was to reduce medical costs related to Medicare and Medicaid. Its focus was to reduce hospital stays and thus reduce hospital costs. The following statistics show some evidence that the Prospective Payment System (PPS) has been successful in achieving that aim:

- Inpatient services have experienced a major growth trend reversal. Admissions are at a 16-year low for patients under age 65 and at a 5-year low for patients 65 years of age or over; inpatient days are at an 18-year low (Hospitals, 1985).
- The Bureau of Labor Statistics reports that the medical component of the consumer price index rose only 6.6 percent between September 1983 and September 1984, compared with 7.5 percent in the same period the previous year and 11.4 percent two years previously (Coddington & Moore, 1987).

- The Health Care Financing Administration reports that for Medicare patients, length of stay decreased from an average of 9.4 days to 8.7 days between October 1983 and June 1984. By 1986 the average length of a hospital stay had dropped to 6.6 days (Coddington & Moore, 1987).

Although the PPS may have served to reduce hospital costs, it does not regulate and therefore has not effected physician fees, pharmaceuticals, and technology, which are all high cost items in the health care industry.

The PPS has also brought about many negative, and costly changes in the health care system. It has resulted in hospitalized patients being more acutely ill and requiring more intensive nursing interventions, which has strained all nursing resources and driven up the cost of nursing care per patient day. There is also a growing controversy over the early discharge of some patients, whether this has contributed to medical instability and worsened health status.

Four Major Changes or Current Restructuring

Today's health care system is characterized by a change in four major areas:

1. Rise in alternative delivery systems (ADS): health maintenance organizations (HMOs), preferred provider organizations (PPOs), and vertical integration of hospitals into multi-service corporations.
2. Fragmentation: excess hospital capacity, and in some areas too many physicians, too little home-based care, too few nursing homes.
3. Competition: increased sophistication in business practices in health care with both good and bad effects. Services are increasingly market driven.
4. Changed medical staff–hospital relations: joint-venture enterprises, increased hospital review of medical practice, increased autonomy of non-physician health providers (Coddington & Moore, 1987).

Ginsberg (1986) argues that the health care industry is not only undergoing a rapid change but also a period of destabilization. If this is alarming to health care providers and lawmakers, they may find some consolation in Coddington and Moore's (1987) belief that social systems seldom remain destabilized for long periods of time, and that markets and organizations adjust to change, and a new set of standard practices, strategies, and assumptions becomes common place.

The current move in health care is toward corporatization and privatization. The provision of health care in the United States is becoming a health industrial complex, in some respects not unlike the military–industrial complex. There is movement of units of service, including hospitals, into multiinstitutional systems. This trend is seen in both investor owned and nonprofit systems (Bauknecht, 1986; Institute of Medicine, 1986; Aydelotte, 1987).

Currently, there are about 250 multihospital systems in the United States (Brown, 1982; Ginsberg, 1986). Some are establishing HMOs and PPOs to tighten referral patterns so that all services in the system are used. Others have developed surgicenters, nursing homes, clinics, various types of outpatient services and emergency centers. The programs these systems offer are highly diversified, including health education, counseling, screening, and public lectures. Some have further diversified by sponsoring insurance plans, hotel services, transportation services, and management agencies. Marketing and advertising, unheard of a few years ago, are accepted practices (Aydelotte, 1987).

Today's health care system is market driven and will become much more competitive in the years ahead. Coddington and Moore (1987) advise to "find a way to differentiate your organization, or face a future of competing as a generic health care provider (a commodity) on the basis of price" (p. 285). They believe this is the bottom line for almost all health systems, hospitals, health plans, and physicians.

THE FUTURE

To try to *predict* the future of the health care system in the United States is not only foolhardy, it is impossible. However, the following may help to explain why the ability to *forecast* the future of health care is so tenuous, at its very best. It should be impossible to make accurate *projections* of probabilities about the future because projections are extensions of trends. If trends are identified and plotted on a curve, the curve is projected to continue in the direction consistent with governmental priorities. Trends are usually guided or determined by recognized problems, which in turn are reflected in rules, regulations, and policies that address those problems. Herein lies the problem. Although certain trends in health care can be identified and plotted; there is a lack of consensus as to national priorities to direct the slope or shape of the curve.

Today's health care system is like a patchwork quilt. A system of diverse programs to try to address target problems. Financing and target problems shift from year to year. There is no national health care policy to direct and guide action. Showstack and colleagues (1979) have described America as a mosaic of public and private programs, each with different rules covering both fees and services. This system has been *allowed* to develop by two very strong forces: (1) the lack of consensus among the American people regarding whether health and health care is a "right" or a "privilege" and (2) the high value placed on "rugged individualism and civil rights." This is exemplified in the deinstitutionalization of the mentally ill. Unless in need of treatment for an acute condition that threatens their safety or others' safety, citizens cannot be forced to be hospitalized and, in fact, must be discharged. This has resulted in thousands of chronically mentally ill persons becoming a "social problem" as homeless residents of our cities. This again demonstrates the intertwining of health and social issues and the unintended political consequences of fragmented policy decisions to improve one aspect of health care—the negative effects of institutionalization of the mentally ill—while ignoring the broader issue of a system of mental health services.

This lack of consensus and high value on rugged individualism and civil rights has resulted in the inability of the legislative and executive branches of government to put together a national health care policy that would serve to guide the development and implementation of health programs and payment systems.

So, without trying to forecast the future, or try to suggest a health care utopia, which would be impossible to achieve anyway, attention is turned to what is actually occurring today and will play itself out in the next 10 to 15 years. From this, knowledge of what might be expected to happen over the next decade or two will be garnered.

Certainly progress in widening access to health care delivery has occurred throughout this century. With this progress the roles and missions of the various health care institutions have also changed. Three distinct eras can be identified as we have moved through the twentieth century: the era of charity, the era of expansionism, and the current era of competition.

This section addresses only the current era of competition. First, this era is characterized by diversification as shown in two sets of activities: (1) adding new services to increase revenue and profits from sources other than inpatient services and (2) investing in a variety of ventures both within the context of the health care industry and outside the health care industry. Coddington and Moore (1987) refer to this as "spreading the risk" (p. 65).

Competitive advantage is the buzz-word of today and the future. Porter (1985) writes that "competitive advantage grows fundamentally out of value a firm is able to create for its buyers that exceeds that firm's cost of creating it. The two basic types of competitive advantage are cost leadership and differentiation" (p. 3). Cost leadership is offering the lowest price—not an acceptable standard for health care choices for most consumers or providers. Porter describes differentiation as "based on the product itself, the delivery system by which it is sold, the marketing approach, and a broad range of other factors" (p. 14). This is the mode chosen by today's leading health care institutions. For success in today's era, Coddington and Moore (1987) have identified ten possible broad strategies for gaining and sustaining competitive advantage in today's health care market. These ten strategies are worth reprinting here:

1. Differentiation on the basis of quality.
2. Alternative delivery systems (HMOs and PPOs): attempting to gain more control over the payers.
3. Diversification: broadening revenue bases both within and outside of the context of health care.
4. Vertical integration: controlling the availability of service through a continuum of care (primary care physicians and urgent care centers to inpatient services to long-term and home care).
5. Aggressive marketing: investing money and effort in seeking to increase market share.
6. Physician bonding: tying physicians to a specific health care plan.

7. Centers of excellence: deliberately seeking to build strong product lines (women's health, open heart surgery, and so on).
8. Networking: joint efforts between not-for-profit and investor-owned organizations.
9. Being a low-cost provider: developing and implementing better over-all systems for reducing costs.
10. Downsizing: finding the optimum level of operation that can be carried out profitably, yet with minimum impact on the quality of care.

It should be noted that seven of the above ten strategies are differentiation strategies.

If diversification is the wave of the future, is it a strategy that most health care systems should pursue? This question obviously has no absolute answer. Coddington and Moore (1987) suggest that diversification should be tempered by knowledge that most new ventures will fail and all require considerable funding before they break even. They believe, however, that there are many opportunities available to aggressive health care systems. They write, "given careful screening and selection, objective marketing and economic analysis, and well-managed implementation, diversification efforts represent a promising alternative and may contribute to the long-term viability of many health care organizations" (p. 126).

So, what is the future of health care and health care policy? Forecasters (Ellwood, 1986; Aydelotte, 1987; Coddington & Moore, 1987) are sharply divided on some issues, and in complete agreement on others—this is expected. None have a crystal ball. To assist the readers in drawing their own conclusions the following is a list of the various predictions of the realities in health care identified by some leaders. Aydelotte (1987) has made seven *predictions* for the future:

1. Many investor-owned multisystem ("supermeds") controlled by a few dozen national and international companies.
2. The systems will reflect a blurring of delivery models, combined to capture the market will be HMOs, PPOs, independent surgicenters, clinics, and other types of health services.
3. Nonprofit health care systems may convert to profit systems or increase the number or kind of subunits that produce a profit. (This is made more complex by the recent discussions about whether "nonprofits" contribute more community service than "for-profits" and, if not, should they lose their nonprofit, tax free status.)
4. The nature of the hospital will change. It will consist of multiple intensive care units offering highly specialized scientific and technological services. Patients will remain in the hospital for short periods.
5. There will be new programs for individuals who wish to maintain their health and to delay the onset of chronic disease.
6. The public hospital as it is today will not exist.

7. The majority of physicians will be employees of chains or in group practices associated with chains (p. 117).

Coddington and Moore (1987) outline 10 *realities* of the health care industry:

1. Health care providers will concentrate on local market or regions.
2. Alternative delivery systems or managed care will dominate the payer market.
3. Teaching and research hospitals will survive.
4. There will continue to be ample financial resources available for the health care industry.
5. Systems and alliances will increase in importance. Significant progress on indigent care and malpractice insurance crises.
6. Better definition of the health care product will emerge.
7. Many existing care ventures and products will merge.
8. Many existing health care ventures and products will be terminated.
9. Physicians will continue to control a major proportion of the market.
10. Many health care systems will find ways to differentiate themselves (p. 278).

Although the predictions are in, they are just that—predictions, and only history will record whether they are right or wrong. Nevertheless, health care policy makers should pay close attention to the current trends in the *need* for health care as well as in health care delivery systems. At this point it is probably not important whether "supermeds" will dominate the health care market, or whether physicians will be employees of corporate chains. The central issue is whether reasonable health care will be available for all Americans at a cost that they can afford. This seems unlikely if the costs of health care continues to spiral upward without a national health policy to help identify the most pertinent aspects of health care and health care delivery.

Ginsberg (1987) reports that for the first time in the history of American medicine, total health care expenditures (including administrative costs) have passed the half-trillion-dollar mark. In 1987 the estimated expenditure of $511 billion will account for 11.4 percent of the GNP. This is an increase of $53 billion in a one-year period, from $458 billion in 1986 to $511 billion in 1987. An advanced knowledge of mathematics is not required to realize that this rate of spending cannot be sustained.

A national health policy is needed to address those issues that can be identified as forces that are shaping health care today. Some of those forces are: A changing health care industry, a continued increase in high-technology, an aging population, an unstable economy, increasing health care insurance costs, and a physician surplus.

Through the creation of a national health policy a monitoring system could be put into place that would monitor the changing forces as a means of accurately projecting national health care needs for the future.

Nurse administrators can play a major role, if not a pivotal role, in helping to shape health policy. This can be done through the active participation in political action organizations—making the needs of practicing nurses and their perceptions of patient needs known. Through the planning and development of marketing strategies aimed at creating and administering cost-effective centers for nursing excellence within their own organizational structure, managing productive, efficient health care programs within the community, and helping to create a competitive health care delivery market.

In a society where health care costs continue to rise, economic and manpower resources continue to dwindle, and fatigue and job dissatisfaction continue to take their toll, nursing administrators not only have a responsibility to address the issues, they have an obligation to act. They have an obligation to become full partners in the development and implementation of a national health policy that addresses all health care issues across all social strata. This role may best be played out by active, aggressive involvement in both the workplace and the political arena.

BIOGRAPHICAL SKETCH

James D. Vail, RN, DNSc is Associate Professor, School of Nursing, George Mason University, Fairfax, Virginia, where he teaches graduate courses in both Research and Nursing Management. He previously served as Director of both the Nursing Research Service and the Nursing Education and Staff Development Service at the Walter Reed Army Medical Center, Washington, D.C. He also served as the Consultant, Nursing Research, Office of the U.S. Army Surgeon General.

Dr Vail has published many articles in professional journals, has spoken extensively throughout this country and in Europe on Quality Assurance, Nursing Research, and Standards of Nursing Practice. He has been active in health care policy formation at every level of nursing throughout his nursing career.

SUGGESTED READINGS

Abramowitz, K.S. (1985). *The future of health care delivery in America.* Barstein Research, Sanford C. Barnstein and Co., Inc.

Aiken, L. (ed.). (1981). *Health policy and nursing practice.* New York: McGraw-Hill.

Aiken, L., Gortner, S. (eds.). (1982). *Nursing in the 1980s: Crises, opportunities, challenge.* Philadelphia: Lippincott.

American Nurses' Association. (1980). *Nursing: A social policy statement.* Kansas City: American Nurses' Association.

American Nurses.' Association. (1985). *Nurses, politics, and public policy,* videotape. Kansas City: American Nurses' Association.

American Academy of Nursing. (1979). *Nursing's influence on health policy for the eighties.* Kansas City: American Academy of Nursing.

American Academy of Nursing. (1982). *From accommodation to self-determination: Nursing's role in the development of health care policy.* Kansas City: American Academy of Nursing.

American Academy of Nursing. (1985). *The economics of health care and nursing.* Kansas City: American Academy of Nursing.

Hirt, E.J. (ed.). (1987). *The health policy agenda for the American people.* The Health Policy Agenda for the American People: Great Northern Design and Printing.

Kalisch, B. , & Kalisch, P. (1982). *Politics of nursing.* Philadelphia: Lippincott.

Milio, N. (1981). *Promoting health through public policy.* Philadelphia: FA Davis Co.

National League for Nursing. (1986). *Integrating public policy into the curriculum.* New York: National League for Nursing.

Rothberg, J.S. (1985). The growth of political action in nursing. *Nursing Outlook, 33*(3).

Solomon, S.B., Roe, S.C. (1986). *Key concepts in public policy: Student workbook.* New York: National League for Nursing.

REFERENCES

Aydelotte, M. (1987). Nursing's preferred future. *Nursing Outlook, 35*(3), 114–120.

Bauknecht, V.L. (1986). IOM study of ''for-profits'' finds care costs not very different. *American Nurse, 18*(7), 3–5.

Brown, M. (1982). Multihospital systems in the 80s—the new shape of the health care industry. *Hospitals, 56*(March 4), 71–74.

Burton, L.E., & Smith, H.N. (1970). *Public health and community medicine.* Baltimore: Williams & Wilkins.

Clark, G. (1980). State government. Where the action is. *The Nation's Health, 10*(4), 16.

Coddington, D.C., & Moore, K.D. (1987). *Market-driven strategies in health care.* San Francisco: Jossey-Bass.

Cray, E. (1970). *In failing health.* Indianapolis: Bobbs-Merrill.

Davis, C.K. (1983a). The federal role in changing health care financing: Part I. National programs and health financing problems. *Nursing Economics, 1*(4), 10–17.

Davis, C.K. (1983b). The federal role in changing health care financing: Part II. Prospective payment and its impact on nursing. *Nursing Economics, 1*(5), 98–104, 146.

Diers, D. (1985). Health policy and nursing curricula—A natural fit. *Nursing and Health Care, 6*(10), 421–433.

Disease Prevention and Health Promotion; Federal Programs and Prospects. (1978). Washington, D.C.: U.S. Department of Health, Education and Welfare.

Duval, M.K. (1977). Provider, government, and consumer. In J.K. Knowles (ed.), *Doing better and feeling worse: Health in the United States.* New York: Norton Publishers.

Dye, T.R. (1984). *Understanding public policy* (5 ed.). Englewood Cliffs, NJ: Prentice-Hall.

Eastaugh, S.R. (1981). *Medical economics and health finance.* Dover, MA: Auburn House Publishing Company.

Ellwood, P. Jr. (1986). Ellwood says "supermed" concept gaining ground, expects up to 10 within a decade. *Medical Benefits, 3*(9), 9–11.

Feingold, E. (1966). *Medicare: Policy and politics.* San Francisco: Chandler Publishing Co.

Gibson, R.M., & Waldo, D.R. (1984). National health expenditures, 1983. *Health Care Financing Review. 8*(4), 1–36.

Ginsberg, E. (1986). The destabilization of health care. *New England Journal of Medicine, 315*(12), 757–761.

Ginsberg, E. (1987). Eight facts of life shaping health care. *Hospitals, 61*(August 20), 80.

Glaser, W.A. (1986). Payment systems and their effects. In L.H. Aiken & D. Mechanic (eds.), *Application of social science to clinical medicine and health policy,* NJ: Rutgers University Press.

Hawkins, J.B.W., & Higgins, L.P. (1982). *Nursing and the American health care delivery system.* New York: The Tiresias Press, Inc.

Hospital Headlines. (1985). *Hospitals,* January 15.

Institute of Medicine, Committee on Implication of For-Profit Enterprise in Health Care. (1986). *For-profit enterprise in health care.* Washington, D.C.: National Academy Press.

Jonas, S., Banta, D., & Enright, M. (1977). Government in the health care delivery system. In S. Jonas (ed.), *Health care delivery in the United States.* New York: Springer.

Jordan, C. (1983). The powers of political activity. In K.R. Stevens (ed.), *Power and influence: A source book for nurses.* New York: Wiley and Sons, p. 83.

Josiah Macy Foundation. (1976). *Physicians for the future: Report of the Macy Commission.* New York: Josiah Macy Foundation.

Kalisch, P.A., & Kalisch, B.J. (1986). *The advance of American nursing* (2 ed.). Boston: Little, Brown, p. 51.

Kaluzny, A.D., Warner, D.M., Warren, D.C., & Zelman, W.N. (1982). *Management of health services.* Englewood Cliffs, NJ: Prentice-Hall, Inc.

Krause, A. (1977). *Power and illness—The political sociology of health and medical care.* New York: Elsevier.

Lewis, D.J. (1983). Evolution of federal policy on access to health care, 1965 to 1980. *Bulletin of the New York Academy of Medicine, 59*(1), 9–20.

MacPherson, K.I. (1987). Health care policy, values, and nursing. *Advances in Nursing Science, 9*(3), 1–11.

Marmor, T.R. (1970). *The politics of medicare.* London: Routledge and Kegan Paul.

Marram, G., Schlegel, M., & Bevis, E. (1974). Primary nursing: A model for individualized care. St Louis: CV Mosby.

Moccia, P. (1984). The nurse as policy maker: Toward a free and equal health care system. *Nursing and Health Care,* 5(11) 481–485.

News from the United States Department of Labor. (1979). Washington, D.C.: U.S. Department of Labor, Office of Information.

NLN Position Statement on National Health Insurance. (1979). NLN Pub. No. 11 1786, New York: NLN.

Porter, M. (1985). *Competitive advantage: Creating and sustaining superior performance.* New York: Free Press.

Reed, D.A. (1988). Nursing shortage: David Reed's top concern. *Hospitals,* August 20, 44–47.

Shaffer, F.A. (1984). Prospective payment: A strategic plan for nursing power. In R.R. Wieczorek, (ed.), *Power, politics, and policy in nursing.* New York: Springer.

Showstack, J.A., Blumber, B.D., Schwartz, J., & Schroeder, S.A. (1979). Fee-for-service physician payment: Analysis of current methods and their development. *Inquiry,* 16, 230–246.

Skaggs, B. (1985). The great shift: Politics at the state level. *Perspectives in nursing—1985–1987,* NLN Pub. No. 41. New York: NLN.

Trafford, A. (1987). With millions of Americans unprotected, national health insurance gains new popularity. *Health—The Washington Post,* July 7, p. 15.

CASE 3–1

The Role of ANA in Legislative Reform of Nursing Homes 1986–1987

Janet Heinrich

Dramatic changes have occurred in the health care delivery system in the past decade, with even more changes proposed for the future. Many of the future changes focus on health care services for the elderly, such as long-term care and insurance coverage of care in nursing homes. The proposals of the Reagan Administration for catastrophic health insurance, proposed legislation, and congressional hearings indicate widespread public interest.

As the largest group of health care providers, nurses are affected by policy decisions regarding health care services made by our elected and appointed officials at the federal, state, and local levels of government. Nurses, because of

This article was prepared on the authors' personal time and was not part of her official responsibilities with nor should it be attributed to the National Institutes of Health.

their numbers and their ubiquitous role in all sectors of the health care system, can be a powerful force in influencing public policy and political outcomes. The American Nurses' Association (ANA), through the governmental affairs program, works to assure that the nursing profession is a major participant in the nation's public policy debates. The staff of this division is responsible for monitoring and influencing the actions of Congress and the federal agencies, consistent with the ANA House of Delegates plan and priorities established by the ANA Board of Directors. The division also works to strengthen nurses' knowledge of the political system, through nurses' involvement in grassroots political action, and understanding of the legislative and regulatory process.

The basic definition of politics, according to Kalisch and Kalisch (1982), "is the authoritative allocation of scarce resources" (p. 31). It is a part of working for change within our communities in every arena and at all levels of government. The study of politics is the study of decision making or put another way how power, influence, and human behavior effect who gets what, when, and how.

Public policy is a chosen course of action taken to address and identify issues and concerns. The policy process includes recognizing and defining a problem, developing programs and allocating resources to address the problem, and implementing and evaluating the impact of the program. Before an issue can move through the arduous public policy labyrinth, there must be a broad consensus on the importance of the problem and the solutions must be developed among many diverse groups. Elected and appointed officials, often leaders without a background in health care, are making policy decisions impacting on nursing practice and health care services. These officials need information from nurses about how the health care system really works.

Tracking a specific issue through the legislative and regulatory process is instructive in understanding how the ANA works to influence national public policy. In 1986 the Institute of Medicine (IOM) of the National Academy of Science reported on its study on quality of care in nursing homes. The study was undertaken at the request of the U.S. Department of Health and Human Services (DHHS), Health Care Financing Administration (HCFA) after consumer groups and professional organizations had strongly opposed a HCFA proposal to change the regulations governing the process of certifying the eligibility of nursing homes to receive payment under the Medicare and Medicaid programs. The American Association of Retired Persons (AARP), the National Senior Citizens Coalition, and the American Nurses' Association were some of the major groups that spoke against the easing of requirements and demanded that nursing home regulations be strengthened to address fundamental weaknesses in the system to assure quality of care.

There have been many studies on nursing home care that identified inadequate care and abuse of the elderly. Robert N. Butler, M.D., received a Pulitzer Prize for his book, *Why Survive? Being Old in America*. In 1977, former U.S. Senator Frank E. Moss documented many of the problems in his book: *Too Old, Too Sick, Too Bad—Nursing Homes in America*. (Moss and Halamandaris, 1977). A broad consensus developed over the years among many diverse groups that government regulation of nursing homes was unsatisfactory because it allowed substandard or marginal homes to continue to participate in the Medicare and Medicaid programs. The IOM study was unique in that it was able to build consensus on recommendations for solutions to the problem.

The IOM study made many recommendations for quality of care and quality of life in nursing homes. The American Nurses' Association had advocated several of these policy changes at regional hearings held by the IOM Committee on Nursing Home Regulations. The following recommendations were of particular interest to the ANA:

> The regulatory distinction between Skilled Nursing Facilities (SNFs) and Intermediate Care Facilities (ICFs) should be abolished. A single set of conditions of participation and standards should be used to certify all nursing homes.
>
> A new condition of participation on resident assessment should be added. It should require that in every certified facility a registered nurse who has received appropriate training for the purpose shall be responsible for seeing that accurate assessments of each resident are done upon admission, periodically, and whenever there is a change in resident status. The results should be recorded and retained in a standard format in the resident's medical record. A new standard, nurse's aide training, should be added to the administration condition. The standard should require that all nurse's aides complete a preservice state-approved training program in a state-accredited institution such as a community college. (Institute of Medicine, 1986, pp. 25–44)

In addition, the ANA took a strong stand on adequate staffing, recommending that there be at least one registered nurse on duty, 24 hours per day, seven days a week.

The ANA, through its Council on Gerontological Nursing and policies put forth by several State Nurses' Associations, had established nursing home reform as a high priority (ANA, 1985). Senior citizen advocacy groups, including the American Association of Retired Persons, the National Council of Senior Citizens, and the Long-Term Care Ombudsman, and professional organizations, including the ANA, and the nursing home trade organization, the American Health Care Association formed the National Citizens Coalition for Nursing Home Reform. Their stated mission was the implementation of the IOM recommendations to improve the quality of care and the quality of life in our nation's nursing homes.

In May, 1986, Senator John Heinz (R-PA), Chairman of the Special Committee on Aging, United States Senate, issued a report of the findings of a two-year study of the quality of care in nursing homes as well as an analysis of federal inspection reports. The Committee found that with 1.5 million Americans utilizing nursing homes, at an annual expenditure of more than $30 billion, almost one-third of the 8852 skilled nursing facilities failed to meet at least one basic federal standard to assure the health and safety of residents in 1984. Many of the violations were in failure to provide 24-hour nursing care (U.S. Senate,

1986). Senator Heinz moved to introduce legislation that would make many of the recommendations of the IOM study law. Congressman Henry Waxman (D-CA) proposed companion legislation in the House. Many of the specific legislative issues remained contentious, especially the issue of adequate staffing. The American Health Care Association was adamantly opposed to any specific registered nurse-staffing requirements due to the increased costs this would impose on the nursing home industry. The ANA was equally adamant that without qualified registered nurses present to provide the necessary care, there would be no quality. The legislation was unable to move through all the necessary committees before the end of the 99th Congress.

With the advent of the 100th Congress, in 1987, new legislative proposals for nursing home reform were introduced. ANA continued to work with other coalition members and the congressional staff of the congressmen and senators on the committees with responsibility for nursing home reform. On the House side this included the Health Subcommittee, Energy and Commerce, chaired by Henry Waxman (D-CA) and the Health Subcommittee, Ways and Means, chaired by Pete Stark (D-CA). Claude Pepper (D-FL), Chairman of the House Special Committee on Aging, also introduced legislation for reforms in long-term care. In the Senate, the Committee with jurisdiction is the Finance Committee, chaired by Lloyd Bentsen (D-TX) with the Health Subcommittee chaired by George Mitchell (D-ME).

Other "must do" issues facing members at the start of the 100th Congress were the budget deficit and Gramm-Rudman, contra aid, the nomination of Judge Robert Bork to the U.S. Supreme Court, budget reconciliation, catastrophic insurance, all 13 appropriations bills, defense authorization, and campaign finance reform. Keeping nursing home reform as a "must do" agenda and the momentum of the last year moving was an issue onto itself.

As Congress was crafting a legislative response to the problems in nursing homes, the Department of Health and Human Services was drafting regulations that would address the problems as well in the hope of adopting changes before legislation could be enacted. HCFA developed new conditions for nursing homes to participate in the Medicare and Medicaid programs, which incorporated several of the IOM study recommendations. These conditions were to replace those established in 1974. The intent of the proposed revisions were to focus on actual facility performance in meeting residents' needs in a safe and healthful environment, rather than on the capacity of a facility to provide appropriate services, and to simplify federal enforcement procedures. The Administration's philosophy was to allow market forces to work and to remove the burden of regulation.

The ANA staff worked with HCFA staff and coalition members to supply information and make formal comments on any proposed rule-making posted in the Federal Register, such as the Medicare and Medicaid Long-Term Care Survey. ANA staff also held meetings with key decision makers such as the Director of HCFA, the Under Secretary DHHS, the Chief of Staff DHHS, and the

Secretary DHHS, to express the views of the organization. They also encouraged other members of the Coalition to do so at times when key decisions where being made by the Administration.

Proposed regulations passed through DHHS to the Office of Management and Budget (OMB) and were published in the Federal Register on October 16, 1987. The proposed rules eliminated the distinction between skilled nursing facilities (SNF) and intermediate care facilities (ICF). They provided that residents' needs be assessed and a plan of care be developed; and added the requirement of nurse's aide training and demonstration of proficiency in patient care. The requirements for sufficient nursing staff were less clear. The stated objective was to assure that nursing homes had adequate nurse staffing to meet the care needs of residents and at the same time to provide maximum flexibility for staffing and to avoid requiring 24-hour nurse staffing. Three alternative staffing requirements were proposed: (1) 24-hour licensed nurses with day shift coverage by a registered nurse, seven days a week; (2) one licensed nurse on the day shift, seven days a week; and (3) waiver of any requirement (Federal Register, October 16, 1987).

The issues of registered nurse-staffing in nursing homes remained unresolved within the Administration. As one official put it: "I am supportive of the need for more nurses in nursing homes but I am unwilling to fall on my pike over the issue." Factual information from studies of indicators of quality of care, such as eating, toileting, and use of restraints was presented to key decision makers within DHHS, OMB, and members of Congress. To address arguments about the additional costs of adding registered nurses to nursing homes, the ANA gathered information on cost per bed by the size of the facility. The cost of adding a registered nurse to a small facility, under 30 beds, was $2.28 per bed and the cost for larger facilities (over 120 beds) was $.50 or less. The cost of upgrading staffing to one licensed nurse around the clock in the state of Texas, a state with a very low ratio of licensed nurses to residents, was $0.08 per resident per day for a total cost to the industry of approximately two million dollars in 1988.

As legislative proposals moved through assigned committees in the House of Representatives, the ANA worked to convince legislators of the need for 24-hour registered nurse staffing in nursing homes. Grassroots activities by nurses, such as phone calls and letters to their Representatives, were orchestrated through state nurses' associations. States with senators and congressman on the health subcommittees are targeted for lobbying on "hot" issues.

Congressman Doug Walgrin (D-PA) pushed for an amendment that would require 24-hour registered nurse staffing, but a tie vote by subcommittee members ended in the exclusion of this provision. Final versions of nursing home reform legislation in both the House and Senate were folded into the omnibus budget reconciliation legislation for 1987. Action on the reconciliation legislation depended on progress on the Gramm-Rudman balanced budget law and ways to reduce budget deficit. There was the possibility that even if Congress were able to reach consensus on the budget and spending legislation, the President would veto the legislation if it included increased taxes.

The Omnibus Budget Reconciliation Act of 1987 was passed and signed into law in late December. It included most of the provisions suggested by the IOM study for nursing home reform including the consolidation of requirements for SNFs and ICFs, resident assessment and plans of care conducted by a registered professional nurse, and required nurse-aide training. Staffing requirements for nursing was stated as "must be provided by qualified persons in accordance with each resident's written plan of care." Specifically, an SNF is required to provide 24-hour nursing service, which is sufficient to meet nursing needs of its residents and must employ a registered nurse "at least during the day tour of duty seven days a week" (U.S. Congress, 1987). The law also allows for state waivers.

The nursing home reform changes will be implemented through HCFA policies over several years and will require close monitoring by interested groups if the intent of the law is to be carried out. Groups, such as the ANA and AARP, will need to continue to provide information, opinions, and negotiate with the nursing home industry over reforms.

Nurses can and do play an important role in shaping health policy. Nursing home reform is only one example. Both the ANA and the AARP have targeted long-term health care as top issues for their future policy agendas. AARP is emerging as one of the most powerful lobbies in the country. They are seen as people who use their time wisely, are well-organized, who vote regularly, and they have launched an $8 million get out the vote effort (Hornblower, 1988). The ANA has a force in shaping the future health care delivery system as well, but it will be important for nurses to work closely with other groups, such as AARP, in defining the problems and articulating the solutions. There are formidable barriers to effective solutions for long-term care benefits not the least of which is expense. Nurses must work with others to define what it is we want to finance and why. The fiscal environment is hostile. Clarification of long-term care is essential to the model of service delivery adopted and financed. Nurses must be visible and articulate about the services they offer and the benefits they provide to the public.

BIOGRAPHICAL SKETCH

Janet Heinrich served as Senior Staff Specialist with the American Nurses' Association government affairs office where she was primarily responsible for monitoring programs and regulations within the Department of Health and Human Services. She is a nursing graduate of the University of Michigan with a MPH from The Johns Hopkins University and a PhD from Yale University. Dr Heinrich has worked in academia, in home health care, and in health planning. She is currently with the National Center for Nursing Research, National Institutes of Health.

SUGGESTED READINGS

Dodd, L.C., & Oppenheimer, B.I. (1981). *Congress reconsidered* (2nd ed.). Washington, D.C.: Congressional Quarterly Press.

Green, M. (1984). *Who runs congress?* (4th ed.) New York: Dell.

Hunter, P.R., & Serger, K.J. (1984). Nurses and the political arena: Lobbying for professional impact. *Nursing Administration Quarterly, 2*, 66–79.

Kalisch, B.J., & Kalisch, P.A. (1982). *Politics of nursing*. Philadelphia: J.B. Lippincott Co.

Make, R.S. (1984). Legislators' opinions about nursing: Results of a pilot study. *Nursing & Health Care, 5*, 204–207.

Mason, D.J., & Talbott, S.W. (1985). *Political action handbook for nurses*. Reading, Mass: Addison-Wesley.

Ornstein, N.J., & Elder, S. (1978). *Interest groups, lobbying and policymaking*. Washington, D.C.: Congressional Quarterly Press.

The Hastings Center. (1985). *The ethics of legislative life*. Hastings-on-Hudson, NY: Institute of Society, Ethics and the Life Sciences.

REFERENCES

American Nurses' Association. (1985). *House of delegates action*. Kansas City, MO: American Nurses' Association.

Federal Register. (October 16, 1987). Vol. 52, No. 200, pp. 38582–38606.

Hornblower, M. (1988). Gray power. *Time, 131*(1), 36–37.

Institute of Medicine. (1986). Committee on Nursing Home Regulation. *Improving the quality of care in nursing homes*. Washington, D.C.: National Academy Press.

Kalisch, B.J., & Kalisch, P.A. (1982). *Politics of nursing*. Philadelphia: J.B. Lippincott, p. 31.

Moss, F.E., & Halamandaris, V.J. (1977). *Too old, too sick, too bad—Nursing homes in America*. Germantown, MD: Aspen Systems Corporation.

U.S. Congress. (1987). *Omnibus Budget Reconciliation Act of 1987*, Conference Report to Accompany H.R. 3545. Washington, D.C.: Government Printing Office, pp. 169–170.

U.S. Senate. (1986). *Nursing Home Care: The Unfinished Agenda*. Staff Report, Special Committee on Aging.

4

Nurse Administrators As Women Managers

Section 1: Stereotyping

Carol M. Ondeck

Women have always cared for the sick, but until the nineteenth century, nursing care outside of the family was provided mainly by members of religious orders or by disreputable women. In the middle of that century, Florence Nightingale created a secular, scientific order of nurses. In a diary entry, in 1850, Nightingale described herself as having an intellectual, passionate, moral, active nature, yet it was women's nurturing, maternal nature that was used to justify their legitimacy and acceptance in nursing (Canedy, 1979).

It appears that, even to the current day, these separate historical influences on the practice of nursing still linger as myths and stereotypes about this most feminine of occupations.

STEREOTYPING THEORY

Through the years the predominant behavior pattern between physician and nurse has been one of dominance and deference. A number of factors contribute to this autocratic relationship, not the least of which is that most physicians are men and most nurses are women. In an analysis of various sources of physician–nurse conflict, Kalisch and Kalisch (1980) explain that to change this relationship the nurse must confront men and "since physicians are not only men but constitute a sort of master race of males, the nurse is in for the fight of her life."

Perhaps, the stereotypes of nurses can be understood best as a subset within the larger set of stereotypes about women and men. A stereotype is a "fuzzy set" or category that includes a number of attributes. Evidence from numerous recent studies points to clearly delineated beliefs about what men and women are typically like. Two distinct clusters of traits are seen as distinguishing men from women (Deaux, 1976) (Figure 4–1). One cluster contains traits reflecting competence such as competitiveness, independence, and objectivity. These traits are perceived as being characteristic of men and the opposite or absence of these traits is associated with women, that is, women are dependent, non-competitive, and subjective.

A second cluster contains traits reflecting warmth and expressiveness such as tact, awareness of other's feelings, and ability to express feelings. These traits are perceived as being characteristic of women, whereas men are viewed as the opposite such as blunt, insensitive and unable to express feelings.

To determine the effects of stereotypes, it is necessary to consider how people use or process this information.

ATTRIBUTION THEORY

The basic paradigm of a *cognitive* theory of motivation is that mental events after the perception of a stimulus determine the response to that stimulus. The cognitive process may be expressed as follows:

$$\text{Stimulus} \longrightarrow \text{Cognitivity activity} \longrightarrow \text{Response}$$

Those familiar with the behavior modification, or the learning theory approach to explaining behavior recognize that this cognitive model differs from the behavioral modification process or:

$$\text{Stimulus} \longrightarrow \text{Response} \longrightarrow \text{Consequences} \longrightarrow \text{Future response}$$

Simply stated, the latter approach states that behavior that has rewarding consequences is likely to be repeated; behavior that leads to a negative or punishing consequence tends not to be repeated. That is the "law of effect" (Stoner & Waukel, 1986). Although the role of cognition versus that of reinforcement may well be a subject of debate, recent research expanding on the model of the cognitive process has yielded interesting results that explain how people process information and the effects of stereotypes. It provides evidence that cognitive

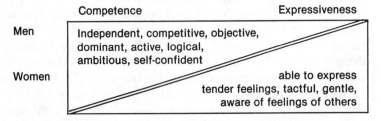

Figure 4–1. Stereotypes of Traits of Men and Women

processes influence anticipations about goal attainment. The anticipation that some action will lead to or be instrumental in achieving a particular result is called expectancy. In addition, cognitive processes influence emotional reactions to a stimulus that creates varying internal arousal states; these are called the affective responses to a stimulus. It has been proposed, therefore, that the cognitive model may be elaborated as (Weiner et al., 1972)

$$\text{Stimulus} \rightarrow \text{Cognitive Activity} \begin{array}{c} \nearrow \text{Expectations} \searrow \\ \\ \searrow \text{Affect} \nearrow \end{array} \text{Behavior}$$

COMBINING SEX ROLE STEREOTYPES AND EXPECTATIONS

An interesting experiment conducted by Deaux and Emswiller in 1974 examined sex role stereotypes as a source of expectations and their effect on what factors people attribute as a contribution to performance. In the experiment, subjects were told that they would be listening to another person perform a task requiring recognition of a common object. Two different classes of objects were used in the experiment. The first was considered to be a set of masculine objects. It included lug wrenches, Philips screwdrivers, and tire jacks. Given the stereotyped belief that men are more competent, particularly at a masculine task, it was hypothesized that subjects would most likely attribute a man's performance to ability and a woman's performance to luck. Not only did this occur, but male and female subjects did not differ in their attributions, confirming further that similar stereotypes are held by both sexes.

Success is consistent with expectancies for men, and when it occurs, it is attributed to the stable, internal cause of high ability. Because failure tends not to be expected, it is attributed to the variable, external cause, bad luck. Given the stereotype of women as passive and dependent, their success on achievement-related tasks is not expected. This inconsistency can be accepted by attributing the success to the variable external cause of luck. Even when women's success occurs on difficult, complex tasks, for example, portfolio analysis or capital budgeting, the attribution is more often to the internal but variable cause of effort rather than to ability. Low expectations for women in subsequent tasks did not change even after successful performance.

A SEX-SEGREGATED OCCUPATION

Nursing has been and continues to be a segregated occupation for women. From a clinical perspective, nurses are considered subordinate to physicians who assume that nurses are carrying out delegated functions or tasks. In addition to societal stereotypes about women in general and nurses in particular, this subordinate status is reinforced by the higher educational levels of physicians and their higher socioeconomic status (Kalisch & Kalisch, 1980).

From an administrative perspective, nurses in hospital settings are the subject of a dual system of authority, receiving orders not only from physicians, but also from hospital administrators.

In a recent review of the role of nursing in hospital decision making, the authors cite Perrow's classic study of hospitals as institutions that have evolved through stages in which trustees, physicians, and finally professional administrators successively dominate (Wisman, Alexander, & Morlock, 1981). The authors conclude that "although hospital decision making is receiving much attention, nursing's role in decision making at the hospital level is a relatively uninvestigated area. Neither the extent of nursing influence relative to other groups nor the areas in which nursing exercises influence has been well documented. . . ." Thus, the role nurse administrators play in hospital decision making is still undocumented. This should be a high priority for nurse researchers.

PROFESSIONAL PRACTICE

As early as 1963 a consultative group in nursing reported to the U.S. Public Health Service's Surgeon General that changes in medical practice should include the delegation of increased responsibilities to professional nurses and the expectation that nurses would increasingly use independent judgment in meeting their responsibilities. An outgrowth of this report was the formation, in 1967, of the National Commission for the Study of Nursing and Nursing Education in the United States. One of the central recommendations of this commission was the establishment of the National Joint Practice Commission (NJPC), joint practice meaning nurses and physicians collaborating to provide patient care. Funded by a Kellogg Foundation grant in 1977, the NJPC conducted four demonstration projects culminating in 1981 with the publication of *Guidelines for Establishing Joint or Collaborative Practice in Hospitals*. The five elements of joint practice included in the project were: (1) primary nursing, (2) clinical decision making by nurses within the scope of nursing practice as defined by the hospital, (3) the integrated patient record as a formal means for nurse–physician communication in the care of patients, (4) joint patient care review, and (5) a joint practice committee to monitor this relationship and recommend actions supporting joint practice (Ritter, 1983). These changes have come slowly and are still not fully implemented in some settings.

ADMINISTRATIVE CHANGE

Earlier chapters of this text have focused on the external environmental influences on health care delivery systems, most notably hospitals. Chapter 6 on strategic planning as well as the current scholarly literature explains that hospital administrators must continually adapt to external pressures regarding regulation, competition, fund acquisition, personnel shortages, and increased clinical effectiveness. In fact, in a study of cost containment policies in hospitals, Provan (1987) suggests that administrators have not only a management orientation, as opposed to a professional one, but also a macro health care delivery perspective rather than the more micro concern for fulfilling individual patients' needs. This perspective is the opposite of clinical staff.

Beginning with the head nurse, nurse managers, at all levels should cultivate both the managerial and macro perspectives based on an appreciation of external pressures. As clinicians they also should bring an appreciation of those perspectives to the management team.

It could be argued that a good staff nurse or clinician is a necessary but not sufficient criteria for a good leader and manager. Promotion to head nurse based on such achievement is a positive factor but the role of nurse administrator is necessarily more diverse and, therefore, requires additional skills. To the surprise of many new nurse administrators assuming managerial responsibilities, this includes assuming a new stereotype that of women as managers.

In a 1978 literature review, Bartol (1978) investigated the "sex structuring of organizations." She reviewed three classes of studies dealing with: (1) leader behavior or style, (2) leader job satisfaction (on the premise that because of their socialization, women might have lower job satisfaction in leadership positions), and (3) job performance. She *found no style, satisfaction, or performance differences based on sex of the leader.* Then why are there few women administrators? Or, "How does it happen that even in organizations with large numbers of women grouped at the lower levels, few women are found at the top?" Bartol states that "in viewing the evidence of three major areas of concern to the study of leadership, it seems unlikely that differential behaviors of job outcomes associated with female leaders can account for significant amounts of the sex structuring of organizations." Yet, that is what exists.

Bartol suggests that Schein's model of career development within organizations provides a useful framework for understanding this filtering of promotions for women in organizations. According to Schein (1971), from the point of view of individual career progress, the organization can be viewed as more of an inverted cone than the traditional hierarchical triangle. The three dimensions of the cone represent three potential types of movement. *Vertical* movement is change in one's formal rank. *Circumferential* movement is horizontal, across division, function, or department. *Radial* movement is toward or away from the core or inner circle of power. Each type of movement is across a type of boundary and at individual transitions or decision points these boundaries act as filters which may or may not be permeable.

The thesis presented is that sexist attitudes and stereotyping are one major explanation of organizational sex structuring. The interplay of personal and social preferences in promotions of women by men is an intriguing conumdrum. Economic considerations concerning geographic mobility, labor force participation and attachment, as well as individuals' investment in education and training have been used, in some cases, to rebut statistical arguments of sexual discrimination in management employment. The search for a single, unequivocal answer is probably as fruitless as it is tempting.

The data reported in these studies are consistent but the causality is open to conjecture. Regardless, increasing numbers of nurse administrators are penetrating the "glass ceiling" by assuming executive positions. Section 2 describes the profiles of successful women administrators. Examination offers suggestions for career planning for aspiring nurse executives.

BIOGRAPHICAL SKETCH

Carol Ondeck is an Associate Professor of Management, School of Business and Economics, at Towson State University. Dr Ondeck was previously a member of the faculty of George Mason University and Director MBA Program at the University of Maryland, College Park. She received her DBA from The George Washington University in 1978.

SUGGESTED READINGS

Nursing as a Stereotyped Occupation

Levine, M., Zacur, S., & Horton, L. (1980). *Professional issues in nursing.* Glen Ridge, NJ: Thomas Horton and Daughters.

Muff, J. (ed.). (1982). *Socialization, sexism, and stereotyping: Women's issues in nursing.* St. Louis: C. V. Mosby.

Collaborative Nursing Practice

Devereux, P. (1981). Essential elements of nurse–physician collaboration. *Journal of Nursing Administration, 11*(5), 19–23.

Norkin, M. (1983, Fall). Collaboration and communication. *Nursing Administration Quarterly,* 1–7.

Women as Managers

Kanter, R. (1979). Men and women of corporation. New York: Basic Books Inc.

Change

Schein, E. (1985). *Organizational culture and leadership.* San Francisco: Jossey-Bass.

REFERENCES

Bartol, K. (1978, October). The sex structuring of organizations: A search for possible causes. *Academy of Management Review,* 805–812.

Canedy, B.H. (1979). Florence Nightingale: Woman with a vision. In Kjervik, D. & Martinson, I. (eds.), *Women in Stress: A Nursing Perspective*, New York: Appleton-Century-Crofts.

Deaux, K. (1976). Sex: A perspective on the attribution process. *New Directions in Attribution Research*, 1, 335–352.

Deaux, K., & Emswiller, T. (1974). Explanations of successful performance on sex-linked tasks: What is skill for the male is luck for the female. *Journal of Personality and Social Psychology*, 27, 80–85.

Kalisch, B.J., & Kalisch, P.A. (1980). An analysis of the sources of physician-nurse conflict. In Levine, M. & Zacur, S. (eds.), *Professional Issues in Nursing: Challenges and Opportunities*, Glen Ridge, NJ: Thomas Horton and Daughters, pp. 64, 65.

Muff, J. (1982). Handmaiden, battle-ax, whore. In Muff, J. (ed). *Socialization, Sexism, and Stereotyping*, St. Louis: CV Mosby, pp. 113–156.

Provan, K. (1987). Environmental and organizational predictors of adoption of cost containment policies in hospitals. *Academy of Management Journal*, 30(2), 219–239.

Ritter, H. (1983, Summer). Collaborative practice. What's in it for medicine? *Nursing Administration Quarterly*, 31–36.

Schein, E. (1971). The individual, the organization, and the career: A conceptual scheme. *Journal of Applied Behavioral Science*, 7(4), 401, 426.

Stoner, J.A., & Wankel, C. (1986). *Management* (3rd ed.). Englewood Cliffs, NJ: Prentice-Hall, p. 429.

Weiner, B., Heckhausen, H., Meyer, W., & Cook, R. (1972). Causal ascriptions and achievement behavior. *Journal of Personality and Social Psychology*, 21, 239–248.

Wisman, C.S., Alexander, C.S., & Morlock, L.L. (1981, September). Hospital decision making: What is nursing's role? *The Journal of Nursing Administration*, 31–39.

Section 2: Successful Women Administrators

Georgine M. Redmond

Research on women in administration has focused on societal, organizational, and personal characteristics. Societal attitudes and sex role stereotyping have already been discussed in the previous section. Organizational concerns for women, as well as the characteristics of successful women administrators are addressed here.

PERSONAL PROFILES OF WOMEN EXECUTIVES

One of the best known studies comparing women executives and middle managers is in Hennig and Jardim's book (1977), *The Managerial Women*. The book is based on their research on the lives of 25 highly successful women executives (corporate women) who held top level managerial positions. Data were obtained by interviews, autobiographical accounts, and a questionnaire. The same questionnaire was administered to a matched "traditional" group with similar background, education, and early career experience, who had remained in middle management positions. The research sought to understand how corporate women managed to depart from traditional female roles to achieve success in a predominantly male organizational culture. This study focused on the personal and professional development of the individual and not on organizational variables. Hennig and Jardim (1977) found remarkable similarities within each group of women studied.

Socialization

One contrast that existed between the corporate and traditional groups was in their family socialization. The corporate woman's childhood was more similar to a traditional boy's than to a girl's. Lynne (1981) describes the traditional father–daughter relationship as one in which fathers tend to treat their daughters with affection, praise, and attention, but do not subject them to the pressure, discipline, and competition their sons experience. He also suggests that the female child lacks assertiveness within the family because she has no need to shift her sexual identification as do her brothers. Chodorow (1978) discusses childhood socialization as related to development of gender identity, which is more than a product of biology. She proposes that mothers treat boys and girls differently. According to Chodorow, girls tend to remain in dyadic relationships with their mothers, whereas mothers push boys to individuate. Chodorow (1978) contends that girls do not require individuation from their mothers as necessary for the development of their gender identity although it is necessary for boys.

Of the 25 corporate women Hennig and Jardim (1977) studied, 20 were eldest or only children. They conclude that position in the family constellation helped these women to develop close relationships with their fathers, thus enabling them to separate from their mothers and become involved in sports, acquire a desire to achieve, and develop the ability to compete (p. 80). Mothers of these women treated them like girls, but their fathers treated them like boys encouraging them to take risks as a consequence of judgment based on experience. Their parents' support allowed them the freedom to question rules (p. 92). These results have been supported in two additional studies of nontraditional career women (Auster and Auster, 1981; Chusmir, 1983). All found that the first-born effect and parental support of career interests were important in women's success.

Morgan and Farber (1982) suggest that aspiring career women, whose mothers presented a traditional female model, need to rely on male relationships within their current environments to counterbalance this original identification and achieve a comfortable nontraditional identity.

In a qualitative study of 29 deans of nursing programs, Redmond (1987) found results that lend support to the above studies. She found that fathers did play a significant role in the early lives of these nursing education administrators but not to the exclusion of the role of their mothers and other successful women in their lives. Analysis of her data revealed a strong pattern of female–female relationships, which provided these deans with models of nontraditional female behaviors like assertiveness, risk taking, and the ability to articulate and speak out on issues.

Sports

Sports, as a factor in the socialization of the sexes, has been described in a study by Lever (1976). She studied 181 fifth graders. The results of her study suggest that sex roles in our society are reinforced by play and games in which children are involved. According to Lever, boys learn to play with all age groups, and they learn the importance of team effort. In addition, boy's games tend to emphasize competition, whereas girl's games emphasize cooperation. Boys learn to resolve their difficulties by interacting as a peer with older boys. Older girls tend to take on the mothering role with their younger followers. Lever concluded that boys develop essential leadership skills through play (pp. 479–484). Diamond (1978–79) agrees that

> the basic lessons of sports—goal setting, team effort, playing by the rules, persisting to master the skills necessary to compete, realizing that success is possible and failure can be overcome—have a definite relationship to the skills needed for management and other leadership positions (p. 60).

Klein (1978–79), in support of the importance of competitive sports for women, notes that sports tend to build self-confidence and that the experiences of both defeat and the need to try again to be successful are important lessons.

Birth Position

Few studies have investigated birth order effects on women. Hennig and Jardim (1977) found that birth position in a family is a significant factor in women's socialization because it affects their relationship with their father. Eckstein (1978) investigated the possible differences in birth order between women elected to leadership or selected for popularity in a college environment. College annuals were used to determine the women who were campus leaders or most popular. All college alumni were canvased to determine their ordinal position in family. The population had balanced numbers of oldest, middle, and youngest children. The results of this study indicate that first borns were significantly over-chosen for leadership and popularity positions. Youngest females were under-chosen for these positions and no significant differences were found in middle children. Sandler and Scalia (1975) investigated the relationship between birth order, sex, and leadership in a voluntary organization. They found that leadership positions were not related to birth order in men, whereas first born women were more likely to serve as organization officers. These studies support Hennig and Jardim's findings.

Education

All of Hennig and Jardim's (1977) corporate women went to college. Most majored in career fields that rejected traditional female choices.

Diamond (1978–79) asserts that an education gives women the "legitimacy needed for security—one of the requirements for leadership" (p. 62). In describing her rise to success as Secretary of State in California, March Fong Eu (1978–79) stated that, if she were to pick out one factor leading to her relative success, it would be her education. She said, "My desire to change my living circumstances motivated my desire for education and to succeed" (p. 63). Education is a prerequisite to competence (Wagner, 1979; Harvard, 1985), which is an essential characteristic of women administrators.

Hennig and Jardim's corporate women (1977) experienced mentoring, first from their fathers and later through their male bosses who helped them move up the career ladder. This was not true of the traditional group.

Traits of Corporate Women

Hennig and Jardim's research has been attacked as a trait theory with little predictive value because it did not investigate the impact of the organizational environment on these traits (Harriman, 1985). Nonetheless, the research has provided information about the differences between corporate women and traditional women and same differences in life-career experiences that appear to be associated with these differences.

Keown and Keown (1982) attempted to replicate part of the research done by Hennig and Jardim (1977). They addressed the following questions: (1) Does the profile of women executives presented in *The Managerial Woman* still hold true today? and, (2) What attitudes and leadership styles appear to affect the success of today's woman executive? Three variables were investigated: (1) inherent characteristics, such as, position in family; (2) extrinsic characteristics, such as, education; and (3) attitudes and leadership styles. The sample was 21 women managers in the San Francisco bay area.

The results of this study indicate that the women were younger; two thirds were under 40 as compared with the study by Hennig and Jardim in which the mean age was 57; 62 percent were the only or oldest child. Only two-thirds of these women were college educated; 43 percent had advanced degrees. Ninety percent were married at least once, the majority before 25. Twenty-four percent had children. They perceived themselves as above average in their ambitions, intellectual ability, and assertiveness.

In the study by Hennig and Jardim (1977) only 50 percent were married (and then in their thirties) and none had children. One of the most significant differences in the samples of the two studies, which could account for variation in the results, is that all of Hennig and Jardim's (1977) women were high up in the organizational structure (corporate president or vice president) whereas only 50 percent of the women in the present study held those positions.

AN ORGANIZATIONAL PERSPECTIVE

Tokenism

Kanter (1977) studied how the organizational structure forms people's sense of themselves and their potential. The focus of her study was on the people within one large organization who ran the offices (clerical and service personnel) and those who ran the administrative apparatus of the organization (corporate executives, managers, professional and technical personnel). In her study (1976) she found that "groups with varying proportions of people of different social types differ qualitatively in dynamics and process" (p. 965). People who are numerically dominant control the group. Those who differ significantly she called "tokens" because ". . . they are often treated as representatives of their category, as symbols rather than individuals" (p. 966). Women often find themselves as tokens in administration. They are visibly different and are frequently put to loyalty tests.

Kanter (1976, 1977) believes that relative numbers are important in shaping outcomes for individuals and that women need to be included in sufficient numbers in the organization to counteract the effect of tokenism. In a recent study of women physicians, Kanter's theory of tokenism was explicitly tested. Sherman and Rosenblatt (1984) examined the effect of proportionate numbers on women physician's role selection (teaching, administration, and research) in 17 medical specialties. They calculated the proportion of women in each role in each of the 17 specialties and used Fisher's exact probability test to determine whether women were overrepresented or underrepresented in the three roles. The results indicated that despite the proportion, women physicians were most likely to be overrepresented as teachers and underrepresented as administrators and researchers. The more powerful position, administration, is still occupied by male physicians, whereas even in medicine teaching remains a women's traditional role.

Queen Bee Syndrome

In discussing the loyalty tests frequently put to women administrators, Kanter (1976) remarked that "For women, the price of being one of the boys is a willingness to turn against the girls" (p. 979). This is discussed in the psychological literature as part of the Queen Bee Syndrome (Berry and Kushner, 1975), which is the stereotype of the anti-feminist who glories in her own success at the expense of other women. Harriman (1985) describes the so-called Queen Bee as "co-opted by the system" (p. 131). For her to survive and flourish, she has taken on the attitudes and behaviors of the predominant culture (male) and enjoys her special position (perks, male attention). The Queen Bee is a woman with traditional male values that believes women have only themselves to blame for their situation and that success is a product of individual effort and achievement and that younger people (male and female) should struggle to succeed, with the fittest surviving. Harriman (1985) believes the Queen Bee is actually not very prevalent, but more of a stereotype.

In contrast, Berry and Kushner (1975) see the so-called "Queen Bee" as characteristic of high achievers who need little reward from the organization, as their behavior is not selling out to the predominant male culture but the result of earlier identification with their fathers, much like that described by Hennig and Jardim (1977). They state that the Queen Bee syndrome is too narrow in focus and fails to take into account many other complex psychological and environmental variables (p. 176).

Marginality

Women in nursing service administration are both tokens and occupy marginal positions. Biordi (1986) points out, "Health work is women's work, controlled by men" (p. 173). She contends that women managers in health care are in marginal positions because of the male occupational dominance in the system. She continues, by saying that the nurse executive's marginality is intensified by the visibility of her work. "Marginality exists when an individual lives in two worlds simultaneously; one of which, by prevailing standards, is regarded as superior" (p. 173). She states that assets for one world are liabilities for another and that the boundaries are permeable between the worlds.

Actually, the nurse executive functions in three worlds: (1) world of femininity and family; (2) world of clinical rank-and-file nurse; and (3) world of male-dominated management. Biordi (1986) stresses that nurse executives need to understand the work standard of each world as these "shape the nature of the work, point to underlying practical systematic knowledge, and are differently embedded visibly or invisibly in the practices and work of their specific work world." Therefore, recognition and understanding will assist resolution of inherent conflicts.

CHARACTERISTICS OF SUCCESSFUL WOMEN ADMINISTRATORS

The characteristics of successful women in administration derived from the literature include competence and the existence of role models, mentors, and networks inside and outside the organization to provide a wide base of support.

Personal Competence

Female administrators studied by Swann and Witty (1980) identify personal competence as a requisite for successful performance in their positions. Personal competence includes both mental and physical health. To maintain health the participants identified a variety of coping strategies for dealing with job-related stress. These include release strategies like support groups and travel; maintenance strategies like positive thinking, self confidence, and humor and, extension strategies like risk-taking behavior and accepting responsibility for decisions made. The importance of self-confidence is frequently identified (Harvard, 1985) as an essential characteristic of the female administrator. Wagner (1979) suggests that it is the job of teachers, counselors, and successful administrators to help aspiring women administrators have confidence so they can achieve.

Professional Competence

The need for women administrators to be professionally competent is essential to their success (Harvard, 1985; Swann & Witty, 1980; Wagner, 1979). This includes both the necessary educational preparation for the position as well as a thorough understanding of the position and the work needed to be done. Maintaining competence involves keeping abreast of issues and topics that impact on one's administrative position through continuing education, professional organizations, and internal committees. Both technical and interpersonal skills are needed. Interpersonal skills include the ability to communicate at all levels of the organization as well as having the ability to develop group consensus and facilitate team play.

A woman's style of management has traditionally been associated with the expressive behaviors of nurturing and helping (Sargent, 1981). Sargent suggests that the focus of management in the 1980s was on both the task (getting the job done) and people (addressing the satisfaction needs of the group) (p. 38). Therefore, effective managers (men and women) need to acquire both instrumental behaviors of rational problem solving and analysis (usually associated with men) as well as the expressive behaviors associated with women. This blending of these management behaviors she calls *androgynous management*.

Implementing androgynous management begins with an awareness of the need to change behaviors on the part of both sexes. Sargent recommends reviewing the current model being used to define "effective management" in one's organization through examining the management behaviors of those being promoted and reviewing the information disseminated in management training programs. Does the model include both people and task management skills? Compare these data with the characteristics of androgenous management and target change as needed.

Administrative Competence

Another component of the competence needed is administrative competence or the ability to carry out the position. Goal setting, planning, and hard work are the most frequently mentioned behaviors needed for successful women administrators. Literature suggests that women must work harder than men to achieve (Kanter, 1977; Harriman, 1985; Harvard, 1985). In addition, the ability to problem solve, make visible decisions, and follow through is essential. As mentioned earlier, cultural awareness and sensitivity to organizational norms is essential. Included is knowing where the power resides, how decisions are made, and building power bases with colleagues within and without the organization.

ROLE MODELS, MENTORS AND NETWORKS

One way for leaders to develop is by following the example of someone they wish to emulate (Diamond, 1978–79). Identification with parents and modeling of various occupational roles are thought to be major elements in occupational choice (Bolton, 1980; Erkut & Mokros, 1984; Noe, 1988).

Moore (1982) studied mentor–protege relationships of leaders in academia and found that most often the mentor was the person who supervised the leader in their first administrative position. She identified three stages in establishing a mentoring relationship: (1) the performance of an important visible task on the part of the protege, such as, functioning on a faculty committee and making a unique contribution; (2) additional "tests" are constructed by the mentor or they naturally occur as the protege carries out his or her responsibilities (this phase does not last long as the mentor makes his or her decision about the protege quickly); and (3) the mentor chooses the protege to work closely with him or her. The protege feels chosen and is put to work. The work, according to Moore, takes many forms, depending on the abilities and values of both mentor and protege.

Vance (1982) defined a mentor as "someone who serves as a career role model and who actively advises, guides, and promotes another's career and training" (p. 10). Moore (1982) defined a mentor as ". . . a long-term, professionally centered relationship between two individuals in which the more experienced individual, the mentor, advises and assists in any number of ways the career of the less experienced, often younger, protege" (p. 47). Bolton (1980), in her discussion of modeling influences on career development, identifies the mentor as a more specific form of career modeling (p. 198). In their discussion of the development of young scholars, May, Meleis, and Winstead-Fry (1982) state: "Mentorship includes role modeling, which in turn provides opportunities for role clarification and role rehearsal" (p. 24). Noe (1988) describes mentoring as a form of career guidance and psychological support to the employee. He states that the majority of mentorships are informal and that the mentor is usually older and more experienced. He does not discuss either the duration or intensity of these relationships. In the foregoing definitions, commonalities exist, as do differences, and mentoring has become a buzz word over the last decade. A major problem is that there is no one accepted definition of mentorship (Bowen, 1986).

Riley and Wrench (1985), in their study of mentoring in female attorneys, developed a *Career Support Scale* from synthesis of six empirical studies and three theoretical views of mentoring. Subjects were asked to list up to five individuals who they felt had played a positive role in the development of their career. The subjects then rated each individual on (1) *provisions*, mentor actively performs a wide range of functions for the mentee; (2) *emotion*, refers to the degree of emotional involvement between the participants; (3) *self-concept*, mentor facilitates development of the mentee's personal and professional self-concept; and (4) *resources*, mentor has higher status than the mentee (e.g., access to resources). Riley and Wrench found that only 35 percent of their subjects met the criterion for being "truly mentored." About 82 percent of the mentored women had at least one male mentor, whereas only 30 percent had at least one female mentor. Only 28 percent of the mentored women had more than one mentor.

Riley and Wrench included a broader and looser definition of mentoring at the end of their scale to determine if the problem that they perceived in reference to definition of mentoring was valid. The question was:

> Individuals who take a personal interest in helping a less experienced person advance in their career have been called 'mentors.' Mentors 'teach the ropes' of a profession, act as sponsors and guides for the mentee, and serve as role models. Have you ever had a mentor? (p. 384).

In response to this question, 67 percent of the subjects said they had one or more mentors. The difference in definition made a tremendous difference in the respondents answers. Those women whose mentoring relationships met the strict criteria did report themselves as significantly more successful and satisfied than those whose relationships did not meet the criterion.

How are mentoring relationships distinguished from nonmentoring relationships? Vance (1982) suggested that we look at the characteristics and functions of the relationship, "particularly its long-term nature and its emotional exchange elements" (p. 12). May, Meleis, and Winstead-Fry (1982) specify the characteristics of the mentor as one who has both the educational experience relevant to the novice's area of interest and the personal characteristics to enhance the mentorship.

Redmond (1987) found that the nursing education administrators she studied did not experience one single mentoring relationship; rather various people (men and women) in their lives and careers took on "quasi-mentoring" roles. These included career guidance, support, and opening doors to advancement within organizations and professional associations. These were not relationships established for a mentoring purpose and lacked the longevity and "emotional-exchange elements" described in the literature.

Women who have been mentored report the benefits of these relationships (Riley & Wrench, 1985; Reich, 1986; Noe, 1988). Because of limited availability of female mentors and problems associated with cross-gender mentoring, however, access to mentoring in the popular sense is limited for women.

Alternatives to informal mentoring may be formal mentoring or preceptorships. According to Noe (1988) successful formal mentoring programs are characterized by support of top level management, careful selection of mentors and proteges, a comprehensive orientation program that establishes realistic expectations and responsibilities for both mentor and protege, and establishes minimums for length and frequency of contact between the mentor and the protege.

Another source of support, information, and career guidance is the establishment of networks through professional organizations both within nursing and outside of nursing. In 1979, Trinchese, discussing her success, cited her participation in professional groups as invaluable to her success. She went on to say, however, that "Women, traditionally nonteam players, have not been encouraged to participate in professional groups" (p. 74). However, this situation is changing today according to Biordi (1986); she says that as nurse executives assume the political and public nature of their role they are building and enlarging their networks of information and mentoring.

In this review of literature on women in administration some themes emerge. Health care is a big business dominated by a predominately male culture. Nurse executives who wish to be successful must be culturally aware of the nuances, biases, and supports within the organization as well as needing to prepare and represent themselves as competent in all areas of their role. These executives must be bi-cultural: use their natural expressive (female) skills to deal with people while incorporating more instrumental (male) behaviors into their repertoire of management skills. Support and career guidance can be sought from role models, formal or informal mentors, and networks established for this purpose.

BIOGRAPHICAL SKETCH

Dr Georgine M. Redmond is the Assistant Dean, Student Affairs, in the School of Nursing at George Mason University. She earned a BSN and MA in New York City at the College of Mt. St. Vincent and New York University, respectively. Her doctoral degree is in higher education administration from Virginia Tech. Her experience during the last 27 years has been in psychiatric–mental health clinical practice and in higher education in both teaching and administration. Dr Redmond's research interest is Women in Administration, which began with her doctoral research. She has written and presented in this area.

SUGGESTED READINGS

Mentoring

Bolton, E.B. (1980). A conceptual analysis of the mentor relationship in career development of women. *Adult Education, 30*(4), 195–207.

Moore, K.M. (1982). The role of mentors in developing leaders for academe. *Educational Record, 63*, 22–48.

Noe, R.A. (1988). Women and mentoring: A review and research agenda. *Academy of Management Review, 13*(1), 65–78.

Women in Administration

Boneparth, E., & Stoper, E. (1988). Women, power and policy. Elmsford NY: Pergamon Books.

Harriman, A. (1985). *Women/men management.* New York: Praeger Publishers.
Shakeshaft, C. (1987). *Women in educational administration.* Newberry Park, CA: Sage.

REFERENCES

Auster, C.J., & Auster, D. (1981). Factors influencing women's choice of non-traditional careers: The role of family, peers, and counselors. *Vocational Guidance Quarterly, 29,* 253–263.

Berry, J., & Kushner, P. (1975). A critical look at the Queen Bee Syndrome. *Journal of N.A.W.D.A.C., 38*(4), 173–176.

Biordi, D.L. (1986). Nursing service administrators: Marginality and the public person. *Nursing Clinics of North America, 21*(1), 173–183.

Bolton, E.B. (1980). A conceptual analysis of the mentor relationship in career development of women. *Adult Education, 30*(4), 195–207.

Bowen, D.D. (1986). The role of identification in mentoring female proteges. *Group and Organizational Studies, 11*(1–2), 61–74.

Chodorow, N. (1978). *The reproduction of mothering.* Berkley: University of California Press.

Chusmir, L.H. (1983). Characteristics and predictive dimensions of women who make non-traditional vocational choices. *Personnel and Guidance Journal, 62*(1), 42–47.

Diamond, H. (1978–1979). Patterns of leadership. *Educational Horizons, 57,* 58–62.

Eckstein, D. (1978). Leadership, popularity, and birth order in women. *Journal of Individual Psychology, 34*(1), 63–66.

Erkut, S., & Mokros, J.R. (1984). *American Educational Research Journal, 21*(2), 399–417.

Eu, M.F. (1978–1979). We've come a long way, baby, but that's only the beginning. *Educational Horizons, 57,* 63–63.

Harriman, A. (1985). *Women/men management.* New York: Praeger Publishers.

Harvard, P.A. (April 1985). Successful behaviors of Black women administrators in higher education: Implications for leadership. Paper presented at the Annual Meeting of the American Educational Research Association, San Francisco, CA.

Hennig, M., & Jardim, A. (1977). *The managerial women.* New York: Pocket Books.

Kanter, R.M. (1976). Some effects of proportions on group life: Skewed sex ratios and response to token women. *American Journal of Sociology, 82*(5), 967–988.

Kanter, R.M. (1977). *Men and women of the corporation.* New York: Basic Books.

Keown, C.F., & Keown, A.L. (1982). Success factors for corporate women executives. *Group and Organization Studies, 7*(4), 445–456.

Klein, J.D. (1978). We must break down the myths. *Educational Horizons, 57,* 84–89.

Lever, J. (1976). Sex differences in the games children play, *Social Problems, 23,* 478–487.

Lynn, D.B. (1981). The process of learning parental and sex-role identification. In L.D. Steinberg (ed.), *The life cycle.* New York: Columbia University Press, pp. 107–117.

May, K.M., Meleis, A.I., & Winstead-Fry, P. (1982). Mentorship for scholarliness: Opportunities and dilemmas. *Nursing Outlook, 82*(1), 22–28.

Moore, K.M. (1982). The role of mentors in developing leaders for academe. *Educational Record, 63,* 22–28.

Morgan, E., & Farber, B. (1982). Toward a reformulation of the Eriksonian model of female identity development. *Adolescence, 17*(65), 199–211.

Noe, R.A. (1988). Women and mentoring: A review and research agenda. *Academy of Management Review, 13*(1), 65–78.

Redmond, G.R. (1987). *Deans of nursing: Pathways to the deanship.* Unpublished doctoral dissertation, Virginia Polytech and State University, Blacksburg, VA.

Reich, M.H. (1986). The mentor connection. *Personnel, 63*(2), 50–56.

Riley, S., & Wrench, D. (1985). Mentoring among women lawyers. *Journal of Applied Social Psychology, 15*(4), 374–386.

Sandler, B.E., & Scalia, F.A. (1975). The relationship between birth order, sex, and leadership in a religious organization. *Journal of Social Psychology, 95,* 279–280.

Sargent, A.G. (1981). *The androgynous manager.* New York: AMACOM.

Sherman, S.R., & Rosenblatt, A. (1984). Women physicians as teachers, administrators and researchers in medical and surgical specialties: Kanter versus "Avis" as competing hypotheses. *Sex Roles, 11*(3/4), 203–209.

Swann, R.A., & Witty, E.P. (1980). Black women administrators at traditional black colleges and universities: Attitudes, perceptions, and potentials. *The Western Journal of Black Studies, 4,* 261–270.

Trinchese, T. (1979). Success: The way there is more fun than the stay there. *Educational Horizons, 57,* 71–76.

Vance, C. N. (1982). The mentor connection. *The Journal of Nursing Administration, 12*(4), 7–13.

Wagner, M.D. (1979). Competency, confidence, courage: Fundamental requirements for success. *Educational Horizons, 57,* 97–101.

CASE 4–1

Head Nurse Preceptor Program at a Community Hospital
Barbara A. Conway

First-level supervision may be one of the most demanding of management roles for nurses today. The direction of 24-hour delivery on a nursing unit requires sophisticated skills in communication, negotiation, and organization. The head nurse position calls for clinical expertise and extraordinary stamina. Yet, the majority of first-level nursing managers receive minimal support and guidance in making the transition into management.

Historically, nurses have been promoted to management on the basis of their clinical competence and seniority with little attention given to their problem-solving skills, creativity, or interpersonal abilities. In many cases, these positions had overlapping responsibilities, unclear authority, and vaguely worded job descriptions. Novice managers often mistakenly assumed that the promotion represented organizational validation and support for their professional ideals (Carter, 1980).

Once promoted, the socialization process of new managers is largely unstructured. Their learning occurs by trial and error, and often in an atmosphere of professional insularity and isolation. According to Darling and McGrath (1983), individuals occupying first-level management positions tend to work at a hectic pace, envision their power and influence as insignificant, yet also perceive a tremendous responsibility for making the system work. They are pulled in conflicting directions by the demands and concerns of their superiors and subordinates.

The need for balance is critical, as the new managers must provide a credible link upward and downward in the organization. They must correctly interpret and communicate the information, needs, and direction of the system as a whole, and their unit in particular. In doing so, they experience role conflict, job ambivalence, and isolation. They express high levels of stress and a fear of failure. It is not surprising to learn that the overall job satisfaction and productivity for these individuals are low in the early months after the promotion. Turnover rates are high. The disruption to operations that results, and the need for continual recruitment and training places high costs on the individuals involved, the clients served, and the organizational interests as a whole. Clearly, some strategies to systematically recruit, socialize, and retain effective new managers for nursing are needed.

One strategy many organizations have instituted is a formal management development program. Most of these seek to improve competency only by imparting the theoretical and functional aspects of management. Such programs address only one component of the new manager's needs. They do not provide the nurturance necessary for role mastery. They do not offer feedback, monitor activity, or foster self-esteem and a sense of belonging. Nor do they address the political realities and informal aspects of the organizational culture. New managers need a coach, a role model and supporter, as they learn new skills for this significant career transition.

The concept of reality shock received wide attention in the 1970s as it became clear that new graduate nurses experienced great difficulties in adapting to the demands of the clinical work setting after leaving a relatively protected academic environment. One successful strategy to overcome reality shock was peer preceptors to assist new graduate nurses in making the transition. Because the transition that new managers and new graduate nurses experience is similar in many respects, our agency decided to institute a preceptor process to ease this transition.

Another strategy is an internship, whereby a newcomer to a role is paired formally with an experienced practitioner for individualized learning experiences. The internship uses many of the concepts of the adult learning model (Knowles, 1973). The model holds the adult learners work best in an informal, collaborative, and supportive climate using participative planning, mutually designed and negotiated learning goals and strategies, and an evaluation by mutual assessment.

Sharmian and colleagues (1984) wrote that preceptorships provide positive role modeling, opportunities for feedback, and marked interdependence between teacher and learner. Although close supervision is available, it is not judgmental, but rather, a part of a mutually agreeable relationship. This relationship in itself can assist in promoting growth and satisfaction by the encouragement it offers to the learner. Other authors, in discussing preceptorships, generally agree that preceptor preparation is essential. Candidates for the role should be mature, capable, and able to communicate easily. They should be individuals who are interested in the teaching process and they should be persons who have successfully integrated their own professional–bureaucratic values; the delicate balance between holding to one's ideals and supporting the needs of the organization.

Preceptorship appears to offer the new nursing manager an important component often missing in other management development efforts. First, it can minimize the sense of isolation often experienced by the beginner, by providing a close contact person. Next, it is a systematic process of educating that capitalizes on the capabilities of the adult learner by participation in the development of learning objectives. In addition, it provides opportunities for role modeling and role rehearsal in an atmosphere that is supportive, but also based within the realities of the organization. Finally, it integrates the newcomer into a peer group and can assist in empowering that group. The relationships established can promote cohesiveness of the members beyond the orientation phase and engender confidence in their capabilities.

It should be emphasized that preceptorship cannot stand alone as the only tool in socializing new managers. Novices certainly need information and skill development as they learn the role. The presence of a strong peer support system enriches the supervision, coaching, and direction by a preceptor and upper management. A third strategy is supervision of the new manager by an immediate supervisor. This relationship is critical in the nurturance and development of new subordinates. From the time of the initial interview and throughout the selection and orientation phases, the supervisor should provide a realistic job preview, communicate expectations carefully, and lend the perspective of history, larger organizational issues, and personal and professional philosophy. The participation of the supervisor also may include preparation of the preceptor, monitoring of the learning process, and provision of feedback to the newcomer and the preceptor alike. Darling and McGrath (1983) point out, "it is upper management's job to create a climate of success whereby new managers are encouraged to be healthy, sturdy, and effective in the mastery of their roles.''

My own interest in the socialization and development of new nurse managers has developed over time. It has been shaped by my personal experience as a new manager, discussions with others as they gained mastery of their roles, and studies or organizational behavior. In addition, while pursuing my graduate studies, I was fortunate to be involved in the planning process for a preceptor program for new head nurses at a nearby hospital.

Only months later, when I took on my current position as Assistant Director of Nursing for seven nursing units at Sibley Memorial Hospital, I had an opportunity to put the theories about socialization and preceptorship to the test. Sibley is a medium-size community hospital in Washington, D.C., with a strong organizational culture, a history of conservative values, and a long tradition of excellent personalized nursing care. At the time I took on my responsibilities, the hospital had undergone significant reorganization and a drive to streamline operations. Moreover, there were two head nurse vacancies to fill within my area at the same time I was learning my own role. Fortunately, the Assistant Administrator for Nursing was well versed in adult learning theory and supportive of the concept of preceptorship. Under her direction, Sibley had used a preceptorship program successfully with new graduates and also with experienced nurses. Most importantly, she recognized the importance of developing our new managers quickly, carefully, and in an organized fashion. We designed a program to use all three strategies mentioned.

Because both units with head nurse vacancies had acting head nurses temporarily in those positions, we had the luxury of a little time to recruit and select candidates carefully and also to orient them properly. Staff nurses on the units provided input into the selection process by participating in group interviews of potential candidates. Once candidates for the unit managers were selected, the selection and preparation of head nurse preceptors was the next step in the program. On the advice of the Assistant Administrator, one of the most experienced of our head nurses was chosen as the first preceptor. Her knowledge of the organization and her clinical and professional reputation were outstanding. When approached, she expressed interest in learning about preceptorship as it applied to new managers and she was also willing to participate in this pilot program. Through a combined process of discussion, guided readings, and an explanation of the process, she offered many suggestions and ideas, and helped me to clarify my own expectations of what might take place. She also precepted the first two new managers. The process has evolved a great deal since then, and the following is a description of the present, one month formal preceptorship for head nurses at Sibley.

Our new head nurses begin their management orientation with a *written self-assessment* that encompasses both clinical and administrative skills. Because the clinical role of the head nurse is extremely visible and highly regarded at Sibley, it is essential that any necessary review of skills be identified quickly and accomplished completely. The administrative portion of the self-assessment includes interviewing, scheduling, personnel issues, and financial management. In addition, it clarifies whether the newcomer is comfortable with the skills and needs only to learn "the Sibley way" or if the issues and concepts are brand new.

The new head nurse is also provided with a *packet of self-learning activities* to be pursued at her own pace and according to her own needs. She is given a number of carefully selected readings that discuss the transition process, a calendar of meetings and events, and a *written orientation plan* that identifies classroom activities, major content areas, and a time frame for the program.

By the end of the first week, it is expected that the self-assessment will be complete and that the newcomer and her preceptor will have had an opportunity to develop a *formal learning contract* based on the self-assessment. The learning contract is a simple tool that states distinct objectives, the strategies to be used to attain them, and the critical indicators that denote their accomplishment. A time frame for completing each objective is specified along with the level of expertise expected.

The role of the *preceptor* is critical in the development of the learning contract. She gently guides the newcomer to those skills that are most essential to master quickly and allays anxieties about matters that can wait until after the orientation period is complete. She suggests resources for the new head nurse to contact for additional assistance and directs her to the most useful strategies. Once the learning contract has been drafted, the new head nurse, the preceptor, and I meet to discuss it. At this time, additional ideas are explored, priorities may be shifted, and activities planned to help meet the objectives. We *meet as a threesome on a regular basis* throughout the month-long orientation period to review and refine the contract and to evaluate progress. In this way, the contract becomes a map that guides and directs the orientation activities, but that is also flexible and geared to the individual's needs. Generally, those items that appear on the first draft alert both the preceptor and me to areas that may be the source of greatest anxiety for the newcomer. Once alerted, we can plan together to provide information, clarify expectations, and develop methods to work through any difficulties.

The next phase of the socialization process occurs on the *home unit of the preceptor.* The newcomer and preceptor make it a point to introduce the new head nurse to her own staff members and assure them of her interest and enthusiasm. It is also made clear however, that the new head nurse must be actively involved in an important learning process before she will be ready to take on her new responsibilities.

For the next ten days, the preceptor and new head nurse spend a great deal of time together involved in learning activities. The new head nurse may observe preparations and leadership of a staff meeting, sit in on an interview, work with the unit secretary to learn charge nurse details, or assist in preparing a schedule. In addition, she may be involved in meetings with the staffing specialist and quality assurance coordinator to gain further insight into the workings of the system. Perhaps most important, she and the preceptor take the time to get to know one another and begin to expand their relationship to others in the hospital. It is a time for exploring the informal organization, the culture, and the resources available for help.

The time spent on the preceptor's unit provides a safe place for the new head nurse to *practice her new skills*. She is perceived as a learner under the guidance of an experienced leader and the atmosphere is a safe and supportive one in which to ask basic questions, make minor mistakes in procedural details, and observe group dynamics and leadership style before taking on the role "for real." While the newcomer practices her skills, the preceptor is presented to her own staff members as a knowledgeable and capable role model and teacher. In addition, as the learning process takes place in a real, as opposed to a laboratory setting, the new head nurse has the opportunity and advantage of integrating theoretical knowledge and information in an actual organizational environment.

By some time in the third week, and often earlier, the new head nurse *moves her "live classroom" to her own unit*. By the time she appears, she will have been introduced to some of her own staff and especially to the person in the acting head nurse role. The acting head nurse helps to conduct the next phase of the socialization process. She meets with the preceptor, the new head nurse, and me briefly to discuss those matters already covered and to make plans for learning activities for the remainder of the orientation period. Sometime within this time, the new head nurse makes it a point to organize her office space, conduct her first staff meeting, and get better acquainted with her staff. In addition, she begins to assume charge nurse functions and perform other clinically visible activities that validate her professional expertise and help build confidence among her staff group and herself.

This phase is, perhaps, the most critical for the new head nurse, for it sets the tone for the first several months of her leadership. Her communication style, her availability, and her assertion of her expectations to her staff. The relationship she develops with the acting head nurse is also a crucial one, and both persons must maintain a fine balance to achieve a smooth transition. The new head nurse is called on to take the reins of leadership without appearing to seize control. She must solicit advice on communication approaches with the staff and develop a sense of their group dynamics. She must gain an early understanding of the culture and sensitive issues within the unit and an appreciation of its history. She must also assist the acting head nurse in making her own transition from a temporary leadership role back into her position as a senior staff member. Perhaps at no other time in her career will the new head nurse be as visible (and feel as vulnerable) as in those first few weeks on her unit. Her every action will be closely scrutinized. Every statement, pronouncement, and off-hand remark is likely to be discussed and analyzed over coffee and lunch breaks. The details of her dress, her speech, and her response to staff overtures will be assessed and noted by her staff.

The new head nurse needs colleagues of her own to depend on at this time and she needs a safe someone in the organization to share her visions, her early impressions, and her uncertainty. Although a *personal journal* can be of some help to her as she sorts out her early experiences, a peer is very important. The *role of the preceptor shifts* in this phase to that of *guide,* confidant, and confidence builder. She and the new head nurse tend to meet briefly and often during this period; sometimes for a quick coffee break or telephone conversation and occasionally for further work on the learning contract. The preceptor accompanies the new head nurse to weekly management meetings and introduces her to other peers. She helps the newcomer to interpret her early experiences, to assess the importance of larger organizational events, and to validate her perceptions and impressions.

By the end of the orientation period, the *new head nurse, preceptor, and I meet one last time* as a threesome to review the learning contract and to evaluate progress. The formal preceptor relationship is terminated, but the informal one generally continues; at least until the new head nurse has had an opportunity to develop her own networks with other colleagues, and often, indefinitely.

Once the orientation period has begun to wind down, the relationship between the new head nurse and myself has also had an opportunity to gel. We will have been in close contact with one another throughout the orientation period and had many informal discussions. Certainly we will have had a chance to assess one another's style and capabilities both in individual and group settings. Depending on the level of "information overload" experienced by the new head nurse (and this is extremely variable), we spend some formal time together discussing unit issues, staff learning needs, leadership and communication approaches, and short-term goals. We set up *weekly meeting times* for informal discussion, questions, follow-up, and general supervision. In addition, the head nurse is appraised of my expectations and my availability for assistance.

Does the system really work this well? Does it have limitations? Can it work in other settings? I believe that it can, it does, and it could. Sometimes the process moves along in beautifully ordered fashion. On other occasions, the personalities, capabilities, and organizational atmosphere color the experience negatively. We have learned, for example, that the system must be extremely flexible. The learning needs of an in-house promotee with no management experience are very different from those of a new head nurse with management experience elsewhere but no knowledge of the system at Sibley.

The match of the preceptor and protegee is critical as well, and not always predictable. The preceptor must be well prepared for her role and must also be available at the time the new head nurse is ready to begin orientation. This means that an ideal preceptor candidate caught up with internal difficulties on her own unit or serious staffing problems may not have the time or the energy to spend with a new manager. It also means that an excellent preceptor match may need to be reconsidered if that person has only recently finished an orientation with another new head nurse. The preceptor role is an intense and demanding one and it is, frankly, much to ask of a manager. But it is also a rewarding experience in many respects, and has been the beginning of many important professional and personal friendships.

Over the past two years, our system at Sibley has evolved in a number of ways. Some parts were discovered to be much too cumbersome in practice.

Other aspects have required more structure. Although the system works well, we have plans for further refinement. First, we are designing a formal orientation manual. Items with key policy statements, lists of resource people, organizational structure and philosophy, and institutional guidelines on such topics as employee discipline, quality assurance, budget monitoring, productivity, and standard reports. Another segment being considered is time management. The new head nurse often feels pressured to "do it all," and therefore, must make careful use of her time to avoid depleting her energies, her patience, and her confidence. At the same time, she *is* called on to accomplish a great deal in a very short period. Some basic tips may ease the newcomer's mastery of this skill.

Another refinement in the system is a more extensive and formal preparation of the head nurse preceptors. We plan to develop criteria for their selection and objectives by which to teach them the role and to evaluate their effectiveness. New preceptors are sometimes anxious about their added responsibilities and deserve thoughtful and well-directed feedback on their performance. At present, preparation and evaluation take place informally, a more consistent and systematic approach will be advantageous.

The program itself has not been formally evaluated at this writing and this is also a need. We have no objective evidence that our head nurses inducted through preceptorship are more effective managers than ones who came into their positions by more traditional methods. There are a great many other variables operating and it would be a difficult task to sort them out. Although informal feedback has been honest, helpful, and generally positive, we recognize that we depend on a number of factors that are intangible and very difficult to measure.

Can the system work in every setting? With some restructuring to fit individual organizational philosophy and style, I believe that it can. It requires, first, a commitment to the careful development of nursing managers. It requires some knowledge and support of the adult learning model. It requires much time, energy, and patience to develop the program and the preceptors. A successful program also requires careful supervision and monitoring by middle and upper management. Most of all, it requires tremendous flexibility and a willingness to evaluate the system and makes changes based on experience and need.

BIOGRAPHICAL SKETCH

Barbara A. Conway, RN, MSN, is Assistant Director of Nursing, Clinical Services, at Sibley Memorial Hospital in Washington D.C. She received a nursing diploma from St. Mary's School of Nursing, Rochester, Minnesota and a Bachelor of Science degree from Metropolitan State College in Denver, Colorado. In 1986 she earned a Master of Science in Nursing from George Mason University. Ms. Conway is a member of Sigma Theta Tau, Episilon Zeta Chapter. Her previous experience includes both clinical and management positions in critical care, medical, and surgical nursing.

SUGGESTED READINGS

Darling, L.A., & McGrath, L.G. (1983). Minimizing promotion trauma. *The Journal of Nursing Administration, 13*(9), 14–19.

Dooley, S.L., and Hauben, J. (1979). From staff nurse to head nurse: A trying transition. *The Journal of Nursing Administration, 9*(4), 4–7.

Everson, S., Panoc, K., Pratt, P., & King, A.M. (1981). Precepting as an entry method for newly hired staff. *The Journal of Continuing Education in Nursing, 12*(5), 22–26.

Friesen, L., & Conrahan, B.J. (1980). A clinical preceptorship program: Strategy for new graduate orientation. *The Journal of Nursing Administration, 10*(4), 18–23.

Garity, J. (1983). Developing head nurses: One hospital's solution. *Nursing Educator, 8*(3), 38–42.

Lanigan, J., & Miller, J. (1981). Developing nurse managers. *Nursing Administration Quarterly, 5*(2), 21–24

Limon, S., Bargagliotti, L.A., & Spencer, J.B. (1981, October). Who precepts the preceptor? *Nursing and Health Care,* 433–436.

Sheridan, D.R., Bronstein, J.E., & Walker, D.D. (1984) *The new nurse manager.* Rockville, MD: The Aspen Systems Corporation.

Turnbull, E. (1983). Rewards in nursing: The case of nurse preceptors. *The Journal of Nursing Administration, 13*(1), 10–13.

REFERENCES

Carter, K.A. (1980). Managerial role development in the nursing supervisor. *Supervisor Nurse, 11*(7), 26–29.

Darling, L.A., & McGrath, L.G. (1983). The causes and costs of promotion trauma. *The Journal of Nursing Administration, 13*(4) 29–33.

Knowles, M. (1973). *The adult learner: A neglected species.* Houston, TX: Gulf Publishing Company.

Sharmian, J., & Lemieux, S. (1984). An evaluation of the preceptor method versus the formal teaching method. *The Journal of Continuing Education in Nursing, 15*(3), 86–89.

CASE 4–2

Feminist Management at a Community Health Clinic
Katrina Clark
Elizabeth Magenheimer

The Fair Haven Community Health Clinic is a 15-year-old community health center that serves the residents of an inner-city neighborhood in New Haven, Connecticut. Over the years, the Clinic has developed and implemented certain practices and policies that challenge the traditional male-dominated hierarchical medical models of health care delivery and management. We have attempted to bring empowerment, nurturing, and education qualities into the administration of health care. We have struggled to structure our work environment to be a model for both patient care and employment.

The Clinic began as an alternative institution, inspired by the early 1970s dream of community people and health care providers working together to make health care accessible and affordable in an inner-city low income neighborhood. For many, the early 1970s were a time of anti-war, anti-institutions, anti-establishment. The founders of the Fair Haven Clinic shared these ideals and quickly found that it was one thing to demand that "health care is a right, not a privilege" and quite another to be confronted with the reality of actually providing those services.

Free clinics, alternative institutions, community health centers sprang up by the hundreds throughout the country in the 1970s. Professionals worked with community people to bring health care into local inner-city neighborhoods. By the mid 1970s, many of these institutions were caught in the squeeze between economic survival and their refusal to comply with bureaucratic demands of public funding and were forced to close.

The Fair Haven Clinic is an exception to that pattern. The Clinic also began as an alternative to city hospital clinics and the associated long waits, high costs, and fragmented, culturally alienating care. The Clinic initiated services by offering care to individuals with episodic problems. Over time new services were added as families began requesting continuing services for family planning, prenatal care, well-child care, and chronic problems such as hypertension, diabetes, and arthritis. Fair Haven health care providers began to look beyond episodic care to life situations influencing their health such as housing and welfare assistance. They came to realize it was more effective to get heat in an apartment than to continue to treat a variety of respiratory complaints.

The Fair Haven Clinic wanted to grow and change to meet the demands of the community and to provide continuity of care. We decided that we could hire clinicians and increase our services without losing the sensitivity to patients that our dedicated volunteer doctors, nurses, and other workers provided. We accepted the challenge of increased paper work, fiscal responsibilities, and intrusive governmental regulations and forms, while maintaining our values. We needed the autonomy of our own building, and the financial security of both public monies and third party reimbursement.

The Clinic staff and Board thought of innovative ways to grow. The Clinic negotiated and became a model practice site for the Yale School of Nursing faculty and student nurse practitioners and midwives to provide comprehensive family-centered primary care. We applied for grants and state contracts to begin prenatal and hypertension programs to meet community health needs. Our volunteer doctors helped us to find specialists in the private sector who would see our patients on referral. We successfully worked with our Health Systems Agency to get our community designated as a Health Manpower Shortage Area so that Fair Haven could apply for National Health Service Corps physicians.

We lobbied the General Assembly of the State of Connecticut to buy us a building. Hard work, hustle, having fun, taking risks, and sharing our vision of what we wanted to become have been the driving forces.

From an original $5000 budget and 1000 visits in a rented storefront and a local elementary school in 1971, the Clinic now has an operating budget of over $1,000,000 with 25,000 visits a year, our own building, and two satellite clinics: one at an elderly housing complex and the second at the local high school. We offer comprehensive primary care services and educational support programs such as the Women, Infants and Children (WIC) Nutrition Program, childbirth preparation and parenting education classes, self-care education, counseling, outreach, and referral services.

The Clinic currently has a staff of nearly 40 salaried employees—12 direct primary care providers (doctors, nurse practitioners, midwives), four administrators (Director, Assistant Director, Financial Administrator, and Coordinator of Elderly Services), seven professional support staff (nurses, social workers, and a nutritionist), five people in the billing and reception office, four people who work as laboratory and clinical assistants, and six people who make appointments, provide outreach, and interpreting. The Clinic is supported by federal, state, city, and private grants, which constitute 60 percent of the budget; the other 40 percent is generated by patient fees through Medicaid, Medicare, private insurance, and out-of-pocket on a sliding scale.

For many of us who work at the Clinic, our salaries are lower than what they might be in a more traditional institution, and the social and economic problems that confront our patients are more frustrating. The rewards of caring for whole families; of working where people are a team and respect one another's opinions, and where providers know that direct care in the examining room is only part of the service provided because it is complemented by the community outreach workers who work "on the street" compensate for the costs.

Education

By educating, we mean that people on all levels of employment share skills and experiences and continue their education to improve patient care. Our emphasis on the importance of on-going education, both formal and informal, constantly reminds each team member they can learn from each other. For example, professionals often are unaware of the cultural differences that stand as barriers to good patient care. When a pediatrician recommends to a Puerto Rican mother that she open the windows at night to let her child with croup get cool air, he loses all credibility with that mother because that mother believes that night air is "dangerous." The Clinic neighborhood worker works both with the doctor and the patient to create a plan of care that is acceptable to the patient and the clinician.

The Clinic promotes an environment that allows people to admit mistakes and improve. We strive to trust others, learn to give and take criticism, and help people to grow.

Formal education is encouraged through release-time and tuition support for staff members who take outside courses. This benefit is offered to everyone.

Staff members are encouraged to use new skills within the organization. For example, the office manager took courses on computing to upgrade her skills and then supervised the introduction of a new automated computer system for the Clinic.

The benefits of education go beyond the individual employee to the entire organization as people assume additional responsibilities and have more confidence in their work; they perform better at their jobs. Even though it takes more time to teach someone new skills rather than to hire someone with them, we feel this policy is also part of our commitment to the community. Our entry level employees are often local women without a high school diploma or technical training, who are single heads of households. They bring knowledge of the people in the community, their beliefs, perspectives, and problems. We train them as clerks, outreach workers, and receptionists. With our commitment to education, we also accept the risk that because we are a small agency without a large promotion ladder, that once trained, workers may move on to larger institutions with more career opportunities.

Another aspect of education within the Clinic is formal in-service education. On a rotating basis, the clinicians present grand rounds to each other every Friday morning. This may be a literature review of a timely issue discussed by a guest speaker, or a discussion of internal productivity, schedules, or clinical protocols. For one hour every two weeks the entire staff meets for a general in-service. This may be a presentation from an outside agency, such as a representative from the Battered Women's Shelter, or one of our own clinicians presenting a medical topic such as asthma, hepatitis, or sexually transmitted diseases. As a goal, some day we hope to offer paid sabbatical leave, exchange programs with clinics in other countries, and/or time off for teaching or travel.

Empowerment

This policy speaks to empower staff and the community. For example, telephone receptionists who answer calls for appointments or clinical assistants who draw blood or weigh a one-month-old are encouraged to view each contact as an opportunity for community residents to learn about their health care. A young parent learns to take and read her child's temperature and a young teen learns to record her menstrual cycle. The entire staff understands that health education is essential for patients to gain control of their lives.

Participative decision making, consensual theory, minimum of reliance on bureaucratic and hierarchical authority, self-management are all terms that are currently popular. The Clinic is an advocate of these ideas. In putting them into operation, we have not erased the hierarchical conflict that exists in any institution, but we have found ways to minimize the stratification and medical task superiority. One example is that managers and clinical providers perform "lower level" support tasks that increase their appreciation and respect of the skills involved. For example, the administrative staff takes turns staffing the front desk, which gives them a better insight into why problems occur and allows a better understanding of how to work toward solutions.

Recently, there were complaints from clinicians that phone messages were not accurate or appropriate. One solution was to have clinicians take turns answering the phones. After that, they not only appreciated how difficult and stressful a task it was, but together with the receptionists made recommendations to improve message taking, respond faster to messages, and educate patients about their role in presenting accurate information. The receptionists then evaluated their own messages for completeness and accuracy to learn from their mistakes.

A positive self-reinforcing cycle is created when people see that they can have an impact, develop an ability to think about and formulate ways to improve the clinic, and are allowed to share in power. It is a slower way to resolve problems, but it seems to reduce the number of problems overall.

The work environment supports cooperation by communicating the importance of each job to the overall functioning of the clinic. An important role of the manager is to show how a job fits into the whole—and how a job well done benefits everyone. Although we do have supervisors, we emphasize that no one is working for an individual boss, but rather for a common purpose. Informally, this is supported by encouraging suggestions that are respected and formally, staff members meet every Friday morning.

The Friday morning meetings alternate between staff meetings of all 40 employees and "flow" meetings, which are task groups that deal with specific issues such as billing, elderly, adolescents, prenatal, or telephone/reception. The flow meetings are designed as task forces to deal in depth and make decisions about specific topics or problems. Members include all the staff members involved in that particular topic or problem. On the alternate Friday, when the entire staff meets, the chair and minutes recorder rotates through the staff to foster leadership skills in everyone. The chair of the meeting must call the meeting to order, read the previous minutes, solicit reports and recommendations from all the flow groups, and go around the room asking each staff member if he or she has anything to say. Individual concerns may range from "who didn't clean the microscope" to a report on an outside meeting or event. Recently, two black clinical assistants wanted to learn more about acquired immune deficiency syndrome (AIDS) and its affect on the minority population. They found a conference on the topic and were sent by the Clinic. After their conference they returned to share the information with the entire staff. Their report sparked an emotional discussion on how AIDS affects the black and Hispanic community with which we work.

At times we question the cost and loss of productivity by closing Friday mornings for rounds, flow meetings, in-service education, and staff meetings. We concluded, however, it is a wise investment that saves us later costs of poor communication, power struggles, and a poorly informed staff.

Another formal extension of empowerment is the role of our Board of Directors, both in the decision-making process and with the staff. Staff representatives serve on each of the Board's committees, and one is an elected member of the Board of Directors. The Board is extremely respectful of staff input and makes a point of soliciting staff's recommendations on important clinic issues that will affect their jobs and patient care. Nearly 75 percent of the Board members are either users of the Clinic or live in the community. Their recommendations, concerns, and power have a direct consequence on their health care and on their neighbors.

Nurturing

Nurturing is the ability to create an environment that is comfortable both physically and organizationally. Unfortunately, women managers often feel that they should eliminate traditionally defined female characteristics, such as nurturing, for fear of being poor administrators. However, many large institutions are now instituting some of the nurturing techniques that the Clinic has been using for years—such as flex time, job sharing, maternity and paternity leaves. Such sensitivity to the whole employee positively contributes to employee retention and productivity.

The Clinic recognizes the necessity of allowing for flexibility in people's schedules to accommodate personal and family responsibilities. We have a commitment to helping people resolve the conflicts of combining a career and a family. Because of our small size, we do not offer day care on site, but are lenient about kids coming to work in emergencies such as when they are sick. All staff, men and women, single or married are allowed to define their schedules within reason (trading 12-hour days for 4 days work, working part-time, working extra evening hours if baby-sitting is a problem) and to align work schedules with school or day care schedules or breastfeeding. This requires people working together to cover clinics and meet personal needs.

The staff turnover at the Clinic is comparatively low when compared with other nonprofit agencies. There are five staff members who have celebrated 15 years with the Clinic and six who have been here 10 years or more. This is reinforced by informal activities that foster strong interstaff relationships and friendships. The Clinic holds an annual Christmas party and a summer picnic, which include past and present staff and their families. There are monthly potluck birthday lunches that are an integral part of work life and includes staff relaxing and celebrating together.

Nurturing is also provided by the comfort of the surroundings inside the Clinic. The Clinic itself is a converted historic building, which is cheerful and welcoming to patients. The building stands as an attractive anchor on the main street of an area that is trying to renovate itself after the emigration of many of the residents during the 1960s and 1970s that left many of the buildings abandoned.

Feminist Administration

In discussing administration at the Fair Haven Clinic, we have reviewed some of the organizational practices and structures that encourage education, empowerment, and creation of a supportive and nurturing environment. One may ask, how is this feminist? Theoretically, there is nothing exclusively female in such management practices. For instance, encouraging equality is not exclusively female—it takes courage and desire for a manager to break traditional hierarchical rules and expectations. We believe women managers have a responsibility to use traditional female qualities that we possess by virtue of our social and cultural roles to create a productive working environment that encourages a team approach in working toward a common goal. We hope men managers will also embrace these qualities and improve not only the quality of work life but also the health care delivered in their organizations.

BIOGRAPHICAL SKETCHES

Katrina Clark has been director of the Fair Haven Community Health Clinic for the past 15 years. After graduating from Cornell University in 1967 as a history major, she joined the Peace Corps and served in Colombia for two years. The Peace Corps experience awakened an interest in health care, and she attended the Yale School of Public Health receiving an MA in Public Health in 1971. She had several jobs at the Yale Medical School before joining the Fair Haven Clinic. Ms. Clark has had a faculty appointment as a lecturer at the Yale School of Public Health since 1980. Ms. Clark has served on numerous community boards and has received several awards for her service to the community including the YWCA's Outstanding Woman of the Year Award in 1981 and the Peace Corps' 25th Anniversary Sergeant Shriver Award for carrying on the goals of the Peace Corps. She currently is a Commissioner for the City of New Haven's Health Department.

Elizabeth Magenheimer has been a family nurse practitioner at the Fair Haven Clinic in Connecticut since 1976. She received her MA in Community Health Nursing from the Yale School of Nursing in 1976. She is also a certified nurse midwife. Before her graduate education, she received her BSN from Villanova University, worked as a public health nurse with the United Farm Workers in California and as a coronary care nurse in a community hospital in New York. Since her graduate education, Ms. Magenheimer has functioned as a FNP in an inner-city community health center. She has dealt with a wide range of medical and social problems in her diverse clinical practice. She is a lecturer at the Yale School of Nursing, lectured widely on issues in family planning and natural family planning, and treats students at the Albertus Magnus College Health Services. Currently, in conjunction with her clinical practice, she is the Director of Nursing at the Fair Haven Clinic.

PART II

Organizational Strategies

5

Organizations as Decision Making Systems

Julianne G. Mahler

Decision making is one of the most intensively studied organizational activities, and for good reason. Organizational decision making offers a forum for discussing values, resolving conflict, responding to new opportunities, designing new structures, clarifying relations with outside groups, and making key personnel or budget changes. But the study of organizational decision making also covers the routine and mundane choices of personnel actions or patient treatment that are largely preprogrammed. All in all, decision making reveals much about an organization, its professional values, power structure, and assumptions about justice and loyalty. Because of the importance and pervasiveness of the activities surrounding decision making, organizations have been viewed as decision-making systems.

This view reminds us that decision making is not an isolated act of choice, but a complex, on-going sequence including several kinds of highly organized activities. There must be some level of agreement on the need to act. Most organizations have some means, formal or informal, for monitoring progress and identifying problems. Evaluation research, continuous management information, productivity reporting, a grapevine that communicates discontent, or a series of conspicuous failures are all examples of the ways in which problems come to be identified.

Other subsystems are designed to gather and process information about identified problems. The information passed through communication networks and management information systems provides the basis for constructing alternative ways of dealing with the recognized problems and making a choice. The distortions in the communication system, such as intentional manipulation, semantic confusion, or information overload, limit the effectiveness of communication and reduce the information base for decision making.

The final act is one of choice. But in theory and in practice there is little consensus about how to make the best decision or choice—when to stop gathering alternatives, how to go about comparing them, and what standard to apply to the alternatives. Rational decision theories advocate making choices that most efficiently achieve some clearly agreed upon goal. Other theorists argue that the best decisions are those that most accurately reflect group preferences. In this chapter we examine these and other views of how to make the best decisions.

Delineation of the means to determine the one best method has been an elusive objective. Recent efforts have focused on finding the type of decision method that is best suited to a particular organizational context. This chapter reviews the strengths, limits, and pitfalls of alternative methods.

METHODS OF DECISION MAKING

The five most common decision-making methods are: (1) the routine or bureaucratic procedures approach, (2) the rational, policy-analysis approach, (3) the "garbage can" or nondecision-making analysis, (4) incrementalism, and (5) aggregative or preference ranking techniques. These are competing views about how organizations do or should make decisions, each claiming to have uncovered principles of choice that will improve organizational functioning. The type of decision is an important difference among these methods. Most researchers and practitioners recognize the utility of bureaucratic procedures for routine decision making in all organizations. The real debates occur over which of the last four methods is best when the question or problem is a novel problem or the circumstances require an innovative solution.

Routine or Bureaucratic Procedures

Administrators in organizations make day-to-day decisions according to an established routine. The majority of organizational problems are not considered unique. The same basic set of circumstances are encountered and decisions are unquestioned. The organization handles such decisions by devising standardized ways for members to classify these routine situations and to respond so that the organization's work is consistent, equitable, and predictable. Little discretion is allowed in this form of decision making. Standardization is accomplished by setting up a complex series of if–then type statements that together comprise the organization's standard operating procedures (SOPs). Because of the rule-governed nature of most decisions made in almost any organization, the vast majority of resulting actions do not disturb the status quo.

In large complex settings where the work of many people is interdependent, a routine, predictable, consistent way of diagnosing and acting is necessary. Without such predictable routines the complex system of interdependent jobs would not work smoothly, and the quality or fairness of treatment might be jeopardized.

Efficiency. Routine decision making is also an efficient organizational response. The organization's resources can be positioned to carry out the decisions, because the resource requirements are predictable. When standardized procedures guide decisions, the resources needed to carry out the decision can be prearranged, saving time and duplicated effort. Organization members can be trained and prepared for their roles in the execution of predictable and consistent decisions. Scenarios can be planned and procedures established.

This approach does mean, however, that the resources of the organization are "sunk" or dedicated to existing scenarios (Downs, 1967). Changing plans or decision rules or even adapting them to new or unusual circumstances is difficult, as Montjoy and O'Toole (1979) demonstrated in studies on the introduction of new policies in governmental agencies. Change and flexibility are very expensive.

March and Simon (1958) describe routine decision making in terms of *decision rules.* These are statements specifying the way to categorize or diagnose a particular situation and the choices or actions that should be associated with each diagnosis. Together they constitute a complex "program" enabling the work to proceed in an orderly and predictable manner. They note further that a great deal can be learned about an organization by scrutinizing the decision rules. To show how important routine decision making is in an organization, Cyert and March (1963) undertook to observe all decisions in a firm, to compile a full set of decision rules for it, and ultimately to create a computer program that could predict the way that organizational executives in the firm made decisions. Achievement demonstrated the high degree of routine decision making in organizations. This method views organizations as machines that can be and are programmed. In practice, of course, few systems of decision rules can operate with that degree of precision. Deviations from the SOPs based on a wide range of personal, professional, or political motivations require elaborate monitoring and control mechanisms to be established and reinforce the use of decision rules.

Examples of the routine decision approach abound in the literature and in organizational life. Research by Paul Nutt (1984) on decision making in service organizations, including hospitals, found that 71 percent of decisions were based on using existing solutions and less than 30 percent were the product of open debate and analysis of new solutions. Allison (1971), in his analysis of an ultimately successful American foreign policy decision, describes the military scenarios and SOPs that limited the responses the government could consider in the Cuban missile crisis. Every organization has stories about rules that either save them time or produce rampant confusion and poor outcomes. This illustrates the double-edged nature of decision making governed by routine.

Advantages and Disadvantages. The most important advantage is efficiency. As noted, the system allows use of personnel and other resources to be planned. But the disadvantage of this decision-making approach, even when the decision rules are fine tuned, is that it tends not to permit deviations from the program for "special cases" or when there is a change in the situations that the rules were designed to serve. If new kinds of cases, new legal requirements, or new treatment routines appear on the horizon, most research shows that the organization tends to resist change. This is an efficient organizational response but not one that is responsive to the real mission and goals of most organizations (Montjoy and O'Toole, 1979), or to the complexity and unpredictability of working situations. Any unrealistic assumptions built into the routines about how cases should be categorized and acted on may lead to bottlenecks and ambiguity about procedures in practice (Morgan, 1986). The dilemma of how to achieve the efficiency of routine, rule-governed decision making, but maintain flexibility and creativity is not easily resolved.

There are several well-researched methods of the routine decision-making approach. Each offers a competing way for the organization to make major, extraordinary decisions.

The Rational-Policy Analysis

The rational-policy analysis approach has several names: the rational method, the economic man approach, and more recently the policy analytic approach. In practice, this highly quantitative and research-oriented technique is used in a variety of decision making situations from technical operational problems to more global policy questions.

The basic logic of the approach is to maximize the utility of the decision maker(s) by analyzing the alternatives and selecting the one that has the best ratio of outputs to inputs. In practice this means that a small number of feasible solutions are compared on the basis of well-researched costs and benefits.

The assumptions of the rational method reflect another version of the machine model of organization in which objectives are clear and stable and a preference among alternatives can be determined. The early time-motion research by Taylor (1967), which looked at job design as a problem of human engineering, is a conceptual antecedent to the rational choice model, which also assumes that one maximally efficient solution can be identified. This orientation tends to redefine decision making as a technical problem rather than a mixture of political, professional, and value issues.

Steps in the Rational Method.

1. Identify the goal.
2. Identify the alternative projects or programs that satisfy the goal.
3. Research the consequences of each of the alternatives.
4. Rank order the decision makers, preferences for the consequences.
5. Select the alternative with the highest ranked assembly of consequences.

Let us examine each of these steps in detail and identify the values and pitfalls at each step.

The first step is to clarify the goal or object of the decision, whether it is a major policy goal or a more mundane operating objective, such as finding a more cost-effective staffing pattern. This step is often more difficult than it would seem. The problem may be only dimly conceptualized and hard to clarify. Each group in an organization may see the problem quite differently due to professional or political viewpoints. Often the goals are defined by a specially empowered group within the organization, such as a board or council, and not by those actually performing the service. Sometimes, especially in public agencies, the goals are set outside the organization through political processes that result in compromise and deliberately ambiguous objectives. There may even be inconsistencies in the stated goals. All this makes a simple statement of goals difficult if not impossible, and suggests a problem in applying the rational analytic method.

The second step is to identify the alternative means to accomplish the goal. In principle, a wide range of feasible options and combinations should be researched so that in the end, the best one can be identified and chosen. Cost of research and political motives, however, reduce the chance that the technically best options will emerge from the process.

The third step is to research the consequences of the alternatives. Intended and unintended, desirable and undesirable consequences must be researched. A system-wide view that permits the identification of indirect effects is also important at this stage. For example, construction projects must look not only at the effects of facility improvements, but also at undesirable environmental or social effects. Research into the productivity of a new staffing pattern must also look for unintended side effects of staff morale and productivity. In reality, many of these side effects are difficult to predict, very costly to research, and politically suppressed by advocates.

Several techniques for analyzing the consequences of alternatives are commonly used. Cost-benefit analysis considers the costs and the advantages of projects in monetary terms. Productivity and efficiency research makes controlled observations of work rates and outputs. Operations research uses mathematical models to analyze the costs and outputs of alternate patterns of workflow, resource use, and staffing. These models have also been used in policy analysis (Stokey and Zeckhauser, 1978). Levine (1980) reviews many examples of these techniques in health care settings.

The fourth and in many ways most difficult step is to find a way of comparing the consequences of the various alternatives. The difficulty comes in finding a way to compare projects that have different types of consequences and ranking preferences for these different types. How do we compare a staffing pattern with high costs but effective treatment results with one with lower costs, slightly poorer patient outcomes, but greater patient satisfaction?

The last step of the rational decision approach is easy, we simply choose the alternative whose mix of consequences we prefer. In practice this often means that we select the policy or project option that shows the highest net monetary benefit or the lowest cost per unit of effective output. The final choice is rational because it has been demonstrated to be the best at reaching the goal with the lowest cost or fewest side effects.

Advantages and Disadvantages. Supporters point out that the method bases organizational choices on evidence of efficiency rather than on tradition or politics. Even if research data are incomplete, it is argued, the method is still better than no analysis because we can always qualify our findings and recommend that they be interpreted with caution.

Critics of the rational method counter with the argument that we tend to have too much faith in quantitative data even when results are known to be incomplete or of questionable validity. Also, the data analysis requirement of the rational method typically leads to a centralized decision process, at odds with efforts to decentralize or widen participation in decision making. Others have noted that there are numerous points in the rational choice process where value judgments may influence technical assumptions so that the most efficient alternative may not be found. Merowitz and Sosnick (1971) illustrate how analysts with various professional or political interests make use of different assumptions about appropriate costs and interest rates, leading to widely different final choices.

March and Simon (1958) in their classic critique of the rational method argue that it is unreasonable to expect any analyst or decision maker to have the imagination or the time to identify a really comprehensive set of alternatives or their consequences. Instead, they propose that we can really practice only bounded or limited rationality, which they termed *satisficing.* The search for improved alternatives continues only until an alternative is found that meets the decision maker's minimum standards for a solution. They contrast their model with the rational method as "the difference between searching a haystack to find the sharpest needle in it and searching a haystack to find a needle sharp enough to sew with" (p. 141).

Some agreement exists about three conditions under which the rational model can be most useful. These are: (1) there is reasonable consensus on the goals to be accomplished or at least no major conflicts; (2) there should be only a limited field of alternatives to study. Time and cost considerations as well as the possibility of selective attention to politically favored alternatives suggests this point. And (3) the consequences of the alternatives under study should be largely quantifiable. These rules of thumb about the method have generally been found to be useful.

Garbage Can Decision Making

The image of decision making as a garbage can was contributed by March and Olsen (1979) and their colleagues to describe the seemingly chaotic side of the process of decision making—the changes in direction midway through lengthy discussions, the apparent absence of clear goals, the way that some solutions seem to crop up again and again and actually shape the definition of the problem. All these observations are in sharp contrast with the rule in rational choice that decision makers first identify a range of options and then choose the best one. March and Olsen (1979) are attempting to describe what happens in some organizations all the time and in all organizations occasionally: that decision making may be an anarchic process, with little order and no clear steps. They are not necessarily prescribing this as a good method, but they do agree that it is a fairly common method and that their model helps us understand some of the choices, satisfactory and unsatisfactory, that organizations arrive at.

Organizational Anarchy. There are several key symptoms of anarchy. Goals may not be clear or there may be conflict over the priorities among goals. There may also be uncertainty or disagreement about the technology of the organization. What is the appropriate work process or procedure? Is the work routine or creative? The absence of clear procedures for some kinds of problems and the lack of clarity about how various parts of the organization fit together may lead to fluid participation in problem solving with various actors moving in and out of the decision process. Fluid participation makes continuity in discussions less likely, therefore, discussions may go in circles. Universities are notorious examples of anarchic organizations, and so are large, complex health care institutions.

In contrast with the logic of the rational choice process, goals are not seen as directing the search for solutions. Goals emerge over the course of lengthy discussions about the merits and flaws of various alternatives. Goals are thus discovered through the decision process as solutions are examined.

The garbage can theorists also show that under conditions of anarchy alternative solutions emerge in a series, each one offered in response to the objections raised to the last one. Anderson (1983) describes this as decision making by objection. The effect of this sequential presentation of ideas precludes comparisons. Without clear goals and a stable set of participants, considerable "drift" is likely. By the time the tenth option is raised, it may be evaluated on completely different grounds than the second one was evaluated.

Decision making thus becomes a forum for the expression of the organization's culture, conflicts, friendships, glory, blame, and myths that reinforce the identity of the organization's members. This complicates the decision process, of course, in ways irrelevant to the efficiency of the solutions under consideration and is thus another point of contrast with the rational model.

The garbage can metaphor reveals some of the assumptions about this theory of decision making:

> A choice opportunity is a garbage can into which various problems and solutions are dumpted [sic] by participants. The mix of garbage in a single can depends partly on the labels attached to the alternative cans; but it also depends on what garbage is being produced at the moment, on the mix of cans available and on the speed with which garbage is collected and removed from the scene. (Cohen, March, & Olsen, 1979, p. 26)

Advantages and Disadvantages. The image of the garbage can and the discussion of organizations as anarchic have some interesting implications. Essentially it rejects the view that organizations are systems or that decision making forms a stable, analytic process within a system. In fact, March and other garbage can theorists go so far as to suggest that the idea of decision making as a coherent planned activity is an organizational fiction. Many of the choices we think of as decisions are actually after-the-fact reconstructions of much more chaotic events.

The uses of the garbage can model are somewhat elusive. March (1979) suggests that the model does have some advantages, notably as a forum for the kind of exploration and learning that can lead to really innovative problem solving. Thus the "foolishness" that characterizes some discussions can be useful, and we should foster some of the positive aspects of the garbage can process.

Other garbage can theorists suggest, however, that the model has a negative connotation from which we learn to diagnose the garbage can process and take steps to impose tighter controls, clearer goals, more stable participation, in hopes of reigning in the anarchy and reestablishing a more rational goal-directed process. The model has received increasing attention over the past decade, and new research using the model to analyze and manage organizations is continually appearing.

Incrementalism

Incrementalism is probably the most common description of actual decision making in most organizations. Decision making occurs by small steps, or increments, so that from 1 year to the next choices rarely depart radically from the status quo. Policies and programs are relatively stable, an advantage according to Lindblom (1959), one of the first theorists of incrementalism. Incrementalism has often been used as a description of choice in political decision-making bodies, such as congressional budget making, but it is also used to discuss the negotiation of decisions by any group, including the key policy makers in organizations.

Bargaining. The incremental process in organizational decision making is a bargaining process in which the participants typically represent different interests, either their own or those of some group or coalition. Thus, one might see department heads bargain over budgets or program authority for their own members, or representatives of professional groups might debate a new organizational structure. Nutt (1984) found in his study of hospitals and service agencies that many of the decisions were incremental.

Typically it is easier to negotiate from the basis of the status quo so any changes are based on variations from current practices with regard to budgets, personnel, procedures, and so on. Skill in persuasion, the ability to find mutually beneficial trade-offs, the subtle use of whatever influence one has to form a temporary coalition or get a favorable rule change are all important in the bargaining. The exchanges, offers, and counter-offers permit the participants to compromise and synthesize their original proposals in such a way that the point of agreement finds all (or almost all) participants better off than they were to start.

By definition the "best" policy is the one that participants can agree on. Such a proposal may not be the most technically or economically efficient. Instead of an economic analysis, a kind of political analysis guides incremental choice. The compromises necessary to arrive at a jointly acceptable solution may, in fact, result in a patchwork of programs that form no coherent goal or policy direction. This is a common complaint about incremental choice processes.

Incremental Political Systems. In contrast with the garbage can theory, incrementalism sees a direction and a systematic process in decision making. What the garbage can theorists see as anarchy is viewed by incrementalists as the normal, healthy pluralism of most organizations. The existence of multiple goals is natural and legitimate, and multiple actors are expected to move in and out of negotiations according to whether their interests are at stake. Discussions that may seem circular are actually the slow working out of a new negotiation. Thus, for the incrementalist, organizations are political systems making political decisions. Decisions are made to balance demands and resources according to the distribution of skill, influence, and organized interests.

A rationale for the approach is argued by Lindblom (1959) who noted that the rational model unrealistically expects participants to have a clear ordering of preferences as a basis for comparing alternatives. In reality, proposals and counter-offers are made not in terms of preferences for abstract goals or values, but in terms of various combinations of concrete proposals. This means that in practice we do not distinguish means from ends or programs from goals.

Another characteristic of incrementalism is the relative lack of innovation in either the proposals considered or in the final choice. As noted, solutions tend not to depart far from the status quo. Innovative solutions represent a drastic rearrangement of the distribution of benefits and therefore are harder to get agreement on. Furthermore, routine procedures of most large, complex bureaucratic organizations do not tend to uncover innovative options, but rather ones that will adapt easily into the existing procedures and programs. Thus, the incremental and the routine decision theories are compatible.

Advantages and Disadvantages. Advocates point out that incrementalism reflects the pluralism of values and interests of most organizations so that all organized interests may be heard. This is also an important value in the larger political system, where many argue it offers the best means of ensuring long-term justice and equity. It also ensures that great dislocations or mistakes do not occur in new policies by restricting change to small increments.

The approach, however, does not promote innovation, even when there is agreement that a real change is needed. Evidence of this can be seen in recent legislation for tax reform, Social Security, and Medicare. With this method, it is also difficult to devise a policy to pursue abstract values such as equity. Participation may be limited to powerful individuals and to representatives of well-organized groups. Lone dissenters, those with little power and unorganized interests, are not heard. Finally, frustrating delay and stalemate can occur as participants become locked in negotiations.

Aggregative Decision Techniques

Structured decision-making methods include (1) the delphi technique, which is often used as a means of forecasting based on group judgments; (2) the nominal group technique, typically used for planning and goal setting; and (3) a variety of preference ranking techniques, such as the planning cell, used here and abroad for determining citizen judgments about technical planning problems. These structured techniques also form the core of the strategic planning process. All of these techniques use consultant intervention, and are recommended by their advocates as ways to improve organizational choice.

The logic behind each of these approaches is to elicit an accurate ranking of preferences from selected participants on the assumption that the best choice is the mathematical aggregation or summing up of individual preferences. There is a similarity to the rational method in the way it rejects a negotiated synthesis of individual options, using instead some form of analysis to determine the highest ranking individual option. Although the aggregative techniques are quite new, they are increasingly used in all types of organizations.

The aggregative techniques respond to some of the perceived weaknesses of the incremental bargaining approach and the rational method. Nominal group technique (NGT), for example, is designed to ensure the full participation of all actors, not just the most influential, and persuasion or bargaining is specifically prohibited. Each phase of NGT tries to, ". . . reduce status barriers among members, encourage free communication, and decrease the tendency for high status individuals to be unduely verbal" (Delbecq, Van de Ven, & Gustavson, 1975, p. 42). These techniques are also designed to promote the discovery of innovative alternatives by using brainstorming and by fostering an atmosphere of acceptance for new ideas. Finally, and most important, the techniques eliminate the possibility of conflict and stalemate by strictly limiting all interaction among group members. The specific procedures for these techniques are discussed shortly.

Aggregative techniques are being used in a variety of settings and for a number of different types of problems. Staff stalemates and ongoing conflicts between staff and external governing boards have been approached with this method (Mahler, 1987). The techniques have also been used for planning and consensus building with large-scale citizen groups (Morgan, Pelissero, & England, 1979), for difficult budget decisions (Gargan & Moore, 1984), and for developing policies to meet the demands of external constituency groups (Christakis, 1985; Mackett, 1985).

Organizations as Group Processes. Organizations are viewed primarily in terms of group interaction processes. Thus, the analysis of functional and pathological group patterns is seen as the key to organizational understanding. The object of decision making within this perspective is to determine individual preferences for the alternatives, undisturbed by any influence, persuasion, or pathological group processes that may emerge. These methods see group choice as simply the sum or aggregation of carefully measured individual choices. This is an important departure from the more traditional interactive approaches, including the incremental method. Interactive methods produce a dialectic process, in which ideas are challenged and a new understanding of options emerges. The result is a solution that reflects the synthesis of proposals in which the ideas of many may be included. The limited interaction permitted under the aggregative approaches reduces the likelihood of conflict and other group pathologies, but sacrifices the potential for a synthesis of proposals.

Other forms of structured group choice are constantly being developed. As an aid to determining public preference structures in the energy policy area, researchers in the Federal Republic of Germany have used a planning cell technique in which randomly selected citizens are given paid leave from work to participate in highly structured process for evaluating energy scenarios. The object of the process, according to Renn and co-workers (1984), is to create a social consensus on a highly technical planning task while still avoiding the political maneuverings of technically well-informed but already committed and self-interested stakeholders.

Advantages and Disadvantages. The major advantages and disadvantages of NGT serve to illustrate some of the issues. The clearest advantage found in research on NGT is that it provides an exceptionally good means of generating innovative alternatives (Delbecq, Van de Ven, & Gustavson, 1975; Casey and co-workers, 1987; Mahler, 1987). Less clear findings have emerged for the claim that NGT provides greater levels of equitable participation in decision making and thus produces higher levels of commitment to solutions.

Because of the absence of direct interaction in the techniques, NGT may be able to reduce the level of overt conflict and stalemate. Research findings are mixed with regard to the claims that participation, commitment, and consensus building are fostered. Questions can also be raised about the potential for manipulating decisions with the technique because of the considerable discretion that the group facilitator has in framing the question, selecting participants, and managing conflict (Mahler, 1987).

COMPARISONS AND RECOMMENDATIONS

Having reviewed a range of commonly practiced techniques, what comparisons and recommendations (Table 5-1) can be drawn? Kraemer and Perry (1983) suggest an appealing way of matching methods to various organizational situations. They suggest we consider three types or levels of nonroutine decisions that organizations commonly make: operational, management, and developmental. Operational decisions have to do with the alternative ways of accomplishing the practices and procedures of the organization's work. What is the most efficient assignment of personnel to this unit? What savings in staff time could be gained? In general the questions at this level are concerned with how *existing* operations could be performed more efficiently, with fewer or less costly re-

TABLE 5-1. KEY ADVANTAGES AND LIMITATIONS OF THE MODELS

Models	Standard problem type	Key advantages	Key limitations
Rational	Efficiency maximization	Detailed research on consequences	Requires clear goals and limited alternatives
Incremental	Goal conflicts among actors	Compromise, synthesis, and political legitimacy	Slow change, little innovation, policy inconsistencies
Garbage can	Ambiguous goals and technologies	Creative, culture-enhancing solutions	Decision drift, inconsistent policy line
Routine	Standardized situations	Stable, efficient	Inflexible, unresponsive to needed change
Preference aggregation	Goal setting for well-understood problems	Innovative alternatives	Limits participation, compromise, and synthesis

sources, or at a higher level of quality or effectiveness. A variety of technical, quantitative methods have been designed, along the general lines of the rational choice model, to address these kinds of problems.

Management decisions raise questions about what programs or procedures the organizations should undertake. Perry and Kraemer (1983) ask, "'How can an existing system be redesigned (or a new one designed) to function better as a whole?'" (p. 258). Questions about how various projects, procedures, or programs fit the organization's mission or professional values may arise. Uncertainties about future needs, demands, and resources must be considered when alternative programs are studied.

Finally, Kraemer and Perry (1983) identify developmental and planning problems as those concerned with the basic goals, mission, or values of the organization. Policy questions are examples of problems at this level, and planning is typically concerned with issues of long-term goals. This level of problem is not always easily distinguished from the program level, as alternative programs may also emphasize different goals or values.

At the operational level, Kraemer and Perry (1983) recommend the rational method generally, in the form of benefit–cost analysis or the more specialized management science models. Mathematical models for analyzing the most efficient staff assignment practices or inventory procedures are examples. Because these methods are designed to identify the most efficient solution, and efficiency is the only value at stake at the operational level of problems, they make a good match.

Programming and management decisions are concerned with efficiency, but also with other qualitative, judgmental aspects of organizational programs and systems. Choices among alternate programs typically are made on broader grounds, so the technical, rational methods are only of limited use. Incrementalism may be especially useful when competing interests must all be satisfied, as that method typically provides pluralistic solutions in which new benefits are distributed among the competing participants. The uncertainties in goals or technologies at the managerial level may also lead to garbage can decision making, with its mixed gifts of ambiguity and new opportunities for creativity.

When the concern is for long-term directions, goals, and values, such as in strategic planning decisions, qualitative methods are the best to identify innovative options. Thus, the preference aggregation techniques may be well suited to planning and forecasting. The delphi technique is often used for judgmental forecasting (in contrast to forecasting based on time series analysis), and NGT has demonstrated its capacity for idea generation. Here again, incrementalism may be useful for compromise and conflict resolution.

Another prescription for identifying which techniques are useful in different situations is mixed scanning (Etzioni, 1967). With this method most problems are dealt with as they are now, using bureaucratic routines and incremental bargaining which fosters slow change and political harmony. But when dramatic change and innovation is deemed necessary, a more thorough examination, using the analytic methods, would be undertaken to capitalize on the thoroughness of technical analysis that the rational method brings.

Hart and colleagues (1985) note an interesting combination of the incremental and preference aggregation methods, in which elements of the preference ranking techniques are used for the idea-generation stage of the decision process, and an interactive bargaining method, such as incrementalism, is used for the evaluation and synthesis of alternatives. This combines the strengths of each method.

On a more theoretical level, Grandiori (1984) reviews many of the models described, analyzing them with regard to their capacities to deal with conflicts of interest and uncertainty, and the consequences of alternative solutions. Her object is to construct a contingency theory of decision-making methods. She finds that the rational model is well suited to situations without conflicting interests and with a high degree of certainty as to the consequences of alternatives. Incremental decision making and an exploratory model, she terms heuristic decision making, are best suited to situations in which there is some minimal agreement on courses of action and enough certainty as to the consequences of alternatives to be able to make comparisons. Finally, with high levels of conflicting interest and virtually no information about the consequences of alternative solutions, even after they have been adopted, the garbage can model fits best.

A final approach to the problem would be to match the choice of decision method to fit the political circumstances of the organization. A high degree of consensus on goals and possible alternatives makes the rational, analytic method politically feasible. Alternatively, high levels of conflict and disagreement on directions may make the garbage can and incremental models more likely, because they permit negotiated resolution of conflict. A long history of incremental decisions with little innovation may leave the organization bereft of new solutions and make the aggregative methods especially attractive and useful.

BIOGRAPHICAL SKETCH

Julianne Mahler is Associate Professor of Government and Politics at George Mason University. She teaches in the public administration program and her research interests are in organizational theory and health policy. Recent articles include research on nominal group technique as a method of decision making in public organizations and research on organizational culture. She co-authored *Organizational Theory: A Public Perspective* with Harold Gortner and Jeanne Nicholson. Her immediate research plans are to work on integrating political, social, and cybernetic conceptions of organizational control.

SUGGESTED READINGS

Decision-Making Process

Bass, B. (1983). *Organizational decision making*. Homewood, IL: Irwin.

Routine Model

Allison, G. (1971). *Essence of decision: Explaining the Cuban missile crisis*. Boston: Little, Brown.

Downs, A. (1967). *Inside bureaucracy*. Boston: Little, Brown.

Rational Model

Stokey, E., & Zeckhauser, R. (1978). *A primer for policy analysis*. New York: Norton.

Incrementalism

Lindblom, C. (1959). The science of muddling through. *Public Administration Review, 19*, 79–88.

Gawthrop, L. (1971). *Administrative politics and social change*. New York: St. Martin's Press.

Garbage Can Model

Anderson, P. (1983). Decision making by objection and the Cuban missile crisis. *Administrative Science Quarterly, 28*, 201–222.

Cohen, M., March, J., & Olsen, J. (1972). A garbage can model of organizational choice. *Administrative Science Quarterly, 17*, 1–25.

Aggregative Choice Models

Delbecq, A., Van de Ven, A., & Gustavson, D. (1975). *Group techniques for program planning*. Glenview, IL: Scott Foresman.

Linstone, H., & Turoff, M. (Eds.). (1975). *The delphi method: Applications and techniques*. Reading, MA: Addison-Wesley.

Freeman, R.E. (1984). *Strategic management: A stakeholder approach.* Marshfield, MA: Pitman

REFERENCES

Allison, G. (1971). *Essence of decision: Explaining the Cuban missile crisis.* Boston: Little Brown.

Anderson, P. (1983). Decision making by objection and the Cuban missile crisis. *Administrative Science Quarterly, 28,* 201–22.

Casey, J., Gettys, C., Pilske, R., & Mehle, T. (1984). A partition of small group predecision performance into informational and social components. *Organization Behavior and Human Performance, 33,* 112–139.

Christakis, A. (1985). The national forum on non-industrial private forest lands. *Systems Research, 2,* 189–199.

Cohen, M., March, J., & Olsen, J. (1979). People, problems, solutions and the ambiguity of relevance. In March, J., & Olsen J. (eds.): *Ambiguity and choice in organizations,* 2nd ed. Bergen, Norway: Universitetsforlaget.

Cyert, R., March, J. (1963). *A behavioral theory of the firm.* Englewood Cliffs, NJ: Prentice Hall.

Delbecq, A., Van de Ven, A., & Gustavson, D. (1975). *Group techniques for program planning.* Glenview, IL: Scott Foresman.

Downs, A. (1967). *Inside bureaucracy.* Boston: Little, Brown.

Gargan, J., & Moore, C. (1984). Enhancing local governmental capacity in budgetary decision making: The use of group process techniques. *Public Administration Review, 44* (November/December), 504–511.

Grandiori, A. (1984). A prescriptive contingency view of organizational decision making. *Administrative Science Quarterly, 29,* 193–209.

Etzioni, A. (1967). Mixed scanning as a third approach to decision making. *Public Administration Review, 27,* 385–392.

Hart, S., Boroush, M., Enk, G., & Hornick, W. (1985). Managing complexity through consensus mapping: Technology for the structuring of group decision. *Academy of Management Review, 10,* 587–599.

Kraemer, K., & Perry, J. (1983). Implementation of management science in the public sector. In Perry, J., & Kramer, K. (eds.): *Public management: Public and private perspectives.* Palo Alto, CA: Mayfield.

Levine, A.L. (1980). Health care delivery. In Washnis, G. (ed.): *Productivity improvement handbook for state and local government.* New York: Wiley.

Lindblom, C. (1959). The science of muddling through. *Public Administration Review, 19,* 79–88.

Mackett, D. (1985). Strategic planning for research and management of the albacore tuna fishery. *Systems Research, 2,* 201–210.

Mahler, J. (1987). Structured decision making in public organizations. *Public Administration Review, 47* (July/August), 336–342.

March, J., & Olsen, J. (1979). *Ambiguity and choice in organizations,* 2nd ed. Bergen, Norway; Universitetsforlaget.

March, J. (1979). The technology of foolishness. In March, J., & Olsen, J. (eds.): *Ambiguity and choice in organizations,* 2nd ed. Bergen, Norway: Universitetsforlaget.

March, J., & Simon, H. (1958). *Organizations.* New York: John Wiley and Sons.

Merowitz, L., & Sosnick, S. (1971). *The budget's new clothes.* Chicago: Markham.

Montjoy, R., & O'Toole, L. (1979). Toward a theory of policy implementation: An organizational perspective. *Public Administration Review, 39,* 456–476.

Morgan, G. (1986). *Images of organization.* Beverly Hills, CA: Sage.

Morgan, D., Pelissero, J., & England, R. (1979). Urban planning: Using delphi as a decision making aid. *Public Administration Review, 39* (July/August), 380–384.

Nutt, P. (1984). Types of organizational decision processes. *Administrative Science Quarterly, 29* (September), 414–450.

Renn, O., Stegelmann, H.U., Albrecht, G., Kotte, U., & Peters, H.P. (1984). An empirical investigation of citizens preferences among four energy scenarios. *Technological Forecasting and Social Change, 26,* 11–46.

Stokey, E., & Zeckhauser, R. (1978). *A primer for policy analysis.* New York: Norton.

Taylor, F. (1967). *Principles of scientific management.* New York: Norton (first published in 1911).

CASE 5-1

A Decision Trail for Implementing a Policy Change
Margaret Fisk Mastal

The following case study describes the several steps of a multidimensional approach pursued by a hospital division of nursing to construct mutually beneficial, cooperative practice–education programs. It examines the interorganizational issues confronted and the types of decisions crucial to program establishment and expansion.

BACKGROUND

Washington Hospital Center is a not-for-profit, 821-bed tertiary care facility in Washington, D.C. Its mission is threefold: (1) to provide health care and health promotion services; (2) to participate in the education of health professionals; and (3) to conduct and facilitate health research.

The Center is not affiliated with any one educational institution but with many. It is a clinical, educational site for medical, nursing, social work, and allied health care students.

The nursing staff includes approximately 1000 registered nurses. The nursing student population averages 250 annually from eight colleges and universities in the Washington metropolitan area. This confluence of faculty, students, and staff was a readily available, rich resource for developing a formal, organized, cooperative practice–education program.

DECISION SCENARIO

Working with 250 students a year from eight different nursing schools was a positive statement about the commitment of the Center's Division of Nursing to provide educational clinical experiences. And yet, at times it was an organizational nightmare. Head nurses, particularly of the heavily utilized critical care units, were inundated by faculty requests for student placements. Accommodating student placement often impacted on unit staffing schedules, as additional staff were needed to assist with the educational process and reduce potential legal liability of students caring for critically ill patients. Furthermore, students and clinical instructors working on medical–surgical units frequently made additional, individual requests for experiences in specialty units such as the operating room, delivery room, emergency room, or trauma unit, contributing progressive complexity to schedules and staffing. Although we enjoyed the challenge of participating in students' education as well as their and the faculty's contributions to patient care, we knew it interfered with organizational efficiency. In short, unorganized placement protocols and accompanying staffing changes were unnecessary costs and were identified as problems the Division of Nursing needed to resolve without losing the benefits that accompanied our participation in nursing education.

In searching for possible solutions, the Executive Committee of the Division of Nursing identified their possible alternatives. We initially speculated on placing a limit on the number of students or schools we could accommodate, but discarded this alternative as premature. Rather, we found two other choices preferable: (1) centralize all student placement requests in one department and (2) develop written protocols governing student placement requests, institutional requirements for mutually successful completion, and a formal plan for fostering more sustained interaction between the faculty and the hospital staff.

The Executive Committee designated the centralized education and research department as responsible for coordination of student placement activities and attendant policies and procedures. Policies were written to clarify expectations. The hospital would provide: (1) one central department to facilitate all requests; (2) a list of required student information that schools needed to submit about their students, such as health and immunization data, malpractice insurance coverage, emergency telephone contacts; (3) forms for the joint hospital–school evaluation of the outcomes of student experiences; and (4) orientation for faculty and students.

The protocols further included that the Division of Nursing expected the schools to provide: (1) appropriate clinical faculty to supervise students' learning activities; (2) information on student levels, educational needs, and learning objectives; (3) verification of acceptable student health status, malpractice insurance coverage, etc.; and (4) faculty consultation in areas of expertise, e.g., in-services or assistance with research or other projects.

To inform the schools about the new policies we considered mailing them an explanatory cover letter or asking them to visit us for individual conferences. Instead, we elected to invite the chairs of undergraduate and graduate programs and clinical faculty to attend an afternoon reception just before the beginning of the fall semester after which the policies were to be discussed.

Greetings, conversational murmur, and laughter pervaded the hospital's first floor classroom during the reception. School faculty and nursing administration representatives renewed acquaintance, retold summer vacation experiences, and plans for the new fall semester.

Duplicated copies of the policies and protocols were distributed to each person present, followed by a discussion of each item. The changes concerning the centralization and coordination of student placement activities and student information data and the formalized evaluation procedures were greeted with general enthusiasm and approval. There was consensus on the need to simplify and organize essential, routine communication. The stipulation for faculty to provide support for hospital in-services and consultation on research or other projects, however, was greeted with mixed reaction.

The hospital's placement coordinators and the majority of the faculty representatives commended the concept, focusing on it as a benefit, an avenue to snare their expertise in specific situations. Others suggested even greater possibilities, such as joint research grants or continuing education seminars and conferences.

A minority of the faculty representatives disagreed. They contended that such a policy was an undue cost and their institution would have to consider such an idea further. The meeting ended with collegial feeling among most of the group and an anticipation of continued joint participation in student nurse education.

In response to the meeting, the Center's Division of Nursing reviewed the policies and protocols and our rationale. We were somewhat concerned that a few of the school representatives perceived them negatively but were heartened that most had positive reactions. In rethinking the policies, we executed a best-case, worst-case analysis, visualizing potential actions by the schools. In the worst case, we kept our policies and dissenting schools withdrew from placing students at the Center, an option considered unlikely. Second, we could open the policies to negotiation with the protesting schools, which could lead to different contracts with each school. We considered this choice unwieldy. Third, the best case, the schools accepted the policies with internal reservations. Considering that the benefits far outweighed the risks, we elected to let the policies stand and wait for official school reaction.

Only one official negative response occurred. The dean of one school of nursing sent a letter stating that their legal counsel advised them that the policies violated the existing contract between our institutions. In a reply letter after receiving advice from the hospital's legal counsel, we stated no violation had occurred and we looked forward to continuing our mutual relationship. No further communication ensued and no schools withdrew.

In the 2 years since the policies and protocols were instituted no sweeping changes have occurred, but joint exchanges have increased. Communication and activities surrounding student placement and clinical experiences to meet learning needs have become more simple, much to the school's delight and ours. In return, school faculty have made valuable contributions to our Division of Nursing, such as providing assistance with the development of a nursing research committee, delivering in-service educational programs to specific groups of nurses, and contributing short articles for Center Nurse, our nursing newsletter. In turn, the Center's nurse managers, instructors, and clinical specialists have served as lecturers, preceptors, and coordinators of graduate courses, holding adjunct faculty positions in several schools. Out of increasing mutual awareness of individual expertise, the Center's nurses and school faculty have participated in each other's continuing education seminars and conferences, generating greater networking and increased revenues for our respective institutions.

We have become more sensitive to each other's organizational constraints as we have explored other institutional exchanges and contacts. We have developed a capacity to negotiate and evolve innovative strategies that maintain the integrity of each institution's different goals while promoting the professional development of faculty and practitioners. For example, the Center recognized a need for their nurses to pursue academic degrees to further their careers and improve patient care. To reduce travel and bureaucratic red tape for hospital employees, we explored having programs provided by a local university at our hospital. When we initially discussed our idea with the university, the Division of Nursing wanted all classes to be held on our site for the staff's easy accessibility. The university, however, had a policy that the majority of credits had to be on its campus. We negotiated a compromise: all courses except science lab and basic nursing lab courses would be given at the Washington Hospital Center; the lab courses would be on the university campus. Each side made acceptable revisions in their receptive policies and expectations to the utility of each.

Complexity and uncertainty were inherent elements in this case scenario. Complexity arose primarily from interorganizational differences. Uncertainty stemmed from the novelty of accommodating separate multiinstitutional goals and policies, while building joint programs. Incremental decisions, made successively, supported joint program development and established collegial relations among nurses from different organizations. Further differences, while partisan in nature, eventually proved an asset: what one agency neglected, the other did not. Distinctly different points of view were valuable. The challenge became making relevant and acceptable decisions.

BIOGRAPHICAL SKETCH

Margaret Fisk Mastal, RN, MSN, CNAA, is currently the Administrative Director of Professional Development and Marketing at the Washington Hospital Center, an 851-bed tertiary care hospital in Washington, D.C. She is a diploma graduate of St. Vincent's Hospital School of Nursing in New York City, received her BSN degree from the University of Nebraska and her MSN from George Mason University School of Nursing. She is presently a doctoral candidate in public administration at George Mason University in the Department of Public Affairs. She was appointed to the 1988 Commission on Nursing by the Secretary of the Department of Health and Human Services.

6

Strategic Planning in Health Care Organizations

Eric Goplerud

RESPONSE TO RAPID CHANGE

Rising costs, shifting service priorities, and erratic funding assure that crises and change are the inevitable forces shaping health services management in the foreseeable future. These rapid changes force health service administrators to examine the goals of their organizations, and to reassess the appropriateness of strategies that have been employed in the past. The process of examining organizational goals, objectives, policies, and strategies and developing plans to guide the organization through its changing environment to achieve prescribed aims is *strategic planning*.

With all of the changes that are taking place in the management of health and human service organizations, it is not surprising that recently there has been a lot of interest in strategic planning. Studies of planning in business and industry have found that planning is most often adopted by moderate size firms when they find themselves in situations where it is difficult to handle rapid external or internal changes by more familiar methods (Thune & House, 1970; Jansson & Taylor, 1978). This certainly describes the situation for many health service agencies (Jansson & Taylor, 1978; Broskowski, O'Brien, & Prevost, 1982; Goplerud, Walfish, & Broskowski, 1984; Broskowski, 1986).

> The single most important generic skill of the future administrator/leader is that of strategic planning: the ability to monitor the multiple environments, seek out and synthesize multiple sources and types of information, and develop and *implement* a plan of action that anticipates trends *before* they are obvious. Some have gone so far as to say that strategic planning implies not only the early anticipation of change, but the *creation* of one's future through the proactive modification of the organization's environments. (Broskowski, 1986, p. 8, emphasis in original)

This choosing of new directions and new strategies is often referred to as *vision*, an essential skill for executives. By this authors are referring to synthesis

153

of information into a long-range goal. One means of identifying such goals is transformational mapping where executives consider the future first and strategies and feasibility later.

EFFECTIVENESS

Fortunately, given the interest in strategic planning, it is reassuring that there is considerable evidence that strategic planning may be effective. Human service and industrial organizations that plan, perform better than organizations with no planning mechanisms. Roemer and Friedman (1971), for example, found that planning and high-quality, effective health care services were strongly correlated. They found that general hospitals that had strategic planning systems made greater use of innovative technologies, maintained better quality control over services, and had lower morbidity rates than did hospitals with fewer planning mechanisms. A longitudinal study of 250 mental health, alcohol, and drug abuse agencies found that organizations that had implemented strategic planning processes were more likely than nonplanning agencies to have increased revenues, client loads, and diversification of services during periods of overall funding reductions (Goplerud, Walfish, & Broskowski, 1985). Thune and House (1970) found formal strategic planning results in superior performance. They compared the performances of 18 matched pairs of medium- to large-sized companies in the food, drug, steel, chemical, and machinery industries over a period of 7 years. They found that firms with formal planning systems significantly outperformed the nonplanners with regard to return on investment, return on equity, and earnings per share growth while equaling or surpassing the performance of the nonplanners with regard to sales growth. They also found that, since the introduction of formal planning, planners significantly outstripped their own prior performance with respect to dollar sales growth, earnings per share growth, and stock appreciation. Pierce, Freeman and Robinson (1987) replicated the study by Thune and House and found less equivocal results. They suggest the need to tighten operational definitions of variables for future studies.

STRATEGIC PLANNING PROCESS

No Single Best Method

Strategic planning is a process. There is no single, uniform procedure adaptable to any and all organizations. Many approaches and techniques have been proposed by various writers. Some of the best surveys of planning techniques are those of Steiner (1969, 1979), Quinn (1982), Tichy (1983), Wrapp (1984), and Gray (1986). A recent article by Georgoff and Murdick (1986) in the *Harvard Business Review* graphically displayed 20 different planning methods. Each was described along 10 dimensions: time required, time span to be predicted, frequency of updates, mathematical sophistication, computerization, cost requirements, requirements for past and future data inputs, stability of assumed relationships, types of output needed, and ability to either reflect or anticipate change.

The complexity of the techniques for planning can be daunting to someone new to planning. The apparent complexity of many methods, however, masks the basic underlying process and goal of all strategic planning—to identify the strengths and weaknesses of the organization. Strategic planners often use the acronym SWOT Analysis (strengths and weaknesses of the organization compared to opportunities and threats of the environment). Whatever the method chosen, it should lead to answers to the 12 questions shown in Table 6-1.

A Universal Process

Strategic planning involves a systematic method for asking and answering these basic questions. Each method includes the three major steps of formulation, implementation, and evaluation. Formulation involves identifying organizational missions and goals, strategic assessment of the internal and external environment, and choice of objectives and strategies for achievement. Implementation involves tactical planning and actions. Evaluation involves control and monitoring activities, analysis, recommendations, and conclusions. Rather than a sequential process, all three steps occur and interact simultaneously (Wheelen & Hunger, 1984). The steps are illustrated in Figure 6-1.

TABLE 6-1. QUESTIONS TO GUIDE STRATEGIC PLANNING

What business are we in?

What are our underlying philosophies and purposes?

What are the agency's long- and short-range objectives? Are the agency's objectives in balance?

What services are going to be obsolete? How and when will we replace/change our obsolete services?

What new services or needs can be identified that fall within the purposes of our organization?

What personnel and skills are needed to meet our objectives? Are those skills likely to be available at reasonable costs?

What will be our funding or cash flow over the next few years?

What and where are our markets? Who buys/consumes our services?

What share of the markets do we wish to get? How will we get the shares we want?

Who are our major competitors and what are they likely to do? Will it be a disadvantage or advantage to us?

What major changes are taking place in our environment that will affect us?

What opportunities or threats exist in the years ahead that we should exploit or avoid?

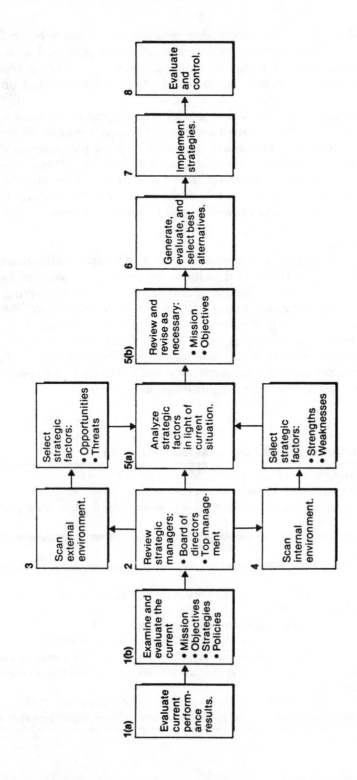

Figure 6–1. Strategic Decision-making Process *(Source: Used with permission from Wheelen, T., & Hunger, J. D. (1986). Strategic management and business policy, 2nd ed. Reading, MA: Addison Wesley.)*

NOTE: **Steps 1 through 6 are strategy formulation.**
Step 7 is strategy implementation.
Step 8 is evaluation and control.

156

LOOKING INWARD: ASSESSING INTERNAL STRATEGIC CAPACITIES

Situation Audit

Strategically oriented managers constantly scan the environment outside their organizations for the activities, market trends, and technological innovations of competitors. Competitive forces present managers with both strategic opportunities and threats. Yet, environmental scanning is worthless if a manager does not understand the internal workings and capabilities of his or her organization. Nurse executives may perceive a unique opportunity to initiate a new service. But if the hospital has a poor reputation for care, if nurses are dissatisfied and morale low, or if competent nurses to perform the new service are not available, then the strategic plan to expand services is crippled before they begin implementation.

George Steiner (1979) suggests that strategically oriented managers undertake a *situation audit*, which includes a careful assessment of internal capabilities and resources. Health services primary resource is professional staff (Harsbarger, 1974). The following questions might guide an internal assessment of professional staff and administrators:

- How do staff feel about who we are as an organization? About its prospects? About their own futures within it?
- How do staff view our purpose? Are there strong disagreements about our purpose or the means to carry out those missions between management and clinical staff?
- What are our staff and administration's most important and dominant capabilities, skills, and relationships? Do they help us meet our organizations' missions? Where do they hinder us?
- What are the strengths and weaknesses of staff in such areas as skills, productivity, turnover, morale, flexibility?
- What are the strengths and weaknesses of management in such areas as leadership, planning, coordination, staff development?

Corporate Culture

The internal workings of organizations are guided by shared values as much as by formal rules. These shared values or "corporate cultures" have been described by Deal and Kennedy (1982) as powerful forces shaping the activities of staff. To understand a corporate culture, managers should examine four basic facets of internal corporate communications: shared values, corporate heroes, rites and rituals, and the cultural network. Values are the basic concepts of beliefs of the people within an organization, the essence of the organization's philosophy for achieving success. These values provide a sense of common direction for all employees and guidelines for their day-to-day behavior. *Values* act as informal control systems that tell people what is expected of them. Values also guide executives in setting priorities for corporate goals and objectives and strategies for achievement that will be the best fit with the corporate culture. Heroes personify those values, showing that the ideal of success in the organization lies within our own capacity. *Heroes* show that success is attainable, provide role models, symbolize the company to the outside world, preserve what makes the organization special, and set a standard of performance. *Rituals and rites* are the systematic and programmed routines of day-to-day life in the organization. Rituals show employees the kind of behavior that is expected of them and the rewards to be gained for performance of desired behaviors. New employee inductions, promotions, retirements, planning retreats, can be rituals that embody the company's core values and beliefs. *Cultural networks* are made up of the communications patterns throughout any organization, carrying beliefs and values across all levels and divisions.

To build and maintain a corporate culture that facilitates strategic management, Hickman and Silva (1984) recommend that managers focus on three areas: commitment, competence, and consistency. A strategic manager focusing on internal processes will seek to instill *commitment* to a common philosophy and purpose, recognizing that employee commitment to a corporate philosophy must coincide with both individual and collective interests. *Competence* should be developed and rewarded in key areas. Foster greater competence by focusing on one or two key skills at a time rather than by addressing a host of skills all at once. Instill *consistency* in commitment and competency by attracting, developing, and keeping the right people.

LOOKING OUTWARD: COMPETITIVE ANALYSIS

Analysis of the external environment allows the organization to determine the market for their services and the direction being taken by other organizations with similar missions. By assessing competitors, managers can identify strategic options and threats to assist them in planning and monitoring their own operations. A framework for competitive analysis was developed by Porter (1980, 1985; Porter & Millar, 1985), which is useful for health service administrators to implement in mapping the strength and character of competition within their industry. Although Porter's research has focused on manufacturing businesses, rather than service industries, the five dominant forces he identified as influencing competition are the same for both types of organizations. By analyzing how these forces affect the mission, goals, and objectives of one's organization, administrators can assess the factors driving competition, the actions competitors are likely to take, the priorities for response, and the direction of evolution likely in their industry.

The five forces, illustrated in Figure 6–2, are (1) threat of entry by potential competitors, (2) threat of substitution, (3) bargaining power of buyers, (4) bargaining power of suppliers, and (5) rivalry among current competitors.

Each of these five forces are briefly described. Through the strategies they adopt, administrators can influence the power of the competitive forces affecting their services and assume the most advantageous position for their organization.

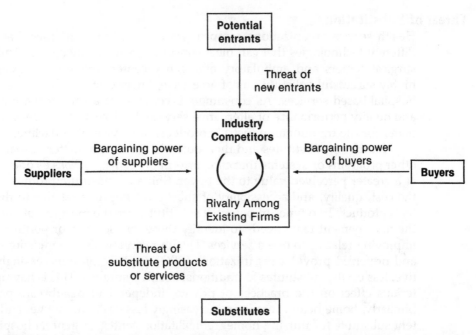

Figure 6-2. Competitive Forces. (*Reprinted with permission of The Free Press, a Division of Macmillan, Inc. from* Competitive Strategy: Techniques for Analyzing Industries and Competitors *by Michael E. Porter. Copyright © 1980 by The Free Press.*)

The assessment framework using the five competitive forces increases the possibility of discovering feasible and effective strategic innovations.

Threat of Entry by Potential Competitors

New entrants to an industry bring new capacity, the desire to gain market share, and often absorb substantial resources. The enormous impact corporate hospital chains such as Hospital Corporation of America, Humana, National Medical Enterprises, and others have had as new entrants within the hospital industry is a case in point. Their success can be attributed to their access to capital markets, their aggressiveness, and their organizational business sophistication.

The seriousness of competitive threats by new entrants depends on the barriers to entry that are present coupled with the reaction expected from existing competitors. If barriers are high and the newcomer can expect sharp retaliation from entrenched competitors, the threat of entry is low for existing service providers. Entry barriers frequently raised in the health care industry include: restrictive Certificate of Need regulations, local zoning ordinances, and difficult and expensive qualifying procedures for access to funding or clients. Low-entry barriers and/or laissez-faire responses encourage competition. When several states in the South and West removed their Certificate of Need regulations for new hospital construction, thousands of new beds were built, many by new entrants to hospital care.

Threat of Substitution

Health service organizations compete with alternative industries that provide different technologies that can meet consumer needs or demands. Ambulatory surgical centers and ambulatory emergency centers are striking examples of highly successful substitutions of accessible, lower cost health care services for hospital-based services. As consumers become more aware of the lower price and quality performance of alternative services the likelihood increases that demand for the traditional industry's products or services will decline.

Identifying substitutes and their potential threat is a matter of searching for other programs or systems that can perform the same *functions* as one's services at a greater perceived value to the buyer. Shifts to substitute products occur as the cost, quality, and accessibility of substitutes improve relative to the industry's product. Two types of potential substitutes are the most threatening. First, the management team needs to identify those whose price or performance are improving relative to one's services. Health maintenance organizations (HMO) and preferred provider organizations (PPO) are becoming increasingly attractive, less costly, substitutes to traditional health insurance. This is having a deleterious effect on the practices of private, independent health care providers. Similarly, home health care is an increasingly less costly attractive, and competent substitute for nursing home, rehabilitation center, or general hospital care. The second important type of potential substitutes are those generated by industries that are earning substantial profits and desire to enter new markets. They can afford to sustain losses in developing new products and services. The vertically integrated health care corporation that opens a home health care agency may be willing to sustain losses to establish a competitive advantage over a group of nurse entrepreneurs operating an established, local agency.

Bargaining Power of Buyers

Buyers increase competition within an industry by forcing down prices, bargaining for higher quality or more services, and playing competitors against each other—all at the expense of industry profitability. Buyers of health care services include direct service recipients, parents and other organized advocacy groups, and third party payers and other aggregate consumers (e.g., insurers, PPOs, HMOs, and federal, state, and local medical assistance programs). The power that buyer groups have on the services and priorities of health care service organizations depends on a number of characteristics of each buyer group's market situation, the relative importance of the buyer group's purchases from the agency, and the share of the market that the buyer group controls. Administrators of health care programs serve a range of buyers whose needs and power differ. Buyer preferences vary in the types and quality of services they desire to purchase, in the current volume of purchases and growth potential, and in the price they are willing to pay for their preferences. Buyer groups also differ in the structure of services and support systems needed to stimulate their purchase of services.

In the case of publicly subsidized programs, such as public health clinics or community mental health centers, the buyer is the state legislature and regulatory agencies. Their power limits the discretion of local administrators and health care consumers. In other words, buyers of publicly supported programs can require the continuation or closing of programs, which vary with local priorities and needs. Administrators of public health programs must recognize that political action is a critical managerial function.

Community agencies, general and specialty hospitals, private practitioners, and courts also influence buyer selection through their roles as referral conduits. Consumers of health services frequently lack the knowledge to assess what services they require and the quality of available alternatives. Managers can exercise a variety of strategic options to attract referrals and control their power over the agency and its programs.

Bargaining Power of Suppliers

Suppliers can exert bargaining power by threatening to raise prices or reduce the quality of goods and services needed by an organization. Powerful suppliers can thereby squeeze quality and quantity of services available in an industry unable to recover cost increases through its own prices. For instance, an insurance company sets a price for a procedure that they will reimburse, which is not adjustable if supply costs change. We usually think of suppliers as other firms selling products such as pharmaceuticals, but labor is also a supplier. Labor exerts great power in health and human service organizations. Scarce, highly skilled employees, or tightly unionized labor can bargain away a significant fraction of potential profits.

Rivalry Among Current Competitors

Rivalry takes the familiar form of jockeying for position, using tactics like price competition, advertising battles, amenity competition, product introductory offers, product differentiation, and increased consumer services. Rivalry occurs because one or more competitors either feels its market share is threatened or sees an opportunity to improve its relative position. Competitive moves by one service provider may incite retaliation by its competitors. If moves and countermoves escalate, then all may suffer and be financially worse off than before.

In any industry, including health service delivery, competitors are mutually dependent. Each acts as a standard others compare themselves against. They are also each dependent on the size of the overall market and its growth patterns. Intense rivalry may be caused by reduced profits due to numerous or equally balanced competitors, increases in fixed costs, a shrinking or slowly growing market, or high exit barriers. For instance, in areas where an excess of hospital beds occurs due to shorter lengths of stay and conversion of surgery from inpatient to ambulatory treatment, intense competition may occur for inpatient admissions. High exit barriers may keep hospitals open that economic logic would lead an analyst to expect exit (closure). High exit barriers may be due to

(1) barriers to conversion, e.g., Certificate of Need requirements to convert unused beds to other uses, (2) high fixed costs of exit due to labor agreements with unions, (3) emotional barriers such as each community wanting its "own" agency or the impact on the career of key agency administrators, (4) political barriers such as regional economic effects or key legislators geographic constituency. Such irrational forces are frequent actors in shaping our fragmented health care delivery system.

FORMULATING A PLAN

Strategic Options

An effective competitive strategy guides managers to actions that create a defensible position against competing demands for resources from the environment. Based on a careful internal assessment and competitive analysis, strategic options can be identified that may include (1) positioning the agency so that its capabilities provide the best defense against the existing array of forces; (2) influencing the balance of forces through strategic moves, thereby improving the agency's market share or offering services to new markets; or (3) anticipating shifts in the forces and responding to them before rivals recognize the trends. Strategic moves that actualize these three strategic options include: widening of service line/area, specialization/niche, vertical/horizontal integration, joint ventures, diversification, retrenchment, and divestiture. Choices among these moves allows health service administrators not only to respond to the demands of their environments, but also to shape the environment in directions favoring the missions and goals of their organizations.

A tentative choice of strategic options and the design of a process to minimize potential planning pitfalls results in formulation of a strategic plan. Before implementing the plan, however, it should be subjected to several tests of its feasibility. Day (1986) suggests seven questions to guide feasibility evaluation:

1. Does the strategy exploit environmental trends and create an enduring advantage?
2. Is it based on realistic assumptions and accurate information?
3. Can it be achieved with available resources? Do people have the skills, resources, and commitments? If not, is there enough time to acquire or develop them before the opportunity passes?
4. Is it internally consistent with other initiatives and goals of the organization?
5. Is it acceptable to the operating managers who will be responsible for implementation?
6. Is it flexible enough to respond to unexpected developments?
7. Will the strategy create economic or political value within acceptable risk limits?

IMPLEMENTATION: AVOIDING THE PITFALLS

Low Incidence of Success

Although there is an awareness of the potential benefits from strategic planning, there are indications that relatively few managers actually engage in strategic planning (Mintzberg, 1973; Jansson & Taylor, 1978; Walfish & Goplerud, 1983). Managers that plan often encounter barriers and traps that derail their planning efforts (Steiner, 1972; 1979; Al-Bazzaz & Grinyer, 1980; Goplerud, Walfish, & Broskowski, 1984). Gray (1986) conducted a survey of business executives that attempted to pinpoint problems in strategic planning systems. He reports that 87 percent of respondents reported feelings of disappointment and frustration with their strategic planning systems and that 59 percent attributed their discontent mainly to difficulties encountered in the implementation of plans.

Need for Strategic Management

Recently we conducted a study to identify critical barriers that inhibit or derail effective strategic planning in health and human service organizations (Goplerud, Walfish, & Broskowski, 1984). Administrators ranked a list of common planning problems developed by Steiner (1972) in order from least to most important pitfalls in their experience. Results very closely mirrored rankings made by a sample of corporate manufacturing executives (Steiner, 1979). Table 6–2 lists the ten most important problems in their rank order.

Among the most important problems ranked by both health service and manufacturing executives was "top management assumption that it can delegate the planning functions to a planner." Several research studies have shown that top management involvement is critical to planning success (Aguilar, Howell, & Vancil, 1970). One survey found that corporate planning is not taken seriously unless chief executives are personally involved (Taylor & Irving, 1971). Another found that chief executive officers of high performance companies are more likely to consider strategic planning a vital part of their job than did executives of sluggishly performing companies (Eastlack & McDonald, 1970). Steiner (1969) goes so far as to assert: "There can and will be no effective comprehensive corporate planning in an organization where the chief executive does not give it firm support and make sure that others in the organization understand his depth of commitment" (p. 88). For a manager contemplating formal planning, one factor is very clear: Either the chief executive officer must become involved, with full authority and prestige, or planning should not be started.

Typically managers at all levels must continuously juggle urgent demands on their time. On the basis of his minute-to-minute analysis of the activities of several executives, Mintzberg (1973) concluded that managers engage in very little formal planning. Rather, he found that managers prefer interactive and reactive modes. Walfish and Goplerud (1983) found that the preference of executives for crisis management was the most frequently reported reason that strategic planning did not take place in health service organizations.

TABLE 6-2. THE TEN MOST IMPORTANT PITFALLS IN STRATEGIC PLANNING IN HEALTH SERVICES

Rank	Pitfall
1.	Ignoring the power structure of the organizational setting in organizing the planning process.
2.	Top management's assumption that it can delegate the planning function to a planner.
3.	Forgetting that planning is a political, a social, and an organizational, as well as a rational process.
4.	Too much centralization of long-range planning in the central administration so that departments feel little responsibility for developing effective plans.
5.	Failure to develop overall agency goals suitable as a basis for formulating long-range plans.
6.	Assuming that comprehensive planning is something separate from the entire management process.
7.	Top management becomes so engrossed in current problems that it spends insufficient time on long-range planning, and the process becomes discredited among other managers and staff.
8.	Failure to assure the necessary involvement of major line personnel in the process.
9.	Failure of top management to review with departmental and divisional heads the long-range plans they have developed.
10.	Assuming that a formal system can be introduced into a human service setting without a careful and perhaps agonizing reappraisal of current management practices and decision-making processes.

Source: Goplerud, Walfish & Broskowski (1984)

Two of the ten most important pitfalls point to the inseparability of planning and decision making: Assuming that comprehensive planning is something separate from the entire management process and assuming that a formal system can be introduced without a careful and perhaps agonizing reappraisal of current management practices and decision-making processes. One of the most important benefits of strategic planning is the process itself. Involvement of the entire management structure in systematically thinking about the organization's goals, its internal and environmental challenges, and internal strengths can foster the development of a consensus that can guide current decision making. As a result, decisions from crisis to crisis, between different parts of the organization, and at different levels of management should be more consistent with the overall aims of the organization. Hrebiniak and Snow (1982) found in a survey of 49 corporations that agreement among top managers within an organization about its strengths and weaknesses was positively related to its economic performance. Agreement on goals and direction appears to reduce uncertainty, provides a consistent basis for organizational action, and reduces the potential stress associated with ambiguity. These factors can increase the effectiveness of important decisions.

Health service organizations exist within very complex internal and external political environment. The most important pitfall described by human service executives was "ignoring the power structure of the human service setting in organizing the planning process." The third and fourth highest ranked pitfalls were "forgetting that planning is a political, a social, and an organizational, as well as a rational process" and "too much centralization of long-range planning in the central administration so that departments feel little responsibility for developing effective plans" (Goplerud, Walfish, & Broskowski, 1984).

One method that can guide executives in being more aware of the multiple groups influencing their organization internally and externally is stakeholder analysis (Freeman, 1984). This method guides management in identifying all of those groups with a stake, or interest in the organization and categorizing them by their type of power. Power categories include formal or voting, economic, and political. Stakeholders include everyone related to an organization: participants, recipients of benefits, competitors, neighbors, and those opposed.

Implementation. Implementation is the crucial change that moves a plan from paper to reality. The key individuals are those actually delivering health services and their immediate supervisors. Throughout the earlier design periods representatives needed to be brought in and consulted as to the feasibility of decisions concerning expansion or cutting back of services.

Responsibility for implementation of the strategic plan lies with operational managers and service providers. Top management should delegate appropriate authority to support implementation. Managers need to devise a realistic timetable and ways to involve all stakeholders in the changes.

The pitfalls suggest some important additional points for managers implementing a strategic plan:

1. Planning must have strong, consistent involvement of top management to be worth undertaking at all.
2. Planning must be viewed as an integral part of management.
3. Planning in health service organizations must take into account the complex organizational, political, and professional forces that affect their strategic actions.
4. Involvement of top management in holding operational managers accountable for implementing plans is critical to a successful strategic planning system.

EVALUATION AND CONTROL

Changing Data to Information

Once a strategic plan is adopted, a manager might wonder how implementation of that plan should be monitored and evaluated. Within health care organizations, management information systems generate vast quantities of data. Yet, senior executives often find that the information presented to them does not fit their needs. Middle managers report frustrations in choosing data to present to senior managers. In the last few years a small amount of literature has emerged on strategic information systems for business managers (Millar, 1985; Porter & Millar, 1985). This section of the chapter focuses on determining the critical data needed for monitoring strategically important areas where poor performance will be disastrous to accomplishing the organization's mission.

Senior managers often respond to briefings and data sent to them in reports with "That's interesting, but that's reality not what I need to see." So the middle managers and management information system (MIS) staff go back, reanalyze that data, develop new indicators, and create another set of charts and graphs. But the next briefing receives the same lukewarm reception. Senior managers know this is not the key information needed but cannot articulate what they need. Information analysts have identified four models of executive information systems and the situations where each is most effective. Nurse administrators should consider their situations in choosing one that best fits their organization.

Interpersonal Approach

Senior managers must work outside, as well as inside, the organization, managing boundaries, and scanning the environment for threats and opportunities. Much of their strategic data is not routine, and cannot be based on regularly collected computer-generated data. The interpersonal approach focuses the attention of managers on sources where information often must be communicated in informal conversations and through other "soft" sources. It does not use a computer. Each manager informally collects information.

A highly intuitive and interpersonally skilled senior manager or management team might use this approach successfully. Businesses favoring the use of this approach include an organization in a highly competitive environment, where there are rapid environmental or technological shifts; a small agency where management is intimately familiar with the internal processes, employees, and its environmental niche; a new, rapidly emerging service where there is little relevant historic or comparable information available; or an organization operating in an environment where success is predicated on satisfying one or two key buyers.

Transactional Report Approach

In most health and human service organizations, senior managers receive routine reports that are either the reporting needs of fiscal authorities or describe internal transactions. The formal information system is essentially a series of regular reports that are inexpensive by-products of systems designed to perform routine transaction processing.

Transaction reports are useful in a stable, noncompetitive environment, where there are few strategic management decisions necessary. These reports are produced with an internal focus. They are useful for meeting external accountability requirements. This approach is often an initial stage in developing a key indicator approach.

Key Indicator Approach

Key indicator systems generate a set of indicators on the health of the business or organization. Data are collected systematically on the status of the indicators, and exception reports are generated on any indicators in which performance is significantly at variance with expected results. Ideally, a key indicator system should be quantitative, objective, and calibrated against some standard(s) that permits comparison within an organization over time and between organizations participating in the program.

A key indicator approach may be valuable if an organization processes a well-designed internal management information system, and reasonably trustworthy indicators have been developed that meaningfully relate to efficiency and effectiveness of services. This approach is also useful when comparisons with other agencies are important for funding or reputation, or when comparisons are required by regulation. Generally it is preferable to a transaction approach as it does reduce the volume of data.

Critical Success Factor Approach

Critical success factors (CSFs) are the few key areas of activity in which favorable results are essential for particular managers to reach their goals. Because these areas of activity are critical, information on their status and progress allows managers to determine whether events are proceeding sufficiently well in each area. At present, most CSF systems require elaborate computer capabilities because MISs are tailored to the unique needs of several top organizational managers (Bullen & Rockart, 1981).

Critical success factors are useful to complex organizations that have identified priorities, where information about progress toward long-term goals is important, and senior managers have sufficient control over resources to be able to make adaptive responses to organizational vulnerabilities or opportunities (Boynton & Zmud, 1984).

Strategic Indicators

Regardless of the information system approach(es) chosen, the identification of what is strategically important data is a critical factor in both monitoring implementation and evaluating the outcomes of a strategic plan. Often, it is valuable to hire a consultant to assist in this identification. This section first discusses sources of strategic indicators and then the process used by consultants to work with management.

Sources. Strategic indicators come from five sources: (1) the structure of the particular industry; (2) the competitive strategy pursued by the organization; (3) environmental factors; (4) temporal factors; and (5) the organizational level of the managers.

Each industry, by its very nature, according to Rockart (1979), has a set of strategic indicators that are determined by the characteristics of the industry itself. These factors are related to commonalities for virtually any organization in that industry. Senior managers of any complex health organization must pay attention to certain factors:

- Predictable flow of resources.
- Basically stable staff, clients, and services.
- Neutral to positive reputation with key individuals.
- Coordination of services between providers.
- Fiscal integrity of the system.
- Physical safety of clients, staff, and public.

The strategies, objectives, and goals for that organization produce organization-specific strategic indicators. For example, many state mental health authorities are pursuing goals to reduce direct state-operated psychiatric hospital services, favoring instead community support services provided by contract agencies (Daniels & Goodrick, 1987). Many community hospitals are reexamining and broadening their missions to include a wider variety of sources of income; this is changing the strategic indicators of success for these organizations.

Organizations must accomplish their goals while riding the tides of environmental changes. Senior managers must constantly scan the environment in which their systems operate. Strategic indicators can emerge from changes in governmental regulations, in the business cycle, or in the demographic and epidemiologic characteristics of the service area. An example of the latter is the impact on health services of the aging of the "baby boom" generation. As this large cohort moves through periods of greatest risk for certain diseases (e.g., schizophrenia and the affective disorders) and through reduced risk for other conditions (e.g., childbirth), the shape of service delivery systems must also shift.

Some areas are significant for the success of an organization for only a particular period of time because of external events, cyclic events, or stage in the organizational life cycle. At other times these same areas may not merit special attention. Some temporal factors recur on regular cycles: state budget preparations and hearings; facility accreditation preparations and site visits; key legislative and executive elections. Other temporal factors are unique, such as class action legal suits, court orders, adverse media exposure of a service. Response to these temporal factors can become strategic indicators for specific managers and for the organization.

Each manager has a set of strategic indicators associated with their location within the organization. In studies of several state mental health authorities, we have found that commissioners generally define their strategic indicators in several areas: (1) good relationships with the governor and key legislators in budget committees; (2) no nasty surprises from the media; (3) positive top management team working relationships; (4) able to monitor and shape legislative initiatives; and (5) balance service system between state hospital services and community service providers. Middle managers would have different strategic indicators associated with their responsibilities in implementing a strategic plan.

Consultation Process

Typically, strategic indicators are identified by means of an interview process between an external consulting team and each top manager. Interviews are usually conducted in two separate sessions with each manager. In the first interview, the executive's goals are recorded and the strategic indicators that underlie the goals are discussed. The interrelationships of the strategic indicators and the goals are then talked about to determine which indicators can be combined, eliminated, or restated.

Four questions are used to elicit strategic indicators during the interview:

1. In what two or three areas would failure to perform well hurt you the most? Where would you most hate to see something go wrong?
2. If you were away for a few weeks, what would you most want to know about the organization upon your return?
3. What are the three or four issues in your health system and its environment that you feel you need to monitor daily?
4. What are the critical vulnerability spots, the places or issues where a problem could develop that would seriously jeopardize your own position or the viability of your organization?

A second session is used to review the results of the first. The manager and the consultant discuss the factors that seem to be emerging in relation to the organization's mission, goals, and objectives and how to "sharpen up" the factors. The consultant also considers the degree to which the manager agrees on factors identified through both interviews. Potential measures and how they will be organized into reports is discussed in depth. The interview process generally takes from two to four hours for each manager.

The consultant team then analyzes all the interviews, refined factors, ways to capture the information, and ways to present the information. The consultant team then meets with the management team and presents its recommendations for strategic indicators for each manager and how results are organized into reports on the implementation of the entire strategic plan.

BIOGRAPHICAL SKETCH

Dr Eric Goplerud is an Assistant Professor of Psychology at George Mason University. He is currently on leave, and working with the Office for Substance Abuse Planning in the Public Health Service where he is responsible for evaluation and strategic planning. Dr Goplerud received his graduate training in clinical and community psychology at the State University of New York at Buffalo, and has published extensively in the areas of mental health administration, program evaluation of human service programs, and prevention among youths at high risk for alcohol, drug abuse, and mental health disorders.

SUGGESTED READINGS

Strategic Planning Methods

Georgoff, D., & Murdick, R. (1986). Manager's guide to forecasting. *Harvard Business Review, 64* (1), 110–120.

Tichy, N.M. (1983). *Managing strategic change: Technical, political, cultural dynamics.* New York: John Wiley & Sons.

External Assessment

Freeman, R.E. (1984). *Strategic management: A stakeholder approach.* Marshfield, MA: Pitman Publishing Inc.

Internal Assessment

Waterman, R. (1982). The seven elements of strategic fit. *Journal of Business Strategy, 2* (3), 69–73.

Health Care Strategic Planning

Fox, D., & Fox, R. (1983). Strategic planning for nursing. *Journal of Nursing Administration, 13* (5), 11–17.

Lukacs, J. (1984). Strategic planning in hospitals: Application for nurse executives. *Journal of Nursing Administration, 10* (9), 11–17.

Rakich, J., Longest, B. Jr., & Darr, K. (1984). *Managing health services organizations,* 2nd ed. Philadelphia, PA: W.B. Saunders.

Implementing Strategic Plans

Young, L., & Hayne, A. (1988). *Nursing administration from concepts to practice.* Philadelphia: W.B. Saunders.

REFERENCES

Aguilar, F.J., Howell, R.C., & Vancil, R.F. (1970). *Formal planning systems 1970: A progress report and prospectus.* Cambridge, MA: Harvard University Press.

Al-Bazzaz, S., & Grinyer, P.M. (1980). How planning works in practice: A survey of 48 U.K. companies. *Long Range Planning, 13,* 30–42.

Boynton, A.C., & Zmud, R.W. (1984). An assessment of critical success factors. *Sloan Management Review,* 17–27.

Broskowski, A. (1986). *Goldfields and minefields: Changing management technologies and resources.* Paper presented at the State-of-the-Art Symposium on Mental Health Administration, Washington, D.C.

Broskowski, A., O'Brien, G., & Prevost, J. (1982). Interorganizational strategies for survival: Looking ahead to 1990. *Administration in Mental Health, 9,* 198–210.

Bullen, C.V., & Rockart, J.F. (1981). *A primer on critical success factors,* Cambridge, MA: Center for Information Systems Research Working Paper, No. 69, Sloan School of Management, M.I.T.

Daniels, L., & Goodrick, D. (1987). *Survey of training needs: State mental health system strategic planning,* Washington, D.C.: Alpha Center.

Deal, T.E., & Kennedy, A.A. (1982). *Corporate cultures.* Reading, MA: Addison Wesley.

Day, G. (1986). Tough questions for developing strategies. *Journal of Business Strategy 6* (1) 60–68.

Eastlack, J.O. Jr., & McDonald, P.R. (1970). CEO's role in corporate growth. *Harvard Business Review, 48,* 150–163.

Freeman, R.E. (1984). *Strategic management.* Marshfield, MA: Pitman Publishing Inc.

Georgoff, D., & Murdick, R. (1986). Manager's guide to forecasting. *Harvard Business Review, 64* (1), 110–120.

Goplerud, E., Walfish, S., & Broskowski, A. (1984). Pitfalls in planning: Contrasting perspectives on mental health and corporate planning. *Evaluation and Program Planning, 7,* 329–336.

Goplerud, E., Walfish, S., & Broskowski, A. (1985). Weathering the cuts: A delphi survey of survival strategies in community mental health. *Community Mental Health Journal, 21,* 14–27.

Gray, D.H. (1986). Uses and misuses of strategic planning. *Harvard Business Review, 64* 89–97.

Harsbarger, D. (1974). The human service organization. In H. Demone & D. Harshbarger (eds.) *Handbook of human service organizations.* New York: Behavioral Publications, 26–29.

Hickman, C.R., & Silva, M.A. (1984). *Creating excellence: Managing corporate culture, strategy, and change in the new age.* New York: New American Library.

Hrebiniak, C.G., & Snow, C.C. (1982). Top management agreement and organizational performance. *Human Relations, 35,* 1139–1158.

Jansson, B.S., & Taylor, S.H. (1978). Top management agreement and organizational performance. *Administration in Social Work, 2,* 171–181.

Millar, V.E. (1985). Strategy execution: The information for motivation approach. *Information Strategy: The Executive's Journal,* 29–32.

Mintzberg, H. (1973). *The nature of managerial work.* New York: Harper & Row.

Pierce, J.A. II, Freeman, E., & Robinson, R.B. Jr. (1987). The tenous link between formal strategic planning and financial performance. *Academy of Management Review, 12* (4), 658–675.

Porter, M.E., (1980). *Competitive strategy: Techniques for analyzing industries and competitors.* New York: Free Press.

Porter, M.E. (1985). *Competitive advantage.* New York: Free Press.

Porter, M.E., & Millar, V.E. (1985). How information gives you competitive advantage. *Harvard Business Review, 63* 149–160.

Quinn, J.B. (1982). Managing strategies incrementally. *Omega,* 613–627.

Roemer, M.I., & Friedman, J.W. (1971). *Doctors and hospitals.* Baltimore, MD: Johns Hopkins University Press.

Rockart, J.F. (1979). Chief executives define their own data needs. *Harvard Business Review, 57* 81–93.

Steiner, G.A. (1969). *Top management planning.* New York: Macmillan.

Steiner, G.A. (1972). *Pitfalls in comprehensive long-range planning.* Oxford, OH: The Planning Executives Institute.

Steiner, G.A. (1979). *Strategic planning: What every manager must know.* New York: Free Press.

Taylor, B., & Irving, P. (1971). Organized planning in major U.K. companies. *Long Range Planning, 3,* 10–26.

Thune, S., & House, R. (1970). Where long-range planning pays off. *Business Horizons, 13,* 81–90.

Tichy, N.M. (1983). *Managing strategic change: Technical, political, cultural dynamics.* New York: John Wiley & Sons.

Walfish, S., & Goplerud, E. (1983, August 29). *Barriers to implementing cutback strategies.* Paper presented at the annual meeting of the American Psychological Association, Anaheim, CA.

Wheelen, T., & Hunger, J.D. (1986). *Strategic management and business policy,* 2nd ed. Reading, MA: Addison Wesley.

Wrapp, H.E. (1984). Good managers don't make policy decisions. *Harvard Business Review, 62* 8–21.

CASE 6-1

Strategic Plan of the Nursing Education Department in a Community Hospital

Karen J. Kelly

When Greater Southeast Community Hospital (GSCH) was in the process of developing its strategic plan in the early 1980s, a window of opportunity was opened for the Center for Nursing Education (CNE) to create its future. During each phase of the strategic planning process, these two questions were continuously considered:

- How can the information collected and conclusions drawn from each phase help the CNE focus its educational activities better.
- What can the CNE do to help the organization achieve the goals set during each phase.

This case study describes the proactive approach used by members of the hospital's CNE during each phase of the strategic planning process and the results realized from this approach.

Greater Southeast Community Hospital (GSCH) is a 450-bed community-oriented acute health care provider facility. Part of the GSCH Foundation System, it is the largest non-public employer east of the Anacostia River. The service area for the hospital is primarily southeast Washington and southern Prince

George's County in Maryland. The 21-year-old facility was opened several years after another hospital, which served the southeast Washington community, moved to its new facility in northeast Washington.

In the early 1980s, hospital administration realized the need to reset the sense of purpose and future direction of GSCH. Administration engaged a consulting firm to help with parts of the strategic planning process and the "planning to plan" process was begun. Management was informed of this activity in the usual manner and key players were identified. Although the (then new) Director of CNE was not a member of the planning team, she was aware of the planning process activities and through formal relationships and informal networks was able to keep pace with the activities, information, and plans. As the organization proceeded through its strategic planning process, the Director of CNE proceeded through the same process on a smaller scale.

The CNE is the provider of the nursing staff development program. This total program effort is designed to assist nurses to develop new competencies and maintain them in their nursing practice. This is accomplished through a variety of learning activities generally described as orientation, in-service education, continuing education, leadership development, skills training, and incidental learning. Dynamic in nature, the staff development process is an integral part of any organization's development and contributes to the growth of professional nursing.

ASSESSMENT PHASE

Although the organization was assessing current and future trends and both the internal and external environment, staff of the CNE was engaged in using that data and developing some of its own.

Current and future trend assessment data collection indicated the following:

- Nurses were beginning to expect the staff development program to meet more of their professional development needs.
- The patient care services expected the CNE to help it meet quality care goals.
- Current administration was progressive and moved quickly to implement new and innovative programs.
- Staff development programming was limited to "good guess" topics without a means of administrative validation for appropriateness and applicability.
- Programs to prepare nurses for staff development practice were non-existent and few nurses could define staff development practice, or would select it as a career choice.
- Proposed changes in reimbursement systems threatened the viability of hospital education departments.

- These same reimbursement system changes seemed to indicate a need for staff to "work smarter."
- Nursing competencies were becoming more complex; determining strategies to help staff learn new competencies was a more complex task.
- No review of hospital and nursing department priorities and imperatives existed to focus staff development programming.

These data were collected from a variety of sources. The CNE Director used primarily interviews with key administrative personnel, informal exchanges with staff, CNE staff member input and validation, professional contacts in the staff development community, and her own 6-year experience in staff development.

Internal environment assessment yielded further data:

- Physical facility, educational equipment, and organizational resources were excellent.
- The location of CNE in the organizational structure limited access to and programming for the primary consumer—nursing administration.
- Budgeted resources for personnel and programming was adequate.
- Few nursing departments had goals related to staff development, education, or training.
- A perception of "CNE nonresponsiveness and dissatisfaction with staff development services was held by nursing administration."
- Roles, responsibilities, communication flow, expectations, and outcomes were unclear.
- Information regarding staff development services, service delivery mechanisms, and standards of practice was not available.
- Record-keeping systems were disorganized and provided little useful data for future programming.
- Little commitment existed on the part of nursing administration in support of programs offered by CNE, a sense of "that's not what we wanted" pervaded.
- No formal overall needs assessment strategy or feedback mechanism existed to plan the staff development program.
- Anticipated changes in health care delivery patterns to home care, ambulatory care, and geriatrics indicated that education programming was needed.

These data were collected from sources similar to those mentioned previously, in addition, sources included a review of the philosophy, purpose, goals, and objective statements and organizational charts of involved departments. Also, exploratory interviews regarding CNE history and expectation were conducted with key individuals. Office records and reports were analyzed. Quality assurance data and risk management information were reviewed and the 20 most common medical diagnoses admissions were examined. The key players involved in the strategic planning process were sought out for information and formal relations were established with the staff members of the marketing and communications departments. Finally, the staff of CNE listened carefully and sought information from the "grapevine."

External environment assessment data collection brought forth the following information:

- Attempts to provide continuing education programs for nurses in the community had met with some success and generated some revenue.
- Nursing staff development departments in the area were providing more continuing education programs.
- The structure, resources, services, and standards of practice of nursing staff development departments varied widely from organization to organization.
- A population of nurses interested in continuing education existed; these same nurses could be tapped for recruitment.
- Regulatory developments for nursing relicensure did not support a mandatory hours of continuing education requirement.
- The value and productivity of many staff development departments was being questioned.
- Changes in reimbursement systems to prospective payment yielded a sicker patient who could spend less time in the hospital.
- A perception of "Greater Southeast, what and where is Greater Southeast?" existed in the nursing community.

The sources for these data included most of those mentioned previously. In addition, hospital ads, advertisements, newspaper, and media coverage was reviewed. Journals, newsletters, and surveys were also read.

POSSIBILITIES AND PROBLEMS

These data provided a rich base of information for the Director of CNE to begin an analysis. Particular consideration was given to the environmental scan of the internal organization. One of the problems in attempting to deliver staff development programs within the existing environment was a lack of credibility. The function of the CNE was severely inhibited and CNE staff motivation and morale were low.

Looking to the hospital's strategic planning process, it was evident that a major marketing effort was needed to (1) change community perceptions and (2) draw a better marketing mix of third-party payors to our institution. The following possibilities and problems in CNE making a major contribution to either goal were identified.

Problems

1. CNE lacked internal organizational credibility as a sophisticated staff development provider.
2. Trends to cut hospital education departments to reduce costs were a threat.
3. A model for success needed to be developed for CNE staff members.
4. New services related to home and ambulatory care required quick and responsive programming.
5. Roles, responsibilities, and lines of communication needed to be clarified and used to set mutual expectations and outcomes.

Possibilities

1. Educational services provided by CNE could be used to assist the patient care services division to recruit nurses.
2. Key activities regarding marketing strategies could be used to change perceptions.
3. Major sources of support could be cultivated.
4. CNE staff members had the capacity to provide excellent programs.
5. The organizational goal to develop new product lines and generate revenue could be contributed to by marketing selected staff development products and programs.
6. Anticipated health care delivery system problems could be addressed through staff development programming.
7. The staff development program should be shifted from a consumer choice approach to an organization training model.
8. Methods to inform all users of staff development services and programs could be developed.
9. Consistent practice standards were also a possibility.

STRATEGY DEVELOPMENT

The analysis and synthesis of the available data and the possibilities and problems created a logical basis for a plan to improve staff development programming and services at GSCH. The impact and feasibility of many strategies was examined. Each strategy was retained or discarded based on this examination and the following three goals were the focus of our strategic plan: (1) establish credibility within the organization as a sophisticated staff development program provider; (2) develop product lines that contributed to organization goals; and (3) create a model staff development program that will draw nurses to GSCH.

Specific strategies to accomplish these goals included, but were not limited to:

Effecting Credibility

- Redefine the role and develop new job descriptions for CNE staff that clearly delineate roles and responsibilities.
- Establish communication charts that assign an education specialist to service every area identified on the patient care services division organizational chart.
- Write standards of staff development practice and develop plans to meet the standards.
- Develop standard needs assessment and evaluation methods to guide the staff development program.
- Meet with key nursing administrative personnel on a regular basis.
- Respond to requests for service quickly and appropriately.
- Develop a CNE practice manual to guide staff members and provide copies to nursing management personnel.

Product line development

- Conduct market research to determine feasibility of providing more continuing education programs for staff nurses and nurses from community.
- Refine program planning and implementation process to guarantee quality.
- Determine a reasonable level of programming for all areas including orientation, in-service education, continuing education, and leadership development.
- Identify other products that might generate revenue.
- Insist that each program developed has an identified organizational source of need.
- Develop a clean, professional image for all marketing and promotional pieces.

Creation of model staff development program. In addition to the above strategies, activities specific to this goal included:

- Develop the application to the American Nurses' Association for accreditation of the continuing education portion of the staff development program.
- Develop positive perceptions of all users of the service through professionalism and responsiveness.
- Develop professional relationships with associations and organizations to provide feedback from another perspective.

- Publish results and accomplishments internally and externally to validate growth.
- Identify further measures to accomplish this goal.

RESULTS

Over the past 5 years the CNE at GSCH has grown in a variety of ways. The strategic plan described helped us accomplish many goals and objectives cited previously. As a testimonial to our achievements, here are a few indicators:

- Identification as one of three of the best managed and most responsive departments within patient care services, both by managers and employees.
- Recognition as a sophisticated and sound continuing education provider in the Washington metropolitan area.
- Accreditation of the continuing education portion of our staff development program by the ANA.
- Use as one major marketing tool for nursing recruitment and retention.
- Major involvement in a subsidiary special project that set up a separate business to sell education programs, consultation, and publications.
- Publication of the CNE practice manual to serve as a model for other staff development departments.
- Increased personnel by 1.0 full time equivalent (FTE) to provide services identified as organizational priority.
- Provision of over 500 staff development programs annually to a staff of 800+ patient care service personnel.

Many other positive benefits were realized, most helped us develop our potential and provide a better service to the organization. The use of the strategic planning process helped us control our destiny and create an environment for nursing staff development practice that is professionally and personally rewarding.

BIOGRAPHICAL SKETCH

Karen Kelly has 12 years' experience in staff development in two different settings, a small community hospital and a large hospital. A diploma graduate, her clinical experience includes staff nursing work in the emergency room, eye, ear, nose, and throat unit, and medical-surgical units. She completed her BSN at the University of the State of New York Regents External Degree Program. Her master's degree was received from Virginia Polytechnic Institute and State University in adult and continuing education with a minor in research and evaluation. She is currently a doctoral student at Virginia Tech. As the Associate Director of Nursing for Education and Research, Karen is responsible for the planning, implementation, and evaluation of a sophisticated staff development program for 800+ nursing personnel at Greater Southeast Community Hospital in Washington, D.C.

CASE 6–2

Strategic Implementation: Some Practical Aspects of Opening a New Continuing Care Retirement Center
Alice Biache

Goodwin House, a nonprofit facility of the Episcopal Diocese of Virginia, is a retirement continuing care center. It has, since its inception 20 years ago, provided an alternative style of retirement housing for persons over 65 years of age. Included in this retirement style of apartment living is the provision of services not readily available when living in the community, e.g., meals served three times each day, maid service, assistance with insurance claims, and a full scope of health services. These health services range from wellness programs for the independent, ambulatory population to 24-hour nursing care for the most frail or acutely ill person.

By 1980, Goodwin House was reaping the benefits of an excellent reputation—a 5-year waiting list of applicants. The Board decided to build an additional facility to meet existing and future needs. It was also decided that sound strategic planning and policy formation had to be used to ensure success of this large venture.

A review of the literature in hospital health care administration reveals that this segment of the economy is many years behind the corporate segment in developing strategic management and strategic planning for policy and management benefits. Strategic management recognizes that "the rational process of planning is only a component of a much more complex sociodynamic process which brings about strategic change." Buller and Timpsen (1986) emphasize that the critical ingredient of successful strategy formulation does not necessarily lead to a successful strategy implementation.

Using the McKinsey Seven-S Framework (Waterman, 1982) (Fig. 6–3), this case application illustrates how the Board of Trustees and the administration developed a strategic plan and implemented it for nursing services for its new facility, Goodwin House West. Each element in the framework is described by Waterman (1982) as follows:

- *Strategy.* A coherent set of actions aimed at gaining a sustainable advantage over competition, improving position vis-a-vis customers or allocating resources.

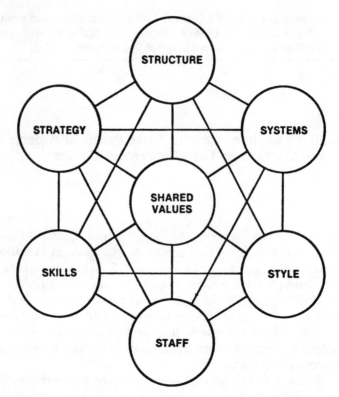

Figure 6-3. The McKinsey 7-S framework. *(Reprinted with permission from Waterman, R.H. The seven elements of strategic fit. Journal of Business Strategy, Winter 1982. Warren, Gorham and Lamont, Inc., 210 South Street, Boston, MA 02111. All rights reserved.)*

- *Structure.* The organizational chart that shows who reports to whom and how tasks are divided and integrated.
- *Systems.* The processes and flows that show how an organization gets things done day-to-day. (Information systems, capital budgeting systems, manufacturing processes, quality control systems, and performance measurement systems each would be good examples.)
- *Style.* Tangible evidence of what management considers important by the way it collectively spends time and attention and its symbolic behavior. It is not what management says that is important; it is the way management behaves.
- *Staff.* The people in an organization. Here it is very useful to think not about individual personalities but about corporate demographics.
- *Shared values.* The values that go beyond, but might well include, simple goal statements in determining corporate destiny. To fit the concept, these values must be shared by most people in an organization.
- *Skills.* A derivative of the rest. Skills are those capabilities that are possessed by an organization as a whole as opposed to the people in it.

In focusing on an organization's use of the framework, Waterman uses the analogy of seven compasses. When all the needles are pointing in the same direction, the company is organized in a way that enhances successful implementation of strategy. When the needles are not aligned, implementation is difficult at best and may not occur even though the strategy may be right (Waterman, 1982).

As this writer views it, the two "S's" that initiated Goodwin House West were strategy and style. From these two basic elements the other five S's naturally flowed.

Strategy

From the moment that Goodwin House West became a possibility, the president of the corporation included the members of the nursing staff in the planning and developmental process. This strategy assured involvement and subsequently a feeling of the staff being vested in the project. Such a strategic approach was felt at the initial City Council meeting when approval for the land use was being sought and continued throughout the implementation of building plans. Nurses were valued through:

- *Item:* The architect consulted countless hours with the Director of Nursing and she, in turn with her staff, to determine such things as the best location on the nursing care unit for clean linen, for utility rooms, and features the nurse's station should contain.
- *Item:* It had long been a dream of the nursing staff that a protected outdoor garden be available for those individuals residing on the nursing care unit. This would add an important dimension to their lives, enabling persons to walk off excess energy, provide a place where those who gain satisfaction from tending flowers could do so, and where the sunshine could be enjoyed. The design of the building precluded the possibility of such a garden being on the ground floor so the architect created a roof garden extending out from the units that filled the stated needs.
- *Item:* In creating the bathing areas for those residing on the units, the president of the organization requested that several manufacturers bring bathtub and shower products to the facility. There, members of the nursing staff stood in the showers, stepped over and sat in the tubs, sat in the chair that raised a person up, over, and down into a whirlpool bath, and tested the grab bars on the walls to determine the best location. The architect also worked with the nursing staff on the placement of the whirlpool tubs to be certain there would be adequate workspace for the wheelchair, resident, and employee to maneuver easily.
- *Item:* The selection of beds was an issue that involved many opinions. Several manufacturers were invited to bring their products so that the nursing staff could compare their features. After months of deliberating, a model was selected that the nursing staff felt would protect the caregiver

from possible back injury, provide the most comfort for the patient, and fall within budget guidelines.

- *Item:* In designing the placement of the oxygen and suction wall outlets the electrical engineer worked in consultation with the nursing staff. The staff held the view that these outlets should be at eye level and in close proximity to the bed so that they would be easily visible. To allow for the differences in staff height, an average was taken to determine the ideal placement. This electrical outlet approach held true for wall sockets as well. Instead of placing them at baseboard level as is done in many private homes, it was a staff decision that 18 inches from the floor would provide easier access, not only on the nursing unit but also in the residential apartment setting. A most important aspect of this decision was the idea of minimizing bending and thereby reducing back injury.

- *Item:* A significant component of the health care service at Goodwin House and one that will continue to be at Goodwin House West is the Health Care Center and Clinic. This area serves those persons living independently in their apartments. Staff members were asked to assist in the designing of the clinic space to ensure smooth traffic flow, privacy, convenience of equipment for the practitioner, and easy accessibility for the resident. Based on staff opinions, the equipment, such as examination tables, cabinets, sinks, and lights drawn in the architect's plans, were selected and installed.

- *Item:* It had been the observation of many staff members that the traditional bathtub is very difficult for older persons to use. The height precludes easy access into the bathtub for arthritic persons and, once seated, it is very difficult to pull oneself to a standing position. It was, therefore, decided to create two options for the resident moving into Goodwin House West: one would be a shower with a molded seat built into its frame and the other, a bathtub with a reduced side height of 14 inches.

Also included in the bathroom design were faucets that would not require wrist action; a feature the staff felt would be helpful for those with limited hand movement.

Style

A large measure of the success of Goodwin House lies in the leadership style of its management. The administration attempts to demonstrate by example a nonpatronizing attitude toward the residents and a do-with, not for, approach when working with them. This genuine concern for each resident extends to the resident's family as well. This special kind of care becomes very personalized over time and such an approach is expected of every employee of this organization.

The concern for others is very evident and extends to employees. Great care is taken in knowing persons by name, recognizing accomplishments, soliciting opinions, and using positive reinforcement. It is felt that these factors of style contribute greatly to the success of the organization.

Structure

As with the original Goodwin House, Goodwin House West provides full services. The organizational chart of Goodwin House West is a replica of the existing organization. Because the site of the new facility is within 1 mile of the older building, a single management team for both facilities is used. Savings are passed on to the clients.

In addition, the management of two facilities under one administration has the very important advantage of minimizing any sense of competition while maintaining uniform quality. Each administrator has an office in each building and travels between the two as needed. Although each facility has its own nursing staff, the PRN pool serves both.

Systems

Quality control is exercised for each facility by a single individual with a nursing background. The position is combined with risk management and works with all departments in both facilities. Employee performance appraisals based on performance standards developed by the nursing department are the same in both facilities. A single continuing education program is offered to both sites.

Other departments, such as dietary, pharmacy, bookkeeping, and environmental services, serve both sites. Again, this plan treats Goodwin House West and Goodwin House as one unit.

Staff

In examining the staff "S" to the Goodwin House organization, one must think of the terms *vested* and *commitment*. The majority of the management staff has been with Goodwin House since its inception 20 years ago or shortly thereafter. Many of the lower echelon employees have had 10 to 15 years of service with the organization. A nucleus of "old" employees will work at Goodwin House West and new employees will work first at Goodwin House to learn the philosophy and management expectations before transferring to Goodwin House West.

The strategy, which is implemented to retain new employees, is a continuation of the existing program including: (1) a built-in career ladder program for all nurse positions that encourages higher education, (2) tuition reimbursement for higher degrees, (3) sending staff to continuing education classes within and outside the organization, (4) rewards for RN certification in gerontology by the American Nurses' Association, and (5) scheduling of work hours to allow for college attendance and personal needs. Several nurse assistants have earned their Licensed Practical Nurse or registered nurse degrees and been promoted.

Skill

Goodwin House West will hopefully develop a skill for decision making involving residents, health clinics, and administration similar to that of Goodwin House.

Shared Values

As can be seen in the previous discussion, the philosophy of the Goodwin House administration is to filter down its style and values to each employee. This aspect of treating each employee as important enough to solicit the employee's opinion and incorporating these opinions into the design and implementation of Goodwin House West provides greater assurance for success in meeting the "shared value" goal.

BIOGRAPHICAL SKETCH

Ms. Biache, RNC, MSN, has spend most of her professional career in planning and implementing care for the elderly. When Director of Staff Development, she developed training programs for staff, facility-wide. In addition, Ms. Biache has served as Director of Nursing and is presently Assistant Administrator of Health Services in a Continuing Care Retirement Community. She has served on the Governor's Task Force for designing the required curriculum for nurse assistants who wish to work in Virginia, and teaches aspects of gerontology on a regular basis for the continuing education program through the University of Virignia. Ms. Biache has published several articles in nursing journals and serves on the advisory boards of the graduate nursing programs at George Mason University and Catholic University.

REFERENCES

Buller, F., & Timpson, L. (1986). The strategic management of hospitals: Toward an integrative approach. *Health Care Management Review, 11* (2), 7–13.

Waterman, R. (1982). The seven elements of strategic fit. *Journal of Business Strategy, 2,* Winter, 333–339.

7

Integrating Marketing Into Health Care Organizations

James W. Harvey

As professionals, health care providers have traditionally viewed marketing as largely conflicting with the delivery of services and were likely to think of themselves as being free from the pressures of business. Several fundamental influences on today's health care delivery system have combined to demonstrate the clear need for new and improved methods of administration. Increasingly, marketing has been recognized as central to these new approaches.

The burgeoning availability of health care marketing research is testimony to growing recognition of its value to administrators. Based on a review of this literature, this chapter is organized in four topics: (1) introduction and overview of marketing; (2) strategic planning and marketing planning; (3) strategy development; and (4) applying marketing to recruitment and retention. Selected examples of recent literature for each of these areas are included.

OVERVIEW OF MARKETING

"Market" is the most frequently used word in business administration and is also common in the everyday language of Americans. Grocery shopping, stock and bond transactions, as well as clever ad campaigns are routinely described with words such as marketing and market. The generally accepted definition of marketing is the analysis, planning, implementation, and control of carefully formulated programs designed to bring about voluntary exchanges of values

Several people deserve grateful thanks for providing background information and proofing earlier drafts. These include Ms. Sue E. Armas, M.B.A. student and Graduate School Research Assistant, George Mason University; Professor Lloyd M. DeBoer, Special Assistant to the President, George Mason University; Mr. Michael C. Rose, M.B.A. student and Marketing Department Graduate Assistant, George Mason University; and Ms. Sunny G. Yoder, Associate Director, Role of Allied Health Personnel, Institute of Medicine, National Academy of Sciences, Washington, D.C.

with target markets for the purpose of achieving organizational objectives. It relies heavily on designing the organization's offering in terms of the target markets' needs and desires, and on using effective pricing, communication, and distribution to inform, motivate, and service the markets.

Understanding the reasons for transactions between organizations and clients is central to marketing thinking and strategy development. For example, in exchange for needed health services, patients give agencies a guarantee of payment and positive recommendations to friends based on satisfaction. Moreover, health care includes many other exchanges between suppliers, boards of directors, volunteers, regulatory agencies, donors, management, insurance carriers, the media, social activists, and competitors. Examples of such exchanges are presented in Figure 7–1.

O'Conner (1982) and Peters (1986) argue that in terms of achieving organizational goals, marketing has been "oversold" to health care administrators. As a result, health care administrators tend to view marketing as a stop gap measure to improve their short-term problems, with primary emphasis on advertising tactics. Both argue that this reliance on advertising cannot be the basis of long run solutions. Rather, effective management is based on a comprehensive un-

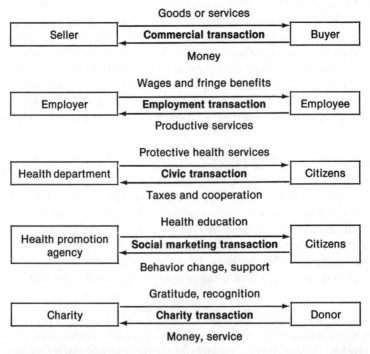

Figure 7-1. Examples of exchange transactions. *(From Kotler, P., & Clarke, R. N. (1987). Marketing for health care organizations. Englewood Cliffs, NJ: Prentice-Hall, 48, reproduced with permission.)*

derstanding of marketing, incorporating the development, planning, and control of all marketing elements, including the traditional "4 Ps" of *product*/service development, *price*, *place*/location, and *promotion* management.

Through the analysis of these multiple and frequently complex exchanges, the health care administrator gains insight into possible courses of action to establish strategies for services. Serving client needs, understanding competitive and environmental dynamics, and developing strategies within the organization's mission and objectives, collectively represent the underpinnings of a *market-driven health care* organization. Figure 7–2 illustrates how health care exchanges often include several parties indirectly related to each other, rather than simple two-way trades.

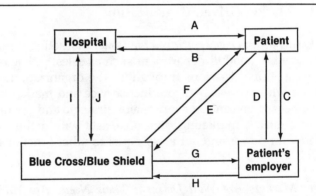

A. The hospital provides health care services to the patient.
B. The patient provides direct payment and/or guarantee of payment from a third party to the hospital. In addition, the patient provides utilization of hospital services, which the hospital seeks.
C. The patient, as an employee, provides productive work services to the employer.
D. The employer provides monetary compensation for work services, plus partial coverage for the employee's health benefits and insurance.
E. The patient provides monthly payments for health insurance, beyond that paid by the patient's employer, to Blue Cross/Blue Shield.
F. Blue Cross/Blue Shield provides guarantee of partial coverage for the patient's medical expenses.
G. Blue Cross/Blue Shield provides a mechanism by which the employer can offer health insurance to the employee group.
H. The employer provides monthly payments to Blue Cross/Blue Shield.
I. Blue Cross/Blue Shield provides reimbursement for services rendered to the hospital.
J. The hospital provides a guarantee that health services will be delivered in a cost-efficient manner so that Blue Cross/Blue Shield will not end up paying out more in reimbursements than it has attracted in payments.

Figure 7–2. Multiple exchanges in health care transactions. *(From Kotler, P., & Clarke, R. N. (1987). Marketing for health care organizations. Englewood Cliffs, NJ: Prentice-Hall, 49, reproduced with permission.)*

To better understand the market-driven health care organization, let us examine other alternatives. Production-driven organizations identify the primary task of managers as assuring production and distribution efficiency, whereas product-driven organizations define and deliver the products and services *managers* believe are wanted by the market, without performing the required research to determine client needs. Furthermore, organizations that are sales-driven seek to persuade possible customers to purchase its existing products and services. In contrast, market-driven organizations orient managers to understand that success is determined by market dynamics; their *first* task is to ascertain the needs of the market and *then* determine if those needs can be effectively served within the context of the organization's mission, objectives, environmental concerns, and competition (Table 7–1).

Indicators of a Market-Driven Organization

Marketing as an Organization-wide Issue. Marketing is not an obscure subfunction buried in another department such as sales, public relations, or communications. Staffing decisions throughout the organization are made on the basis of those who possess both product/service and market knowledge. Marketing personnel are present on every major strategic and operating committee in the organization. A marketing division exists within the organization, which is vested with power and authority equal to other functions throughout the hierarchy.

Target Markets Are Well Defined; Their Needs Are Understood. Attention is given to the identity of the health care organization's customers: patients, physicians, other providers, insurance companies, and service employees. An ongoing commitment is made to defining, profiling, listening, and responding to existing and potential clients. The organization's responsibility to the customer extends beyond the immediate transaction of services to include providing information that encourages informed decision making assuring customer satisfaction. Markets are divided into discrete segments, rather than treated uniformly. Clients are seen as goal-directed problem-solvers with different needs at each

TABLE 7-1. INDICATORS OF A MARKET-DRIVEN HEALTH CARE ORGANIZATION

1. Marketing is seen as an organization-wide issue.
2. Target markets are well defined; their needs are understood.
3. Strategy development is based on provider/market relationships.
4. Strategic objectives are explicit.
5. Clear market identity is established.
6. Marketing strategies recognize unique aspects of the service industries.
7. Services are seen as solutions to consumers problems.
8. Location and layout are key to provider choice.
9. Prices are based on value to customers.
10. Promotion plays a limited specific role in overall strategy.

Adapted from Andreasen (1982) and Kotler (1985).

stage of their decision process. The organization is prepared to alter its offerings and methods to meet changed client needs and to address competition.

Strategy Development Based on Provider/Market Relationships. Organizational success is acknowledged to be based *collectively* on market need and provider capability. Administrators in a market-driven organization do not view the offering as inherently desirable and lack of market response is not automatically attributed to consumer ignorance or lack of motivation.

Strategic Objectives Are Explicit. Commitment to long-term and short-term planning pervades the organization. The environment is continually scanned because market success is recognized as having a limited time dimension and its causes are frequently not self-evident. Strategic planning and strategy development begin with a statement of clear and quantifiable objectives, within a time frame and in the context of target markets and competitors. Efforts are made to understand and manage market place processes, as failure to do so will likely lead to loss of control of the service enterprise's future.

Clear Market Identity Is Established. Market positioning and establishment of differential advantage are based on organizational strengths. Multiple strategies are tailored for multiple markets. A portfolio of offerings and market segments is developed that maintains the organization's distinctive advantages and is consistent with its mission. Growth occurs by "edging out" from organizational strengths, avoiding weaknesses, and not by trying to be all things to all people or by adopting strategies better suited to the skills of its competitors.

Marketing Strategies Recognize Unique Aspects of the Service Industries. Literature and practice clearly indicate that professional services marketers face problems unlikely to be addressed by other industries. The intangible nature of offerings, the inseparability of provider and recipient, the inability to store exchanges, and the provider's role as inextricably determinant of consumer satisfaction are unique issues encountered by service providers. Health care's position as a profession further underscores the differences in its marketing practice. Provider-specific and industry-wide issues, such as third-party accountability, client uncertainty in evaluating service performance, the need for greater provider experience and quality control, as well as limited opportunity for service differentiation, are examples of the unique characteristics that must be addressed in professional services marketing. Health care is also unique in that client options are often restricted, with the choice of service being funneled through providers who act as gatekeepers.

Services Are Seen as Solutions to Customers' Problems. Clients are seen as active problem-solvers who want specific results, such as long life, weight loss, and freedom from pain, who differ in the way they assess their health needs. Competition from other industries is based on the consumer's willingness to substitute alternative solutions to the decision maker's health care needs. For example, some may choose health spas, nutrition centers, or religious meditation as alternatives to health services.

Location and Layout Are Key to Provider Choice. Site location, buildings, and architectural design are recognized as bridges to the market as well as opportunities to be close to and influence the customer. Thus, customer travel time, comfort, and convenience are closely monitored. These intermediary factors frequently determine whether or not market transactions take place and are, therefore, chosen and monitored carefully.

Prices Are Based on Value to Customers. Frequently, pricing is problematic because of regulation, cost guidelines, and confusion as to who is the customer. Is the customer the payor, the referral gatekeeper, or the patient? When pricing decision is under control of management, prices are based both on value to the customer and the objectives of the organization, while not ignoring costs and margins.

Promotion Plays a Limited, Specific Role in Overall Strategy. The promotion mix is one of the last strategic considerations. First it is essential to determine: What are we selling? To whom? What are the benefits of the offering? What are the information needs of the targets? What are the best ways to reach them?

Ethics of Marketing Health Care

Many professionals argue that marketing health care is unethical; others point out that marketing has increased sensitivity to consumer needs and desires, increased awareness of services, while not sacrificing industry standards or client trust (Bloom, 1984).

The American Marketing Association's Academy for Health Services Marketing has developed a set of professional ethics for health care marketing professionals, which encourages them to: (1) respect the primacy of patient and customer welfare; (2) ensure the competitiveness of their organization; (3) provide communications that inform and persuade but do not deceive; (4) compare competitive offerings in ways that are fair and can be substantiated; (5) never enter relationships that constitute a conflict with existing client interests; (6) respect the privacy and confidentiality of patient, customer, and client relationships; and (7) be vigilant in encouraging the application of these standards (*Marketing News, 1985*).

Incorporating Marketing into the Health Care Organization

Once the marketing approach is understood, one of the greatest challenges to an organization is integrating this perspective into the enterprise (George & Compton, 1985; Clarke & Shyavitz, 1987; Miaoulis et al., 1985). Once the need is recognized, frequently a primary problem in implementation is a lack of marketing expertise. For example, Witt and McRoberts (1983) report in a survey of hospital marketing executives, that, at first, their organizations tended to mandate that current planning staff become marketing specialists despite the fact that three-fourths of them had no marketing background. This is an example of failing to make staffing decisions based on those who possess knowledge of both marketing and products/services, an indicator of an organization that is not market-driven.

In setting up a marketing department, Marshall (1980) notes that marketing is not just designing public relations programs and communicating with the media. Health care marketing involves building strong relationships with the community, recruiting providers, attracting board members, maintaining productivity, planning for the future, ensuring the financial position, and working with all primary constituencies. A common method of classifying constituents is: (1) external constituencies—those who support, control, or create an outside influence on the organization, including suppliers, regulatory agencies, community leaders; (2) internal constituencies—those who work in or for the organization, such as boards of trustees, employees, physicians, volunteers; (3) clients—existing and potential clients who use or benefit from the health provider's services; and (4) colleagues—those who provide similar services and work with or compete against the provider, such as other professionals, private practice physicians, private laboratories, independent clinics, and public health departments. Each represents a target market requiring strategy development.

Restructuring to Incorporate Marketing

Anticipating organizational resistance to the introduction of marketing, Kotler and Clarke (1987, p. 140) summarize four strategies to begin to develop a market-driven organization: (1) board appointments of qualified marketing personnel to guide the introduction, (2) contracting for a study of a specific problem by qualified outside personnel to acquaint administration with the value of marketing, (3) executive development seminars to acquaint key staff with marketing knowledge, and (4) adopting a committee approach to marketing.

Once the practice of marketing is accepted, four alternative approaches to the organizational structure are available: (1) the *functional* approach, which creates a marketing department, by combining the previously separate activities such as public relations, promotion, service development, distribution and the various research groups; (2) the *product/service line* management approach, which assigns the responsibility of one related group of products or services to one administrator, who receives the support of centralized staff in developing needed activities of public relations, promotion, and research for that product/service line across all consumer groups; (3) the *customer-centered* approach, which assigns responsibility of each customer group by location, age group, or other category to a different administrator, who develops and coordinates all functions required to support the products and services used by this single group of customers; and (4) a *mixed* approach, which combines features of these three alternatives to best meet the needs of the organization. Figure 7–3 summarizes these four approaches. Each approach has its strengths, limitations, and

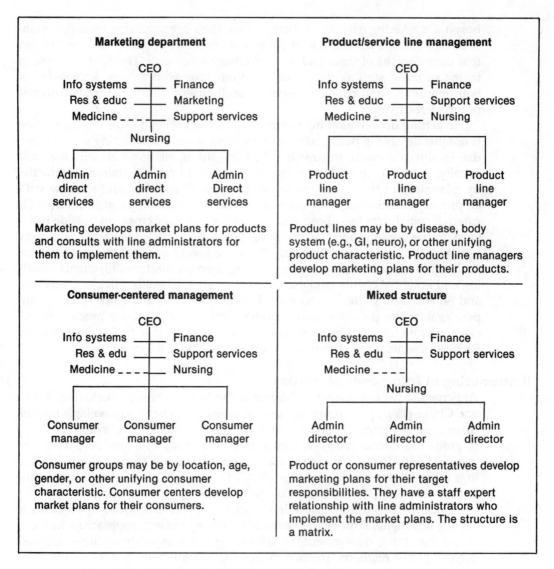

Figure 7–3. Alternative Marketing Structures *(Res & Edu-research and education.)*

situations when one is more appropriate than the others (Kotler & Andreasen, 1987, Chapter 9).

Health Care as a Unique Marketing Challenge

Health care institutions represent a unique challenge to marketing in that no single existing marketing perspective or stream of research applies to it without some modification. Concerns unique to health care organizations include (1) the distinctive problems posed by services and professional services marketing; (2)

their status as either nonprofit or mixed profit and nonprofit entities; (3) a high level of public, community, and political scrutiny compared with other organizations; (4) their need to engage (in varying degrees) in fund raising; (5) the unique nature of consumer demand and price sensitivity, the result of access controlled largely by providers and fees mainly underwritten by third-party payers; (6) the extent of federal and state regulation, which frequently limits strategic choices; and (7) an inherent struggle for power and authority between administration and providers, which may lead to major conflicts in the design and delivery of organizational strategies (Lovelock and Weinberg, 1984; Kotler and Clarke, 1987). Despite these concerns, marketing is making a significant contribution to the current restructuring of health care delivery.

MARKETING'S ROLE IN STRATEGIC PLANNING

A strategic plan consists of four sets of related decisions, usually performed by top-level administration: (1) defining the business, (2) determining the mission or role of the business, (3) formulating functional strategies, and (4) budgeting.

The approach to planning emphasized by marketing puts the consumer at the beginning of the process by first defining relevant market customers and determining how their needs are currently being served (Abell & Hammond, 1979; Nichols, 1986; McDevitt, 1987; Hunter, 1987). Next, current offerings are analyzed in terms of customer needs and exchanges. Similarly, competition is analyzed in terms of the alternative methods provided to facilitate these exchange relationships. Once this is accomplished, the organization makes a commitment to develop a plan that may call for restructuring or developing new services. An audit of the effectiveness of the plan is instituted both in terms of satisfying the needs of the target market and of achieving organizational goals.

Marketing supports strategic planning through: (1) competitor analysis; (2) consumer analysis, including client satisfaction and market segmentation; (3) self-assessment; and (4) strategy development. The first three topics use market research to gather data. Strategies can only be as good as the quality of the data collected. Thus, marketing managers need to be knowledgeable and proficient in research methods.

Competitor Analysis

Competition arises from both direct and indirect sources. Direct competition stems from other health care institutions that participate in the same industry, using similar methods (Jensen, 1986). Indirect competition, often neglected in strategic analysis, but quite important to understand, comes from prospective clients choosing industries and technologies other than mainstream health care. For example, although many Americans are involved with a limited number of health care activities and institutions of any form, most use a variety of folk and fad techniques. Trends, such as the use of family recipes to create elixirs, bracelets for arthritis, and crystals that sell for up to $150,000 to stimulate the immune system, improve positive thinking, improve sleep, reduce tension and meditate, all compete with traditional health care providers for the potential client's money and loyalty (Robert Wood Johnson Foundation, 1987; *Time*, 1987b).

Competition occurs indirectly among all providers of the benefits consumers seek. For example, Figure 7–4 illustrates the many possible services of health devices as they are perceived by consumers to provide care along the dimensions of the benefits of transactions costs (convenience) and degree of specialization. Services and devices that are located in close proximity to each other in this figure are thought of as near substitutes by consumers, as they are seen as possessing similar combinations of desired benefits. Furthermore, those located

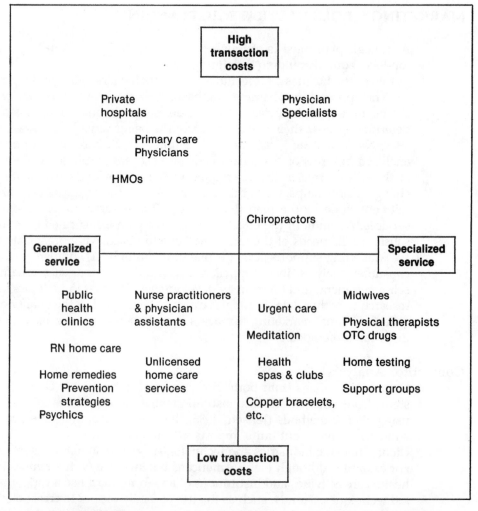

Figure 7–4. Graphic representation of direct and indirect health care competition.

some distance from each other are less likely to be seen as substitutes. This analysis shows, for example, that many consumers would prefer an over-the-counter diet pill to a professionally supervised program of weight reduction because of its lower transaction costs.

This method of analysis helps to demonstrate to planners the need for identifying the benefits that are the basis of competition, understanding the combination of benefits offered by each rival, realizing which organizations are most intensely competitive, and seeing the options available in redefining competitive positioning through altered combinations of benefits.

Potential Consumer Analysis

One of the first problems confronting health care administrators wishing to assess the need and preferences of their consumers is the identification of whether their consumers are the users of their services (patients), the users of their facility to provide medical services (physicians), or the payors for their services (insurance companies, government programs, patients). The answer is all three.

The most sought after patient group for most hospitals is the privately insured primary care patient. Hospitals have traditionally used four approaches to attract these patients: (1) physician-based, (2) client-focused, (3) physician and client; and (4) the "turtle" approach (Sturm, 1984). In the first approach, the physician is the key customer. This approach emphasizes increasing medical staff size and assumes that the share of services delivered will increase proportionately. The two weaknesses of this strategy are that physicians practice at multiple sites and that fewer people have primary physicians. The second approach focuses directly on the "great American consumer." For hospitals, this type of strategy tends to fail as it ignores the fact that physicians influence access and consumer choice. This approach, however, has had more success with urgent care services and other direct access health services (Kroger & Perry, 1983). The third approach combines appeals to both physicians and clients. This strategy involves team-building within the medical staff, coupled with concern for user satisfaction and promotion of name recognition and centers of excellence. This is the most successful method for hospitals. The last approach, referred to as the turtle strategy, postpones promotional activities and takes a cautious wait-and-see attitude of how the environment is evolving before choosing a strategy. This is the riskiest strategy, good only for those with firmly entrenched market positions and deep reserves.

An example of consumer analysis is offered by Inguanzo and Harju (1985b), who report that although four of five consumers have a hospital preference, fewer than half stated that their preference is very strong. Most facility loyalty is associated with those living in the eastern U.S., in medium-size cities, aged 55 and older, with household incomes under $15,000. Those with lowest facility loyalties are more likely to be from the western U.S., younger, college-educated, and have family incomes of $25,000 to $40,000. Findings from the study indicate the following reasons for facility loyalty: (1) good medical care, (2) location (proximity to home), (3) tradition (where usually gone), and (4) physician's recommendation. These findings point to the need for administrators to determine the extent of such loyalty and the factors determining choice in their market area.

Inguanzo and Harji (1985b) also found that good medical care means something different to different groups of people. One type of client reported that the availability of specialists was most important. Another group defined "good care" as based on personalized care, whereas a third group of health care consumers insisted on the latest technology and equipment. This study points out several important findings: (1) it identifies the criteria that determine hospital choice, (2) the study underscores that the importance of these criteria varies by consumer segment, (3) it emphasizes the need for the facility to perform market research in its local area, (4) the physician's recommendation is more important than client preferences in deciding hospital choice, and (5) consumer preferences also play a major role in many other aspects of health care choices.

Consumer Satisfaction

Patient satisfaction is an integral component of the marketing program (Swan et al., 1985). Costello (1985) notes that patients have an enlarged role in health care decision making, and a well-defined set of expectations against which service performance is assessed. Costello outlines the primary sources of patient dissatisfaction: discourteous nurses, discourteous staff attitudes, confusing billing statements, and room appearance. Health organizations need to measure these potential sources of dissatisfaction using patient surveys and to take remedial action where indicated. Patient satisfaction is key to repeat business and positive word-of-mouth referral.

Market Segmentation

Identification of discrete subgroups within the market for health care services and responding appropriately to differences in their health care needs and preferences represents one of the most effective approaches to marketing. This process of identification is called market segmentation. Market segment analysis assists health care organizations to better understand that they serve multiple sets of clients who possess different wants and needs and to deliver services that are congruent with these diverse values and desires.

Segmentation analysis has traditionally relied on demographic, geographic, situational, life style, and behavioral differences. For example, demographic segmentation would focus on the fact that women use more health care services than men (Coe, 1979). In contrast, the geographic segmentation approach would examine regional differences in health care needs and utilization, for example, urban versus rural or suburban clients. The health needs of travelers or those preferring home care would offer a basis for situational segmentation, creating a target market uniting otherwise diverse groups (Edmondson, 1985a). A hospital located in an area with many international travelers might position itself as sensitive to particular needs of visitors and reach them through hotels and embassies/consulates.

The self-care market is a life style market segment. As summarized by Edmondson (1985b), it is 69 percent female, has a median age of 35, with an upscale income and education. Those with a self-care life style are willing to spend money for prevention and fitness supplies, vitamins, supplements, health foods, diagnostic software, and self-assessment equipment. An administrator targeting this group would offer different services and use different methods of persuasion than if a different segmentation approach had been used or another target group had been identified.

The final traditional market segmentation method is the behavioral process approach, such as the role of referral agents in the client decision processes. For example, Legg and Lamb (1986) found that the recommendations of experts, such as physicians, ministers, and school counselors, were mentioned well over twice as often as any other group.

Haley (1985) notes, however, that each of these methods of segmentation has distinct disadvantages because they are based on frequently arbitrary categories of descriptive factors. They do not reveal why people choose a service, only the characteristics of users and nonusers. This lack of causality is the basis for the relatively poor performance of demographic segmentation in predicting future behavior, such as receptivity to persuasive communication and product/ service changes. To improve the lack of causality inherent in segmentation strategies, many have turned to the use of benefit segmentation. Defining markets on the basis of benefits sought by consumers identifies groups of people with fairly homogeneous preferences for product/service attributes or combinations of attributes. Although this technique was first documented to have been used by industry in 1961, little publicly documented evidence exists of the use of benefit segmentation in health care.

In one such study, Steiber and Boscarino (1983) identified five health care behavioral segments: (1) doctor knows best—consumers who abide by the physician's recommendation and who tend to be older as well as less educated; (2) repeaters—brand loyal clients who are more likely long-time residents of the community; (3) convenience—busy professionals who want accessible facilities; (4) high tech—well-informed consumers who insist on the latest medical innovation; and (5) image—people who want new and reputable facilities, who tend to hold blue collar occupations, and are more easily influenced by media (Wotruba, Haas, & Oulhen, 1985). More recently, Finn and Lamb (1986) found four benefit segments for hospitals: (1) take care of me—clients who were very interested in the physical comforts, including good food, comfortable room, and suitable bathroom; (2) cure me—people who see a hospital stay as serious and personal and want quiet and privacy; (3) pamper me—a group who wants personal attention and psychological comfort; and (4) explain to me—patients who want good medical procedures and much explanation of procedures and practices.

Self-assessment

Competitor analysis and consumer analysis focus on external factors in developing marketing strategies. Also essential to strategic planning is the examination of internal organizational strengths and weaknesses, indicators of resources, effectiveness of activities, constituency and support groups, and market position (Crompton & Lamb, 1983; Salvatore 1984). For examples of an internal and external marketing audit for a health care provider, see Walter (1981).

One critical aspect of an internal self-assessment is the examination of the organization's array of services. This appraisal leads to decisions concerning adding, pruning, divesting, and discontinuing the organization's offerings in the context of the market served (Wood & Singh, 1986).

Service Portfolio Analysis

One of the best known methods for evaluating the service array is portfolio analysis, originally developed by the Boston Consulting Group (BCG). Each service is classified into one of four categories, as defined by two dimensions. First, the relative share of the market already captured by each service (high/low), and second, the prospects for growth of that market (high/low). This matrix is illustrated in Figure 7–5. The rationale for this fourfold typology is concern for current performance (market share) and prospects for the future (market growth). Moreover, market share provides the organization with cash through sales of the service, whereas market growth absorbs cash, necessitated by adding facilities, staff, and supplies needed to meet increased levels of activity.

For example, a hospital may be a local leader in delivering babies (high share), but because of the aging of the nearby population, the growth rate for the need for such services is low (low growth). As a result of this analysis, obstetric services would be classified as a "Cash Cow", due to its high market share and low market growth. Cash cows provide more cash than they absorb, thus, the hospital will want to hold its market share position, by neither allowing the success of obstetrics to deteriorate, nor expanding these services, which would build useless capacity. Alternatively, "Question Marks" demand large amounts of cash to finance the market growth being experienced, but provide very little revenue, due to low market share. Cash cows are needed to provide cash to subsidize services classified as question marks. Question marks, in turn, are needed, as they represent the organization's opportunity for future cash from growing markets.

Services that struggle for share in low growth markets represent opportunities to spend scarce resources elsewhere. These are classified as "Dogs" and should be divested, unless they can be shown to be tied into the success of other services. For example, a new program of teenage counseling may not be meeting organizational goals, but may represent a method for identifying clients for a successful drug abuse service. "Stars" generate as much money as they spend and thus finance their own growth.

Although BCG analysis fails to consider long-term community needs, image value, services required for the public good that are unprofitable (e.g., indigent

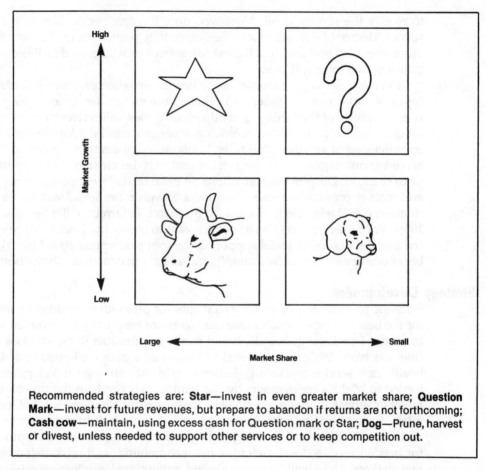

Recommended strategies are: **Star**—invest in even greater market share; **Question Mark**—invest for future revenues, but prepare to abandon if returns are not forthcoming; **Cash cow**—maintain, using excess cash for Question mark or Star; **Dog**—Prune, harvest or divest, unless needed to support other services or to keep competition out.

Figure 7-5. Service portfolio management. *(Source: Adapted from the concept developed by the Boston Consulting Group, Boston, MA.)*

care) or other subjective criteria, portfolio thinking does encourage administrators to evaluate the financial contribution of each service in relation to the organization's overall offering of services. An expanded portfolio analysis could be used more comprehensively to compare the services a health care organization offers. Key factors might include the BCG type; the consumer's likely assessment of the risk with each service; and the traditional 4 Ps of marketing—product (service), place of distribution, price, and promotion. A matrix to display this information could then be constructed.

Each factor could then be assessed as to how it affects the financial success and identification of the key decision maker in choosing this service. For instance, perceptions of risk to the client receiving the service have been shown to vary across medical procedures, with high risk motivating individuals to search for more information, compare prices, and spend more time deliberating decisions to receive the service at all. Moreover, once the receiver decides to accept the service, degree of risk influences the degree they participate in choosing the provider–specialist and facility. Highest risk service providers and facilities are typically selected by physicians.

Price is a deciding factor in many health care choices. Price includes three types of costs: money, time, and other nonmonetary issues such as personal comfort, image of the facility, and other intangibles, often referred to as the amenities of health care. Different pricing strategies can be adopted for different combinations of services ("no frills," unbundled pricing, or "posh" pricing) to serve various segments of the market that may be more or less responsive to price changes. Despite the restrictions on price flexibility imposed by regulation and market pressures, these decisions are even more important in the future (Inguanzo & Harju, 1985a; Swanson, Swanson, & Jarrett, 1985; Segal & Smith, 1986). Price may be classified as not relevant to choice (no issue); not relevant to the user because of financial support of the user's insurance (third party); possibly affecting user choice (sensitive?); and a factor in consumer choice (sensitive).

Strategy Development

Strategic plans must also include strategies for promoting services. In searching for the best strategies, health care managers are frequently encouraged to think in terms of packaging, brands, brand managers, product lines, and loss leaders (*Business Week*, 1985). It is a mistake to translate a packaged goods mentality to health care service marketing. Better insight into strategy development is afforded to health care planners by comparing their needs to the problems faced by other service marketers. Small banks share many characteristics of local hospitals. Encouraged by advertising agencies, many small banks purchased time and space in mass media serving wide geographic areas, rather than purchasing for needed service development, employee training, and advertising targeting key markets. The result has been wasted promotional monies that attracted few additional customers.

There are five important ways health care marketing differs from packaged goods marketing (Mindak, 1986). First, the decision process for purchasing health care services is quite different. Health care services are intangible, high risk for the wrong choice, high priced, uncommon life events, and involve technology that the user lacks the expertise to evaluate. These characteristics make sampling the service in advance of a major purchase difficult and evaluation of quality problematic. Consequently many users rely on expert referrals of physicians.

The second difference between health care services and packaged goods is that the latter is distinct from the provider or the store selling it. Manufacturers focus efforts primarily on product recognition, preference, and distribution and are frequently able to be less concerned with the transactions in acquiring it. Compared with a health care service where satisfaction is heavily determined by the transaction experience, people are less likely to judge a product by the store that sold it. Interpersonal relations in the service encounter are critical (Czepiel, Solomon, & Surprenant, 1985). Health providers must carefully evaluate individual transactions, as they can have such a strong generalizable effect. For example, a competent nurse can affect the consumer's perception of the entire organization. Interactions with other health care employees, such as receptionists, triage clerks, escorts, and cashiers, can affect satisfaction.

Third, loyalty in health care services is more complex than in packaged goods marketing. Brand loyalty to a packaged good product motivates the customer to shop wherever the merchandise can be obtained. Conversely, studies have shown patients may develop long-term relationships with a primary care physician, such as a pediatrician, which is continuous over many years and across different services. Such loyalties may result in turning to this provider even when services are needed that are not offered, resulting in a referral to another physician who then may admit the patient to one of several hospitals. "Provider loyalty" only indirectly results in use of a hospital for needed services and that hospital may not be one where the primary care physician practices.

Fourth, packaged goods are bought directly by the user, the decision maker, or the purchasing agent. In health care, the consumer is frequently not the decision maker, is always the recipient of the services, but is usually not the payor. Consequently, hospitals must be concerned with satisfying users, providers, and payors. The insurance company, employer, or government agency paying for the service may have criteria for satisfaction and continued support that differs from those of consumers or physicians.

Fifth and last, packaged goods are frequently distributed nationally, whereas hospitals engage primarily in local or regional competition, stressing special services and competencies. Therefore, careful market targeting and differentiated services are key to a health care organization's success. Effective promotional strategies are more likely based on face-to-face communications with decision makers and on direct mail, coupled with limited media advertising.

Positioning

The final set of strategies chosen results in what marketing experts refer to as *positioning* (Aaker & Shansby, 1982; Ackerman, 1986). An organization seeks to have a market position that is distinct and positive in the minds of its consumers. For instance, Orlando Regional Medical Center discovered that white collar residents thought it was a poor people's county hospital when it is actually the largest private, nonprofit hospital in all of Florida. This finding led to an advertising campaign directed at changing how it was seen by its community.

Administrators seeking to position their facilities need to ask themselves: (1) what do we stand for? (2) what are the objectives of our marketing plan? (3) how can we identify our strengths and weaknesses? (4) what type of client mix is desired? (5) what type of service should we focus on? and (6) what is our competition doing? On the basis of research and insight into questions such as these, a market position that maximizes the organization's strengths and minimizes its limitations is adopted. Underlying a strong position is the recognition that an institution cannot successfully be all things to all parts of the market (Pena, Jamison, & Rosen, 1986).

Adapting Porter's model for positioning opportunities (Porter, 1980, 1985; *Fortune*, 1987), Autrey and Thomas (1986) show how health care providers can build differential advantage using any mix of three basic strategies: (1) cost leadership—offering the lowest price; (2) differentiation—creating uniqueness by technology, equipment, staff, services or quality offered; and (3) focus—concentrating on a particular type of client.

THE MARKETING PLAN

The strategic plan defines goals for the organization and the strategies executives have chosen to achieve them. The next, and often most crucial step, is the implementation of this plan through actions by middle management, first line management, service providers, and support people.

Promotion Planning and Development

Marketing ideally is matching client needs and preferences to maintenance and development of organizational products and services. Promotion plays a key role in this process, by achieving the communications objectives, consistent with organizational goals. Promotion management is particularly challenging to health care administrators, due to consumer avoidance of the topic (Bertrand, 1979). These promotional methods include advertising, personal selling, and public relations (Malo, 1987).

Advertising

The push for name recognition in a market-driven environment is responsible for dramatic increases in hospital marketing costs, an estimated $1.1 billion in 1986, up from $700 million in 1985. In their current form, however, the effects of these expenditures appear to be mixed (Hitt & Cavusgil, 1985; Powills, 1986). A recent study of 200 health care ads reveals that the following seven themes and appeals were used: (1) the services offered, (2) technology available, (3) physician referral for prospective clients, (4) geographic appeal and local accessibility, (5) satellite locations that underscore accessibility and community involvement, (6) cost/quality, especially cost-reduction with a reason, such as ambulatory surgery, and (7) image, feel good, advertisements (*Hospitals*, 1987).

Advertising is an extremely powerful and effective method of achieving organizational goals. There are, however, also examples of successful marketing campaigns in which advertising played a minimal role. Mindak (1986) cities Humana's Women's Center's use of education and word-of-mouth to help nearly quadruple the number of babies delivered. He notes another example from Florida where 19 hospitals cooperated, in a "trade show" to develop a

"Shopping for Wellness" exposition at local shopping malls. With a total budget of $20,500 and one 30-second public service announcement, 25,000 people were attracted to the health show. The size of the promotional budget is not the only key to success. An advertising budget contains inherent waste, as by the nature of its broad-scope character, it reaches many irrelevant groups, as well as the consumers who represent the primary objective of the communication. However, the "shotgun" feature of advertising is beneficial when the character of the target audience is somewhat unclear or when the goal is to create image and positioning beliefs for the general community, using general interest media, such as newspapers, radio, television, and magazines. Furthermore, much advertising can be targeted to specific populations through careful choice of media, such as newsletters sent to specifically desirable groups and specialty magazines with clearly identified readers.

Personal Selling

Many administrators perform personal selling functions by visiting important customers, such as physicians, other referral agents, community leaders, insurance executives, and suppliers. These visits are important opportunities for administrators to explain current initiatives, outline future plans, and provide symposia on current issues facing the health care industry. Brochures that highlight available staff and services, as well as business cards and other promotional literature, are usually left with the potential customer for future reference. Such marketing visits are becoming an increasingly common expectation of health care administrators.

Public Relations

Confusion often exists as to the difference between personal selling, advertising, and public relations. Personal selling and advertising are techniques that have narrowly defined objectives, ultimately to stimulate the demand of a target group. Alternatively, public relations methods are those that are used to encourage broad community support. These techniques are designed to educate, inform, introduce, and create favorable images of the organization, either directly or indirectly, and include means such as institutional advertising, publicity, and personal appearances.

Public relations techniques developed to influence more directly community attitudes include speeches made by staff, open houses, and seminars to introduce the community to available services and programs.

APPLYING MARKETING TO RECRUITMENT AND RETENTION

Nurses represent a key element in the success of health care organizations. Far beyond providing essential health care, skilled decision making, and needed organizational capabilities, nurses play a pivotal role in client satisfaction and the achievement of organizational goals. Nursing as a profession has undergone considerable change in recent years resulting in wider roles or roles beyond direct patient care.

Currently there is a critical shortage of nurses in America, which is predicted to worsen. Curran, Minnick, and Moss (1987) report that in 1986 an average RN vacancy rate of 11 percent was found at sampled hospitals. The larger the hospital, the greater the percentage of vacant RN positions. Overall, the shortage of nurses is predicted to be 400,000 by the year 1990, and grow to 500,000 in the year 2000. The authors conclude that recruitment, increasing the supply, and retention are the three issues that a health care agency's marketing plan must address. Many agencies now have full-time recruiters responsible both for marketing the agency to potential employees and for making recommendations concerning retention strategies that are based on employee surveys, competitor practices, and research findings. Fundamental to the success of these efforts is an understanding of the sources of attraction of this profession (London, 1985).

BIOGRAPHICAL SKETCH

James W. Harvey is Assistant Professor of Marketing, George Mason University. He received his PhD from Penn State University and is active in the study of consumer behavior and strategic planning for service and nonprofit institutions, including philanthropy and health-care. He has published in *Journal of Consumer Research, Journal of Public Policy and Marketing, Long Range Planning, Business and Society, Advances in Consumer Research,* and in various conference proceedings. He has also been recognized for teaching excellence. As consultant to philanthropic organizations, he has been involved in over 50 research studies and is also faculty member, National Academy for Voluntarism.

SUGGESTED READINGS

Berkowitz, E.N., & Flexner, W.A. (1978). The marketing audit: A tool for health service organizations. *Health Care Management Review,* (Fall) 55–56.

Bloom, P.N. (1984). Effective marketing for professional services. *Harvard Business Review, 62*(5) 102–110.

Crawford, M. & Fisher, M.L. (1986). Marketing: The creative advantage. *Journal of Nursing Administration, 16*(12), 17–20.

Ferrell, O.C., Madden, C.S., & Legg, D. (1986). Strategic planning for nonprofit health care organization funding. *Journal of Health Care Marketing, 6*(1), 13–21.

George, W.R., & Compton, F. (1985). How to initiate a marketing perspective in a health care organization. *Journal of Health Care Marketing, 5*(1), 29–37.

Kotler, P., & Clarke, R.N. (1987). *Marketing for health care organizations,* Englewood Cliffs, N.J.: Prentice-Hall.

Lovelock, C.H., & Weinberg, C.B. (1984). *Marketing for public and nonprofit managers,* New York: Wiley.

Porter, M.E. (1985). *Competitive advantage.* New York: The Free Press.

Strasen, L. (1986). Promoting entrepreneurship in the acute care setting. *Journal of Nursing Administration, 16*(11), 9–12.

Van Doren, D., Smith, L., & Biglin, R. (1985). The challenges of professional services marketing. *Journal of Consumer Marketing, 2*(2), 19–27.

REFERENCES

Aaker, D.A., & Shansby J.G. (1982, May–June). Positioning your product. *Business Horizons,* pp. 56–62.

Abell, D.F., & Hammond, J.S. (1979). *Strategic market planning: Problems and analytical approaches.* Englewood Cliffs, NJ: Prentice-Hall.

Ackerman, L.D. (1986). Optimizing identity: A marketing imperative for health care management. *Journal of Health Care Marketing, 6*(2), 49–56.

Andreasen, A.R. (1982). Nonprofits: Check your attention to customers. *Harvard Business Review, 60*(3) 105–110.

Autrey, P. & Thomas, D. (1986). Competitive strategy in the hospital industry. *Health Care Management Review, 11*(1), 7–14.

Bertrand, J.T. (1979, July). Selective avoidance of health topics: A field test. *Communications Research,* pp. 271–294.

Bloom, P.N. (1984). Effective marketing for professional services. *Harvard Business Review, 62*(5), 102–110.

Business Week. (1985, Sept. 2). A high powered pitch to cure hospitals' ills. pp. 60–61.

Clarke, R.N., & Shyavitz, L. (1987). Health care marketing: Lots of talk, any action? *Health Care Management Review, 12*(1), 31–36.

Coe, P. (1979). Morbidity in the United States. In Jaco, E.G. (ed.): *Patients, physicians and illnesses.* New York: The Free Press, pp. 30–52.

Costello, M.M. (1985, Oct. 25). Patient satisfaction is often ignored by health marketers. *Marketing News,* p. 8.

Crompton, C.L., & Lamb, C.W. Jr. (1983). Distributing public services: A strategic approach. In Kotler, P., Ferrell, O.C., & Lamb, C. (eds.): *Cases and readings for marketing for nonprofit organizations.* Englewood Cliffs, NJ: Prentice-Hall, pp. 210–221.

Curran, C.R., Minnick, A., & Moss, J. (1987, April). Who needs nurses? *American Journal of Nursing,* pp. 444–447.

Czepiel, J.A., Solomon, M.R., & Surprenant, C.F. (1985). *The service encounter.* Lexington, MA: Lexington Books.

Edmondson, B. (1985a, April). The home health care market. *American Demographics*, pp. 29–51ff.

Edmondson, B. (1985b, June). The market for medical self-care. *American Demographics*, pp. 35–51ff.

Finn, D.W., & Lamb, Jr. C.W. (1986). Hospital benefit segmentation. *Journal of Health Care Marketing* 6(4), 26–33.

Fortune. (1987, November). The case of Michael Porter, superstar. 9, 44.

George, W.R., & Compton, F. (1985). How to initiate a marketing perspective in a health care organization. *Journal of Health Care Marketing*, 5(1), 29–37.

Haley, R.I. (1985). *Developing effective communications strategy.* New York: John Wiley and Sons.

Hitt, C., & Cavusgil, S.T. (1985, Sept.). Study shows consumers receptive to hospital ads. *Marketing News*, 19, pp. 21–22.

Hospitals. (1987). Study outlines six hottest ad strategies. pp. 39–40.

Hunter, S.S. (1987, May). Marketing and strategic management: Integrating skills of a better hospital. *Hospital and Health Services Administration*, pp. 205–216.

Inguanzo, J.M., & Harju, M. (1985). What makes consumers select a hospital? *Hospitals*, pp. 90–94.

Jensen, J. (1986, March). Healthcare alternatives. *American Demographics* pp. 36–38.

Kotler, P. (1985). The role and development of marketing in today's health care institution. *Health Care Strategic Management*, 3, 24.

Kotler, P., & Andreasen, A.R. (1987). *Strategic marketing for nonprofit organization.* Englewood Cliffs, NJ: Prentice-Hall.

Kotler, P., & Clarke, R.N. (1987). *Marketing for health care organizations.* Englewood Cliffs, NJ: Prentice-Hall.

Kroger, D.A., & Perry, F.L. (1983, May–June). Physician-centered marketing: A practical step to hospital survival. *Hospital and Health Services Administration*, p. 43.

Legg, D., & Lamb, C.W. Jr. (1986). The role of referral agents in the marketing of home health services. *Journal of Health Care Marketing*, 6(1), 51–56.

London, F. (1985, January). Why choose nursing? *American Journal of Nursing*, p. 114.

Lovelock, C. H., & Weinberg, C.B. (1984). *Marketing for public and nonprofit managers.* New York: John Wiley & Sons.

Malo, E. (1987). Decision points for hospital-based health promotion. *Hospital and Health Services Administration*, 32(1), 49–61.

Marketing News. (1985, June 7). Ethics for emerging field a key topic before 1,000 attending health services marketing symposium. pp. 20–21.

Marshall, D. (1980). Setting up a marketing department: Why? How? *Hospital Progress*, pp. 60–62.

McDevitt, P. (1987). Learning by doing: Strategic marketing management in hospitals. *Health Care Management Review*, 12(1), 23–30.

Miaoulis, G., Anderson, D.C., LaPlaca, P.J., Geduldig, J.P., Giesler, R.H., &

West, S. (1985). A model for hospital marketing decision processes and relationships. *Journal of Health Care Marketing, 5*(2), 37–45.

Mindak, W.A. (1986). Comparing packaged good and industrial product analogues for hospital marketing strategies. *Journal of Health Care Marketing, 6*(4), 44–49.

Nichols, P. (1986, Summer). Market oriented strategic planning, revisited. *Health Management Forum,* pp. 47–55.

O'Conner, C.P. (1982). Why marketing isn't working in the health care arena. *Journal of Health Care Marketing, 2*(1), 31–36.

Pena, J.J., Jamison, T.R., & Rosen, B. (1986). Marketing: A necessary art under DRGs. *Hospital & Health Services, 31*(4), 55–63.

Peters, M.P. (1986). Innovation for hospitals: An application of the product development process. *Journal of Health Care Marketing, 6*(3), 52–59.

Porter, M.E. (1980). *Competitive strategy.* New York, NY: The Free Press.

Porter, M.E. (1985). *Competitive advantage.* New York, NY: The Free Press.

Powills, S. (1986, January 5). Hospital advertising invisible to consumers. *Hospitals,* p. 66.

Robert Wood Johnson Foundation. (1987). *Access to health care in the United States: Results of a 1986 survey.* Special Report Number Two, Weisfeld, V.D. (ed.). Princeton, NJ: Robert Wood Johnson Foundation.

Salvatore, T. (1984). Competitor analysis in health care marketing. *Journal of Health Care Marketing, 4*(4), 11–15.

Segal, R., & Payn Smith, D. (1986). Pharmacists, beliefs and values about advertising patient oriented services. *Journal of Health Care Marketing, 6*(1), 35–41.

Steiber, S.R., & Boscarino, J.A. (1983, October). Qualitative forecasting tools help to pinpoint health care segments. *Marketing News,* p. 4.

Sturm, A. C., Jr. (1984, May). Selling the medical staff and hospital as a package. *Hospitals,* pp. 98–101.

Swan, J.E., Sawyer, J.C., Van Matre, J.G., & McGee, G.W. (1985). Deepening the understanding of hospital patient satisfaction: Fulfillment and equity effects. *Journal of Health Care Marketing, 5*(3), 7–18.

Swanson, K.J., Swanson, J.A., & Jarrett, S.L. (1985, March). Physicians and patients benefit when product, price, distribution, and promotion variables are manipulated. *Marketing News,* p. 10.

Time. (1987, Jan. 19). Rock power for health and wealth, p. 66.

Walter, C.M. (1981, August 15). Academic medical center features image analysis in marketing audit. *Hospitals,* pp. 91–100.

Witt, J.A., & McRoberts, N.L. (1983, April). Lack of expertise, funding shackles marketing moves. *Modern Healthcare,* 75–78.

Wood, V.R., & Singh, J. (1986). Strategic planning for health care markets: A framework and case study in analyzing diagnosis related groups. *Journal of Health Care Marketing, 6*(3), 19–28.

Wotruba, T.R., Haas, R.W., & Oulhen, H. (1985). Marketing factors affecting physician choice as related to consumers extent of use and predisposition toward use of physicians services. *Journal of Health Care Marketing, 5*(4), 7–17.

CASE 7-1

Marketing Principles Applied by Nurses in an Outpatient Psychiatric Service
Carol A. Patney

Perhaps the single most difficult challenge facing a service delivery group is to maintain the quality of care, meet community needs, and ensure that, economically, the practitioner or organization remains in the black. Additionally, in investor-owned organizations, stockholders seek a prospectus that indicates a considerable return on investment.

Marketing departments and strategic planning are vital to health care organizations wishing to remain viable and profitable in the twenty-first century. Health care administrators, as well as individual clinicians, must learn a new language and become conversant with terms such as market penetration, market segmentation, relative market share. Marketing is the responsibility of every employee within a health care organization, from the C.E.O. down to the laundry technician. Thus, nurses have a marketing responsibility not only to the organization in which they practice, but to the nursing profession as a whole. This is not a new role, but rather a new emphasis cloaked in a new language.

Nurses have promoted products when they have assured patients that Tylenol would ease their discomfort, Triaminic would relieve nasal congestion, and Metamucil would ensure regularity. They have professionally endorsed providers when they recommended Physician A instead of Physician B to friends or family. One nurses' association, aware of the power professional endorsement can carry, recently received compensation for endorsing one brand of disposable diaper on national television while also increasing public awareness of their nursing specialty. Pause for just a moment to ponder the diversified roles that nurses can assume in promoting health care delivery, products, and other. Possibilities are almost limitless.

The purpose of this case application is to present one example of how marketing principles were applied by nurses. Marketing and business terminology are used throughout in an effort to assist the reader in becoming more comfortable with these terms.

Certain conditions must exist in an organization before it is ready for a marketing program. The organization must define its mission and goals, develop an appropriate strategy to reach these goals, build an appropriate organizational structure that will carry out this strategy, and equip the organization with effective systems of information, planning, control, and reward to get the job done (Kotler, 1984). All successful health care organizations have these conditions.

In addition, the successful organization also contains the following four soft strengths: (1) *Style,* the employees share a common style of behaving and thinking (Kotler, 1984). Successful companies exhibit a distinct and widely shared culture that fits its strategy (Deal & Kennedy, 1988). (2) Appropriate mix of *skills,* which is needed to carry out the company's strategy. (3) *Staffing*, the company has hired able people and has put them in the right jobs to exercise their talents. (4) *Shared values*, the employers share the same guiding values and goals as the organization. Today, these soft strengths are becoming more identifiable in the health care field.

An investor-owned psychiatric hospital in a large urban, metropolitan tri-state area decided to improve its reputation in the community by providing some new *product* (service) that could be made available to all community members regardless of economic status, and would simultaneously be economically beneficial to the hospital. It was hoped that increased visibility and a demonstration of concern for community problems would increase the hospital's *market share.*

The Vice President for Nursing (VPN) and Director of Marketing (DOM), as part of the strategic planning management group, were charged to identify a product that would meet community needs, to create a marketing plan for this product, and then to present their plan for top management approval. The VPN convened key nurses and the DOM to brainstorm. This VPN was quite progressive; she had been introducing marketing concepts to her staff for some time. Many of the nurses already realized the importance of these concepts to the hospital and their profession.

The first meeting began with a statement of the task. Next the group reviewed the mission statement, goals, and objectives of the hospital. The group agreed on the following summary: This is a private, free-standing psychiatric hospital that provides quality psychiatric care to members of the community who meet admission criteria. The hospital's *business domain* consists of those individuals (1) who have a psychiatric illness not responsive to outpatient treatment and (2) who are free from medical disorders warranting care in a general hospital setting. All DSM-III R diagnostic categories can be treated at this facility. The organization's main goal is to provide quality psychiatric care, remain profitable, show continued growth, see market-share improvement, have the ability to diversify, and remain innovative in the health care industry.

The group identified the hospital's *distinctive competency* as the psychiatric care delivered across all psychiatric diagnoses. The DOM agreed and translated the nurses' product-oriented definition of what they did into a consumer-oriented definition, that is, they offered the best hope in the area to individuals with problems. The DOM also summed up the hospital's mission more succinctly: To improve service to customers and to increase return on investments.

One of the nurses noted that "individuals living in the suburbs are reluctant to come into the city for treatment, especially since they knew very little about the hospital." Another nurse added, "very few people really know anything about mental illness or mental health." A third observed that "people are afraid to go into a 'shrink's' office." After several minutes of discussion the VPN offered an idea. The group expanded this idea to include nurses offering emergency evaluations that were convenient and required no appointment.

The group continued to brainstorm. Nurse therapists could perform several functions: (1) they could provide community education programs with no fee, a community service sponsored by the hospital and (2) patients seen by nurses could be evaluated for short-term crises and, if needed, referral for crisis intervention by the nurse therapists, outpatient treatment by doctors affiliated with the hospital, or referred directly for inpatient treatment in a hospital.

The hospital would provide both education and psychiatric treatment in the suburbs and nurse therapists would be the link between the hsopital and the community. Nurses would be the staff for this service as they would be less threatening, holistically oriented, and less costly. This idea was presented to top management and was accepted. The green light was given for step two, the *marketing plan*. The *marketing management* process put into action consisted of analyzing market opportunities, researching and selecting target markets, developing marketing strategies, planning marketing tactics, and implementing and controlling the marketing effort (Kotler, 1984).

A *target market* was selected from an analysis of demographic data provided by the state health departments, county offices of Research and Statistics, and hospital admission demographics. County A was identified as having a high incidence of drug abuse, a well-insured population with few admissions into our private psychiatric hospital. *Full market coverage* would be given to County A: the full spectrum of services offered by the hospital would be promoted, as well as a new service cluster, crisis evaluation and referral and education.

A *marketing strategy* was formulated for the new service cluster. Marketing strategy consists of making decisions on the business' marketing expenditures and marketing allocations in relation to expected environmental and competitive conditions (Kotler, 1984). This is accomplished through the four P's of marketing—*product, price, place,* and *promotion*.

A master's prepared psychiatric nurse therapist would staff one suburban evaluation and education office. Secretarial support and phone coverage would be provided at the main hospital. *Pricing* included no charge for evaluation, a sliding scale for short-term follow-up, and no fees for the indigent. Revenues generated by the hospital admissions from this service were planned to offset the costs of the nurse's salary, office supplies, lowered outpatient revenues due to indigent care, and sliding scale fees. A private psychiatrist offered a site (*place*) at no cost in exchange for the appropriate referrals of patients to his practice. The site for the office was convenient to public transportation and centrally located. *Promotion* for this product (service) consisted of local newspaper advertisements and a press release, interviews by the nurse therapist on radio and television programs, and personal appearances with selected target groups in the community (Table 7-2). These target groups were local suburban private practices of psychiatrists and family physicians, and occupational health nurses and employee assistance counselors in local businesses. The nurse, in addition to raising awareness of the evaluation and educational services, would also mention treatment programs at the private psychiatric hospital.

The marketing plan was presented by the DOM to top management and implementation of the first suburban evaluation and education office was approved. Gatekeepers were identified and the promotion activities directed toward them. We decided that face-to-face contacts would be more productive than just phone calls or letters. A schedule was devised for the number of community contacts expected for the nurse therapist each month (Table 7–3). Over time the number of expected visits decreased. It was assumed that as outreach efforts were successful, time spent speaking and making calls would decrease. A quarterly reporting form was devised to report the progress and productivity of the office (Table 7–4) to the supervisor. The hospital agreed to fund this experiment for 1 year.

Initially the nurse staffing this service was not comfortable with a marketing role but over time and when results of marketing contacts began to pay off in referrals she became more comfortable. This pay-off did not occur immediately, it took 4 months before results could be seen. The nurse did not become discouraged, however, as she believed in her product and received support from her supervisor.

The first two quarterly reports were promising. Feedback from the community about the presence of the service was positive and encouraging. A consumer survey conducted by the hospital marketing department compared with a similar survey done before this "experiment" showed a significant increase in consumer recognition of the psychiatric hospital. The third quarter report indicated at least eight direct admissions through this service and eight indirect admissions. The final (or first annual) report of the first year showed a total of 12 direct admissions and 14 indirect admissions. Referrals for admission from Employee Assistance Programs (EAP), guidance counselors, and emergency rooms (target groups for the nurse therapist to market) were up by 65 percent. The revenues generated by these admissions far offset the expenditures for the project. As a result, the management group decided to open at least three more suburban offices. Many people, including other professionals, began to see nursing in a new light. Just as major corporations must understand and effectively use marketing, the nursing profession must seize this time to move to the forefront with innovations in the delivery of care. The future of the profession depends on decisions made today. Those who desire to lead in nursing must become experts, not only in clinical care, but also in all aspects of management and corporate operations.

BIOGRAPHICAL SKETCH

Carol Patney received her basic nursing education at the Mercy Hospital School of Nursing in Wilkes-Barre. She then earned her BSN from College Misericordia in Dallas, PA, and her master's degree as an advanced practitioner in Mental Health Nursing from the University of Pennsylvania. On completion of graduate work Ms. Patney joined the United States Army. While stationed at the Walter Reed Army Medical Center, she designed and functioned in the role of Psychiatric Liaison Nurse. For her performance of duty at Walter Reed she was awarded the Meritorious Service Medal (the peace

TABLE 7-2. FIRST-YEAR MARKETING PLAN

Type of Marketing Effort	1st Quarter	2nd, 3rd, and 4th Quarters	Results
Personal Contact Nurse Therapist	Marketing visits to physicians, businesses, and other target groups to be interspaced with patient appointment times.	Number of visits to each group will be formulated with supervisor and marketing.	1st Qtr. – 0 Admit. 2nd Qtr. – 3 Admit. 3rd Qtr. – 3 Admit. 4th Qtr. – 4 Admit. 1st Yr. Tot. = 10 Admit.
Education	Open luncheon conference for each target group. To be set up by Marketing Representative and Nurse Therapist. Three luncheons in 1st Qtr.	Educational workshops for identified group. 2–3 presentations per quarter to be set up by either Marketing Rep. or Nurse Therapist and staffed by both.	
Media Print: PIW Inkblot	News blurb with location and directions to new office and additional information as determined by Marketing. News item will be placed by marketing.	Each quarter up-date on offices with relevent articles provided by nursing staff. Marketing will review article and place in Inkblot.	
Yellow Pages	Marketing to place ad as early as possible to include small maps if not cost prohibitive.		

Introductory Letter and Brochures	Letter prepared by nurse to be mailed with brochure to all Mental Health Professionals and Groups, along with non-psychiatric M.D.'s in defined geographic area that office will service. To be sent during first month of operation by marketing.	Direct mailing each month of newsletter to group identified in first quarter. Mailing list will be expanded by appropriate referral names as supplied by PIW personnel. Nurse will provide newsletter, marketing will do mailing.
Radio: Talk Shows	Marketing will target station that specifically serves defined geographic area. Nurse for that office and Nurse Administrator will do shows.	One show per quarter by nurse. Marketing will set up time and station. Special attention should be directed toward holiday seasons and summer months.
	One paid ad at local station	Repeat one each quarter if first airing is successful.
Press Release:	Press release at least 8 x's by marketing. Paid ad 1 per week first month and then 2 per month in local publications.	Press release - 4 per quarter
	Bus and Metro Ads, marketing will assume resp. for this.	
Research	Information Base: Develop list of M.D.'s offices and Health Care Agencies for each catchment area.	Update regularly.

Used with permission of The Psychiatric Institute of Washington D.C.

TABLE 7-3. TARGET POPULATION AND CONTACT FREQUENCY

First Quarter

Week		1	2	3	4	5	6	7	8	9	10	11	12
Phone Calls to Community		40	30	25	20	20	15	15	15	15	10	10	10
Physician Contact		3	3	3	3	3	3	3	3	2	2	2	2
Community Contact	Personal Contact	2	3	3	2	2	2	2	2	2	2	2	2
EAP's		3	3	2	2	2	2	1	1	1	1	1	1

Second Quarter

Week		13	14	15	16	17	18	19	20	21	22	23	24
Phone Calls to Community		10	10	10	10	10	10	10	10	10	10	10	10
Physcian Contact		2	2	2	2	2	2	2	2	2	2	2	2
Community Contact	Personal Contact	2	2	2	2	2	2	1	1	1	1	1	1
EAP's		1	1	1	1	1	1	1	1	1	1	1	1

Third Quarter

Week		25	26	27	28	29	30	31	32	33	34	35	36
Phone Calls to Community		8	8	8	8	8	8	8	8	8	8	8	8
Physician Contact		2	2	2	2	2	2	2	2	2	2	2	2
Community Contact	Personal Contact	1	1	1	1	1	1	1	1	1	1	1	1
EAP's		1	1	1	1	1	1	1	1	1	1	1	1

Fourth Quarter

Week		37	38	39	40	41	42	43	44	45	46	47	48
Phone Calls to Community		8	8	8	8	8	8	8	8	8	8	8	8
Physician Contact		2	2	2	2	2	2	2	2	2	2	2	2
Community Contact	Personal Contact	1	1	1	1	1	1	1	1	1	1	1	1
EAP's		1	1	1	1	1	1	1	1	1	1	1	1

Used with permission of The Psychiatric Institute of Washington D.C.

TABLE 7-4. QUARTERLY REPORT

To: Nursing Administrator of Outpatient Services
Form: Nurse Therapist's Name
Subject: Quarterly Progress Report For: _____ Crisis Center Covering _____
          to _____.

QUARTERLY REPORT OUTLINE

This report documents the progress of the _____ Crisis Center during the _____ quarter of operation from _____ to _____. Included you will find information related to four primary areas: 1) marketing; 2) clinical service; 3) finances; and, 4) conclusions and directions for the future.

MARKETING

Summary paragraph (Report on follow-up of needs identified in previous report)
Referral Development Record

Date of Contact	Name of Organization	Contact Person	Outcome

Source of referral information for clients admitted to Crisis Center between _____ and _____.

Name of Referral Source	# Referred

Summary comments related to statistical significance of marketing information (i.e., number of referrals (percentage of referrals) from various referral sources; percentage of referrals resulting from nurse therapist's marketing, E.A.P. referrals, Hopeline, etc.)

CLINICAL SERVICES

Summary to clinical statistics for _____ quarter and year to date

	MONTH	MONTH	MONTH
Number patients admitted			
Number patients discharged			
Number patients followed end of month			
Phone consults:			
A.M.			
P.M.			

Summary to clinical statistics for _____ quarter and year to date

	MONTH	MONTH	MONTH
Hospitalizations:			
P.I.			
Other			
Outpatient Disposition:			
(Name of group assoc. with C.C. office)			
M.P.G.			
Community			
D.A.A.			
D.I.			
D.S.C.			

Summary paragraph explaining any special circumstances related to clinical statistics (i.e., R.P.I. - refused, no medical back-up times 1 week so centers closed to new admits etc.)

_____

_____

_____

Summary paragraph addressing percentage of admissions to C.C. admitted to P.I., referred to community, seen in C.C.I.S. etc.

_____

_____

_____

Demographic data on clients admitted to Crisis Center during the quarter.

Sex:
    Female   _____
    Male   _____

Race
    White   _____
    Black   _____
    Oriental _____
    Hispanic _____
    Other   _____

Age:
    13–18   _____
    19–25   _____
    26–35   _____
    36–45   _____
    46–55   _____

Age:
    55–65   _____
    65–75   _____

Marital Status:
    Single   _____
    Married   _____
    Separated   _____
    Divorced   _____
    Widowed   _____

Chief Complaint:
    Chemical Dependency—Self   _____
    Chemical Dependency—Family Member   _____
    Depression/Chemical Dependency/Stress   _____
    Depression/Co-Alcoholic   _____
    Family Violence   _____
    Grief   _____
    Multiple Stresses/Personal Crisis   _____
    Developmental Crisis   _____
    Marital Dysfunction   _____
    Family Dysfunction   _____
    Adolescent Behavior Problems   _____
    Affective Disorder   _____
    Anxiety   _____
    Sex Offence   _____
    Other   _____

Summary paragraph(s) addressing any pertinent clinical issues:
_____
_____
_____

FINANCES

Insurance coverage of clients seen in the Crisis Center during quarter.
No coverage _____
Has insurance but doesn't know name of company _____
Alphabetical listing of insurance companies _____ number patients involved by Co.

    1. _____ _____
    2. _____ _____
    3. _____ _____

Summary paragraph(s) commenting on percentage of patients admitted to Crisis Center with insurance, percentage of insured patients with inpatient/outpatient mental health coverage, employers providing insurance benefits with poor mental health coverage.
_____
_____
_____

Income generated by the _____ Crisis Center during _____ quarter.

Hospitalizations at P.I.	$ _____
Crisis Center visits—evaluations only	$ _____ plus
Crisis Center visits—brief treatment	$ _____
	_____
Total revenue generated by _____	$ _____
Crisis Center _____	

Summary paragraph(s) reporting number of hospital patient days or particular unit at per diem rate; also comments on numbers of hospitalizations and cost of hospitalizations resulting from nurse therapists' marketing efforts, E.A.P.'s, Hopeline, etc.

_____
_____
_____

CONCLUSIONS AND DIRECTIONS FOR THE FUTURE

Summary paragraph(s) highlighting pertinent issues presented in report. Comment on progress of Crisis Center from your perspective. Identify any clinical, marketing, administrative concerns that need to be/will be addressed in our next quarter. (list)

_____
_____
_____

cc: President/Medical Director
      Administrator
      Director of Patient Services

Used with the permission of The Psychiatric Institute of Washington D.C.

time equivalent of the Bronze Star). On leaving the military Ms. Patney began working for the Psychiatric Institute of America. Initially, she was employed at their Norfolk, VA, facility and is currently employed at the Psychiatric Institute of Washington. Ms. Patney has functioned in positions of increasing administrative responsibilities of the institute. Under her supervision, the Crisis Service of the Psychiatric Institute grew from an inner city service to a multi-site operation servicing the entire D.C. metropolitan area. For her work at the Institute, Ms. Patney was awarded the Distinguished Service Award by the D.C. Hospital Association. Since working at the Psychiatric Institute of Washington, Ms. Patney has completed the certification program in nursing administration at George Mason University. Ms. Patney is also certified by ANA as a certified specialist in psychiatric/mental health nursing. She is currently a doctoral student at the University of Virginia. She is listed in the Who's Who of American Nursing and belongs to numerous nursing organizations.

REFERENCES

Kotler, P. (1984). *Marketing management*. Englewood Cliffs, NJ: Prentice-Hall.

Deal, T., & Kennedy, A. (1988). Corporate Cultures: *The Rites and Rituals of Corporate Life*. Reading, MA: Addison-Wesley.

CASE 7-2

Initiating Marketing in a County Health Department
Joanne M. Jorgenson

Here we were—six of us—attending a 2-day workshop on marketing. We are members of the management team of an official health agency whose services were primarily focused on preventive care to a cross section of a large suburban community. We wondered why we were devoting precious time to learn about a corporate business activity. We did not need to increase our service demand and we had little choice in the products we offered. Two days later, we returned to our agency, excited, enthusiastic, and committed to share what we had learned with anyone who would listen! Publics–features–target–benefits–product promotion–marketing. Words applicable to public health! Internal marketing versus external marketing? Could marketing be used to work smarter rather than harder? We agreed staff could not work much harder; service demand already exceeded service supply; resources were limited. We envisioned no new resources. How could we "market" what we had learned to our supervisors, to our co-workers?

Aware that marketing endeavors must have support from the top, we agreed that our first task was to gain total administrative support. Using our newly learned marketing principles, we decided the key to a successful presentation rested on the "benefits package." To convince the Agency and Divisional Directors that investing in marketing would bring valuable benefits, we incorporated the values, beliefs, and preferences of administration into a marketing proposal. Our first endeavor was a success! A marketing steering committee was authorized to begin the process of incorporating marketing principles into our service activities.

The second task was more difficult—to "market" marketing to our co-workers. We realized that this was a formidable task. For services, we needed to follow all the steps of marketing, no shortcuts could be taken, the timetable could not be rushed.

Our first endeavor would be to present marketing concepts to the staff. It was not feasible or practical to present a 2-day workshop to all staff. So, how could it be abbreviated but not lose any essential content? How could we present the information in a way that it would make sense to the nursing service staff?

"Packaging the product in the target's terms," one of the nine steps in marketing, was the key. We would use what was already familiar—the nursing process—identify, assess, plan, intervene—as the cornerstone process.

Phase I. Introduction of Marketing:
"To Market, To Market"

The "Marketing Team," as the steering committee became known, took their workshop on the road—to staff in each of the five field offices. A 1 1/2-hour workshop on the steps in marketing using the nursing process framework was presented (Table 7-5). We emphasized marketing strategies used in the business world making the marketing terms real and recognizable.

The objective of phase I was to increase the awareness of staff regarding the marketing steps and their results. Success would be evaluated by the degree staff could mentally apply what they had learned to their own activities over the following 2 months. The time frame for phase I—from our original workshop to the completion of the final field office presentation was 3 months.

Phase II. Application of Marketing Principles in the Work Setting:
"100% of 10%"

Two months after completion of Phase I, the "Team" met again with staff in each field setting. The meetings were informal. We gathered information and responses from staff regarding their ideas and reactions to using marketing concepts in the work setting. Suggestions were solicited from the staff regarding marketing techniques that could help them feel better about their work. Many ideas were implemented during the course of this phase; such as, procurement of personalized calling cards for each staff person, agency sponsorship to attend courses on development of audiovisual aids, and initiation of a staff newsletter. A spark had been ignited within our staff—the interest, enthusiasm, and excitement of the workshop possibilities caught on!

Keeping in mind a marketing concept that it is better to reach "100% of 10% rather than 10% of 100%," we requested that interested staff volunteer to serve on agency-wide, program-based marketing committees. Our agency already had a matrix structure with staff assigned by service area in each geographically defined office. Each service area was, in marketing terms, a product line: adult health, maternal/child health and school health. The charge of each marketing committee was to identify a service problem and develop a market plan, using the nine steps of marketing learned in the workshops.

Throughout Phase II, which lasted approximately 1 year, staff in each office were involved in creating, implementing, and evaluating a marketing plan. In doing assessments of target populations, they learned where to find demographic survey data, and to supplement it with interviews and surveys they designed. The nurses gathered general information about their target population and validated with clients the definition of the service problem and solicited their solutions. This often lead to fresh perspectives on old problems. For exam-

TABLE 7-5. MARKETING FRAMEWORK

Nursing Process	Marketing Process	Marketing Plan

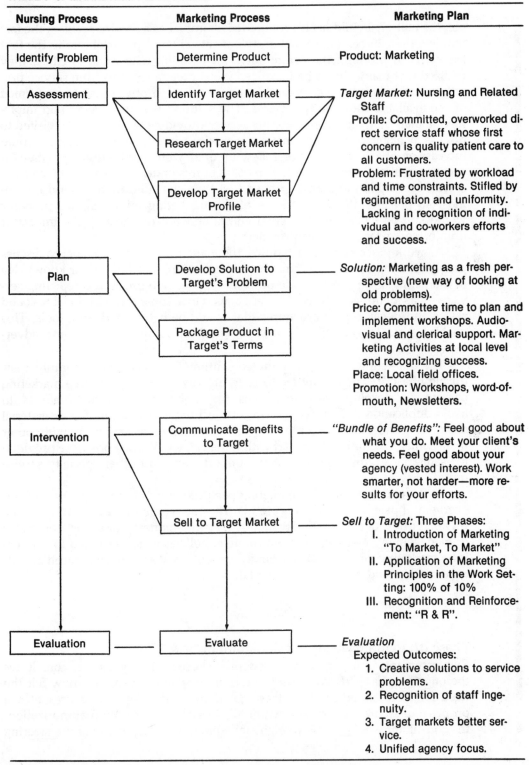

Identify Problem ——— Determine Product ——— Product: Marketing

Assessment — Identify Target Market ——— *Target Market:* Nursing and Related Staff
Profile: Committed, overworked direct service staff whose first concern is quality patient care to all customers.
Problem: Frustrated by workload and time constraints. Stifled by regimentation and uniformity. Lacking in recognition of individual and co-workers efforts and success.

Research Target Market

Develop Target Market Profile

Plan — Develop Solution to Target's Problem ——— *Solution:* Marketing as a fresh perspective (new way of looking at old problems).
Price: Committee time to plan and implement workshops. Audiovisual and clerical support. Marketing Activities at local level and recognizing success.
Place: Local field offices.
Promotion: Workshops, word-of-mouth, Newsletters.

Package Product in Target's Terms

Intervention — Communicate Benefits to Target ——— *"Bundle of Benefits":* Feel good about what you do. Meet your client's needs. Feel good about your agency (vested interest). Work smarter, not harder—more results for your efforts.

Sell to Target Market ——— *Sell to Target:* Three Phases:
I. Introduction of Marketing "To Market, To Market"
II. Application of Marketing Principles in the Work Setting: 100% of 10%
III. Recognition and Reinforcement: "R & R".

Evaluation ——— Evaluate ——— *Evaluation*
Expected Outcomes:
1. Creative solutions to service problems.
2. Recognition of staff ingenuity.
3. Target markets better service.
4. Unified agency focus.

ple, the maternal/child health committee identified as a service problem the fact that less than 25 percent of maternity patients entered prenatal care in the first trimester. In profiling the community and defining who came to clinic, they realized that many clients had received initial pregnancy tests from service providers external to the agency, and had not been promptly referred or informed of the available community services. The solution was to develop and implement a plan by which these external service providers would each be visited to discuss available community maternity services; in addition, the agency would increase emphasis internally on follow-up of all women who tested positive for pregnancy in our own services. The result of this endeavor increased maternity service registration and an improved first trimester utilization of service to almost 40 percent. Without the use of the marketing approach, we probably would still be focusing on internal efforts and not recognizing the impact of uninformed external service providers.

As work proceeded in each office, the marketing committees met to discuss problems, keep up momentum, share information, and build their knowledge of marketing. One agency-wide problem—inadequate brochures depicting services—was identified. The committees agreed to assume this additional task and revise and develop new brochures that would be better marketing tools. This enabled them to get "first-hand experience" at using promotion and advertising.

The marketing steering committee continued to meet on a monthly basis during phase II. The committee focused on ways to assist the three marketing committees develop additional tools for their use, coordinate efforts to avoid duplication and determine ways to secure necessary funding or material resources. The steering committee also functioned as a liaison with other management/administration staff within the agency. Workshops were provided for sanitarians, administrative staff, support staff, and other specialty service units.

At the end of 1 year the marketing perspective was becoming a part of our everyday business. Marketing terms became commonplace—"What's the B.O.B. (bundle of benefits)?" frequently followed requests for action from peers or management. New services, procedures, policies were presented to staff using a marketing format, that is, product, benefits, features that enhanced acceptance, understanding, and implementation.

Phase III. Reinforcement and Recognition: "R & R"

Reinforcement, building on knowledge and recognition of efforts, constitutes the ongoing phase III. We introduced basic marketing ideas; we now felt the need for more expertise. The steering committee developed and presented a proposal to secure a consultant within the existing budget. With authorization, the consultant was hired who originally tapped the imagination of the steering committee 18 months previously in the 2-day workshop. He helped analyze our product: service; he helped us to emphasize that when the product is service, providers of the service are an integral part of the product. The consultant also helped us to look objectively at our progress, recognize our limitations, and develop a long-range plan. With his assistance we chose "agency image" as our focus. The first stage was another round of workshops in each field office given by the consultant on our new marketing plan.

The total agency is now involved in marketing endeavors. A community education committee, comprised of representatives of all divisions of the agency, has been established. The image of the agency is the focus of this group, and how to project it positively to our various "publics." Development of an agency logo and slogan is in progress.

The initial marketing plan implemented by the six excited, enthusiastic nursing management staff was a success! Integration and internalization of marketing concepts was accomplished, on a much wider basis than originally envisioned. Marketing has become an integral component of our agency:

- A marketing module is included in the orientation of all new employees.
- Community assessments are now routinely done before initiating changes in service delivery.
- Clients are now surveyed regarding satisfaction with our services and ideas for improvement.
- Agency brochures are continually critiqued as marketing tools.
- "Bundle of benefits" are identified for various services by staff initiative.
- Marketing activities are included in the pay for performance standards.
- An agency newsletter with reporters in each field office keeps marketing efforts visible and provides recognition for creativity.

"Word of mouth," one of the best promotion techniques, became real as the requests came in from other parts of the state: would we be willing to share with other jurisdictions what we were doing with our staff? The "Team" went on the road! Workshops were presented in six areas of the state. The enthusiasm was contagious; health department staff learned that marketing not only benefits the client and the agency, but it also adds an element of fun to work as it allows creativity and ingenuity to flow freely.

The marketing process received official recognition by the local government in the form of the highest award given to a public employee—the Health On-thank Award—when the Steering Committee Chairman was nominated and selected as a recipient. The award was accepted on behalf of the staff involved.

We began with six managerial staff having an interest in incorporating marketing techniques into a large suburban health department. After attending a workshop where we learned basic marketing ideas, we had to "sell" the need for marketing to our superiors, peers, and staff. We developed a market plan to be implemented in three phases over a minimum of a 3-year period (Table 7–6):

TABLE 7-6. MARKETING BEGINS WITH ME: PHASES AND TASKS

	Tasks	Responsible Party	Time Frame
Phase I: Introduction of Marketing Principles: *"To Market, To Market"*	1. Proposal to Health Officer 2. Design and schedule workshops for field staff 3. Conduct workshops and allow 2 months for integration of ideas	Steering Committee	3 months
Phase II: Application of Marketing Principles in the Work Setting: "100% of 10%"	1. Meet with field office to gather information and level of integration achieved 2. Implement suggestions from staff 3. Appoint marketing committees for each program area 4. Marketing committees develop and implement a market plan to solve mutually indentified service problem; involves program peers in process 5. Conduct workshops for other divisions within agency	Steering Committee Steering Committee Interested Staff Steering Committee	12 months
Phase III: Reinforcement and Recognition: "R & R"	1. Secure consultant to add depth, evaluation and agency-wide coordination/focus 2. Establish community education committee 3. Recognition—activities, staff, successes, and failures	Steering Committee Division Directors All via newsletters, awards, articles, etc.	Ongoing

- **Phase I:** Introduction of staff to marketing principles
- **Phase II:** Application of Marketing principles to work activities
- **Phase III:** Reinforcement and expansion of marketing principles to total agency

We envision that the consultant obtained in phase III will provide periodic guidance and assistance indefinitely as the administrative staff identify areas of need.

BIOGRAPHICAL SKETCH

Joanne M. Jorgenson is currently Director of Nursing with the Fairfax County Health Department in Fairfax, Virginia. A graduate of South Dakota State University and the University of Minnesota School of Public Health, she has held a variety of positions in public health nursing during her career. She is an active member of the professional association (Virginia Nurses' Association and American Nurses' Association) holding offices on the local and state level. In addition to membership in the Virginia Public Health Association and Sigma Theta Tau, she is Chairman of the Public Health Nurse Leaders of Virginia.

PART III

Structuring Health Care Organizations

8

Organizations As Open Systems

Jacqueline A. Dienemann

Nurse administrators work within complex bureaucratic organizations. They require considerable organizational savvy to perform their work. Viewing organizations as open systems can provide administrators with a valuable perspective, a way to step back for a moment and look at the whole organization beyond their department, position, or present dilemma.

Organizational development (OD) is a field of organization theory that uses open systems models for organizational assessment, diagnosis, and planned change. The OD models vary widely in their sophistication and theoretical bases. Some merely identify types of organizational structures, others identify critical elements and processes within various structural types, and still others identify relationships among elements using diagrams of interactive processes (Burke, 1987). This chapter describes four open systems models—the systems model, congruence model, professional bureaucracy model, and contingency model. It also describes the influence that life cycle stage has on organizational structure and management strategies.

OPEN SYSTEMS MODELS

Open systems models derive from the concepts of general systems theory; therefore, they share a holistic view of internal processes and the same basic analytical elements. Many times elements are differently named due to independent development of general systems models in different disciplines. Moreover, each model offers a slightly different perspective and emphasis on different elements or processes. Nurse administrators need to be aware of the emphasis when choosing a model for analysis of a problem.

The major concepts of general systems theory applied to organizations are summarized in Figure 8-1. The basic elements include: *inputs* from the environment that cross the organization boundaries; a *transformation process* that changes

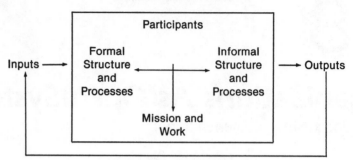

Figure 8-1. Major concepts in general systems theory.

- *Open systems.* Permeable boundaries exist between the system and its environment.
- *Holism/ synergism/ organicism/ Gestalt.* The *whole* is greater than the sum of its parts and is the focus of study.
- The four major analytical components of the transformation process are: *participants, formal sociotechnical structure and processes, mission and technology or work, and informal structure and processes.*
- Components/ subunits/ subsystems are interconnected and *interdependent.*
- *Input—Transformation/throughout—output* process is goal oriented.
- *Feedback,* inputs, and feedforward provide information for self-regulation/dynamic equilibrium/cybernetic system.
- Systems are *resource dependent* on their environment.
- *Change/ adaptation/ homeostasis/ steady state* processes are dynamic and ongoing.
- *Equifinality* of varying strategies to reach the same goals.
- Over time, systems *division of labor/internal elaboration* is reorganized and increasingly complex.

the inputs and transfers them to the environment as *outputs;* and *feedback,* which is information on outputs and the organization received through multiple channels. Desired inputs, transformation processes, and outputs are defined by the organization's mission and stated as goals. General systems theory has been described as cybernetic due to how interpretation of feedback leads to internal adjustments in the transformation process to adapt outputs. General systems theory emphasizes the importance of the *structure of work and people,* and the formal and informal *interaction processes among work and people* as the critical analytical elements for understanding what happens within organizations. Early general systems theory had a "closed" perspective emphasizing how internal processes resisted change and promoted internal stability. Recent general systems theory has an "open" perspective emphasizing the dependence of the organization on its environment and the importance of rapid adaptation for survival (Scott, 1987). The organizational models described in this chapter are open systems models.

Other concepts of general systems theory that apply to all open systems models are listed at the bottom of Figure 8-1. They include a holistic view, interdependence of internal elements or components, constancy of change, multiple ways to accomplish the same output or equifinality, and periodic restructuring and increasing complexity as organizations grow.

Open systems models promote better understanding of organizations. It is impossible to depict all the interactions among people within and across the boundaries of an organization. The multitude of factors impacting organizations are impossible to map and interpret. Open systems models simplify reality allowing a person to analyze critically what would otherwise be too complex to comprehend. Morgan (1987) describes models as "metaphors of reality" that assist us to understand our world by extending to new situations what we already know. Thus, models provide one means for administrators to focus on the mission of the whole, to recognize the interconnectedness of internal components, to value feedback and equifinality, to devise strategies to shape proactively the environment, to seek multiple channels of information, and to plan systematic change.

Open systems models used in OD were developed within the human relations school of management theory, which began in the late 1920s with the Western Electric studies. These studies were the first to identify the presence of work group norms and the importance of worker motivation in determining productivity levels. Management research within this perspective focuses on motivation, values, traits, and other psychological and social characteristics of workers and managers. Consultants using this perspective promote humanistic, participative management. The OD approach became well established in the late 1960s and early 1970s as academic behavioral scientists began to work more and more with management of large firms to develop interventions to implement research findings to increase job satisfaction and productivity among workers. This applied field of organizational assessment, diagnosis, intervention, and evaluation uses open systems models as their theoretical basis. Interventions continue to focus primarily in job design, team building, participative management, communication and sensitivity training for management, and design of reward and compensation systems. The joint involvement of scientists and managers in the entire process is emphasized.

SYSTEMS MODEL

The systems model of Noel Tichy and Richard Beckhard (1982) is shown in Figure 8-2. It was developed to assist health care administrators to (1) establish core missions to guide strategic decisions, (2) understand and map environmental pressures, (3) develop more sophisticated planning processes, (4) set operational objectives at each level of the organization, (5) design functional structures, (6) manage consensual decision making, (7) manage multiple tasks, (8) cope with

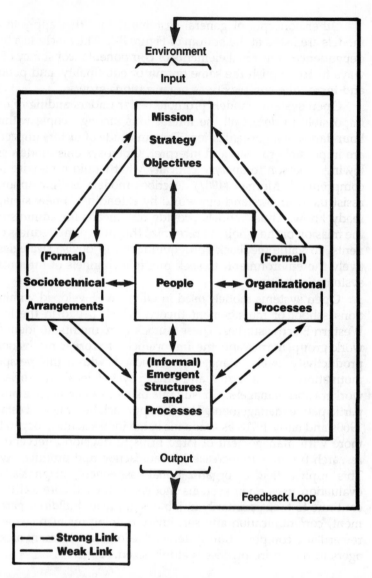

Figure 8-2. Systems model. *(Source: Used with permission from Tichy, N., and Beckhard, R., Organization development for health care organizations in* Health Care Organizations, *Marguilies, N., and Adams, J.D. (Eds.). Reading, MA: Addison-Wesley Publishing Company, 1982.)*

internal conflict, (9) motivate and manage professionals and, (10) manage change (pp. 27–128).

This open systems model uses the general systems theory concepts of inputs, transformation within organizational boundaries, outputs, and feedback. As illustrated in Figure 8-2:

The *environment* provides *inputs* of tangible resources such as potential organizational participants, financial credit, affiliations and networks, physical plant, machinery and other capital assets, and consumable supplies. There are also intangible resource inputs such as regulations by governmental and accrediting bodies, credit, image and reputation, the market and competition for services, public accountability, locale, job satisfaction of employees, and quality of client relations.

- *Transformation* occurs through interaction of mission, people, sociotechnical arrangements, organizational processes, and informal structures and processes.
- *Mission, strategy,* and *objectives* define the purpose of the organization and the administration's plans to effectively achieve its objectives.
- *People* refers to the characteristics of employees, attending physicians, volunteers, and patients that participate in the work of the organization. What are their skills, abilities, and motivations? How does their personal life, cultural heritage, and goals affect their work? What leadership characteristics and learning and coping styles do they exhibit?
- *Sociotechnical arrangements* refers to work design. The technology or work to be done including the machines, equipment, skills of workers, and number of different people needed to provide health care services to each patient. The social structure created to carry out the work—share of the hierarchy, degree of interdependence and temporal sequence of work, and degree work arrangements are formal, centralized, specialized, departmentalized, and standardized.
- *Organizational processes* manage and control work flow. They include the budget processes, information systems, quality assurance, risk management, accreditation and licensing process, formal conflict management systems, reward systems, communication systems, and designated planning and decision making processes.
- *Informal, emergent structures and processes* are supplements to sociotechnical arrangements and organizational processes. They include: organizational history, small group dynamics, corporate culture, networks and political coalitions, and other social patterns among organizational participants.
- *Outputs* are the result of the transformation process. They include research results, patient health status on discharge, medical procedures completed, educational certification of students, quality care indicators, financial status reports, satisfaction of patients, physicians, and employees, employee turnover and absenteeism, and environmental information. Outputs are fed back as an input through the *feedback loop.*

The most complex factor in the systems model is the environment. As health care agencies integrate and restructure complexity is added. It is becoming increasingly common for health care agencies to be a part of larger corporations that act as environmental controls. A corporate hospital may be autonomous in many ways, such as developing its own contracts with suppliers, professionals, and others, and maintaining a separate board of directors, but it still must act as a part of the larger corporation. The parent corporation supplies and delimits member hospital's financial resources, policies and new ventures as it coordinates the image, mission, and financial health of the whole.

The extent to which the external environment is relatively stable, dynamic, or even turbulent significantly influences the functioning of the four internal analytical elements. The dependence of health care agencies on an uncertain environment is of increasing concern to administrators as recent changes in funding and payment mechanisms and the nursing shortage have dramatically demonstrated.

The systems model directs nurse administrators to include a variety of work and working factors when assessing organizational problems. The model also assists them to recall how interconnected the key elements are with one another and the environment and that action directed at one element always impacts on all others.

CONGRUENCE MODEL

David Nadler and Michael Tushman (1982) refer to their organizational model as a congruence model because it directs the user to assess the fit between an organization and its environment at the levels of system functioning, work group behavior, and individual behavior (Fig. 8–3). They also suggest using more specific models or submodels to examine the fit between pairs of transformation components. For instance, designing jobs that tightly fit work tasks with motivational needs of workers using the core job dimensions analysis of Hackman and Oldham (1975).

The four-key inputs to the congruence model are (1) *environment;* (2) *resources,* which the organization has access to; (3) organizational *history;* and (4) *strategy* or stream of decisions to meet the demands, constraints, and opportunities presented by the environment.

Environment and *resource* inputs are the same as in the systems model described previously. The environment is further described in the discussion of the contingency model. *History* is an input not highlighted in the other open systems models. It includes the factors of age, size, complexity, patterns of leadership, patterns of key past decisions, and sacred cows. Each factor is a unique characteristic of an organization. For example, sacred cows are those aspects of the organization that are taboo subjects for discussion to outsiders or consideration for change such as the placement of a certain person in the hierarchy or how parking spaces are designated. A newcomer often encounters sacred cows as illogical informal rules or incongruent actions of others that "old timers" may know the history of but most co-workers merely accept as an idiosyncrasy of that organization.

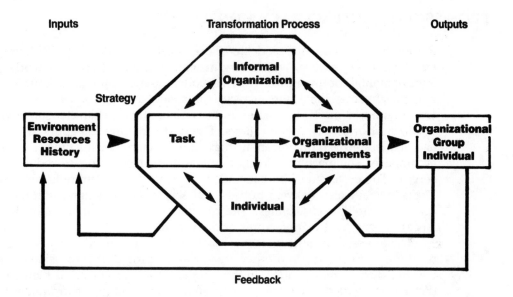

Figure 8-3. Congruence model. *(Source: Hackman, J.R., Lawler, E.E., & Porter, L.W. (eds.)* Perspectives on Behavior in Organizations. © *New York: McGraw-Hill, p. 121.)*

Strategy includes identification of the core mission, marketing plans, objectives for performance, and supporting systems for performance. Organizations vary widely in the degree that strategy is a formal process, but a historical pattern for each may be identified through retrospective analysis.

These four inputs shape the interactions of the four major components within the organizational boundaries: *tasks, individuals, formal organizational arrangements,* and *informal organization.* The outcomes of the transformation process are *outputs* and *feedback.* These elements are standard for all general systems models.

The congruence model differs from the systems model by (1) moving the mission, strategy, and objectives under the subheading of strategy as a force driving the transformation process, (2) separating the environmental components into environment, resources, and history, (3) highlighting the importance of the technology or work of the organization by having it as a separate transformation component. Conversely, Tichy and Beckhard (1982) highlight organizational processes within the transformation process by identifying them as a separate component. Finally, (4) this model depicts a more complex feedback process.

Keep in mind, that the authors of both models warn the reader that information being fed back as an input does not infer that reception will result in adaptive action. Due to distortion, time lapse, filtering, and mistargeting much feedback is received but never used in decision making.

PROFESSIONAL BUREAUCRACY MODEL

Rather than applying one model to all organizations, Mintzberg (1979) proposes five alternative models, which vary in work technology, type of worker, and environmental contingencies. The five models are: entrepreneurial, machine bureaucracy, professional bureaucracy, adhocracy, and divisionalized form. The entrepreneurial model is simple, undifferentiated, and characteristic of young, small, craft or service organizations. The next three models apply to medium-age, moderate-sized organizations that differ primarily by the type of work they accomplish. The machine bureaucracy manufactures a standardized product or service. The professional bureaucracy delivers a complex unpredictable service. The adhocracy also delivers professional services that require interdependent action by multiple disciplines. The divisionalized form organization is older, largest in size, and manufactures or delivers diverse products or services.

The professional bureaucracy is most commonly applied to health care organizations, universities, and other organizations providing professional services within a bureaucratic context. In these organizations, the work is highly unpredictable and varied, the workers are professionals, and the environment is relatively stable. Since 1979 the environment of health care and many other professional service organizations has become much less stable but the characteristics of the work and the workers that Mintzberg described have remained constant. Many health care organizations are now in the process of restructuring into matrix organizations or, as Mintzberg labels them, adhocracies. Droste (1988), however, notes that hospitals reporting restructuring into matrix organizations using product line management are frequently merely reorganizing without changing their financial or authority structures. Droste found most hospitals still traditionally organized as professional bureaucracies with the addition of improved financial operations and marketing to specific market segments such as the elderly or women.

All Mintzberg's models include the same critical elements configured into five different shapes depending on which element has the greatest "pull." Figure 8–4 illustrates the professional bureaucracy model (p. 348). The five critical elements are: strategic apex, technostructure, support staff, middle line management, and operating core. These are analyzed using five perspectives or "overlays," which are: formal authority; regulated flows of information, decisions, and staff information; informal communication; work constellations; and ad hoc decision processes. This model does not appear, at first, to be an open systems model because the diagram only shows the structure of work and people; the processes among them are not depicted. Mintzberg chooses to refer to the processes as overlays. Inputs, outputs, and feedback are described in his discussions of the model but not always drawn in the diagram. Thus, Mintzberg's models draw the reader to focus more on structure and how it is changed by different work, workers, and environmental factors. His diagrams are more complex and the reader must conceptually add overlays, inputs, outputs, and feedback.

Looking back to Figure 8–4, the *strategic apex* is the executive management

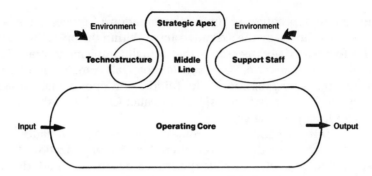

Figure 8-4. Professional bureaucracy model. *(Source: Mintzberg, H.* The Structuring of Organizations: A Synthesis of the Research. © *1979, pp. 20, 355. Reprinted by permission of Prentice-Hall, Inc., Englewood Cliffs, N.J.)*

level of the organization. People in these positions spend much of their time and energies focusing outside the organization onto the environment and future strategies for the organization, to serve its mission in an effective way. They spend very little in maintenance activities or operational decisions. In a professional bureaucracy this is a relatively small number of people. Only recently have nurse executives moved to this level of strategic management, requiring many to adopt new skills in strategic planning, marketing, and finance.

Technostructure workers are analysts in staff, as opposed to line, positions. They design and monitor work flow for the implementation of strategic plans, provide all internal education and training, and design and use the management information systems to gather information to measure quality, unit performance, financial soundness, and so on. Their purpose is to standardize work processes, outputs, or personnel skills. In a professional bureaucracy this group is also relatively small in size due to the standardization of work through lengthy training of professionals and self-monitoring activities of professionals in committees and ad hoc task forces. Other factors restricting the technostructure's size in the nonroutine nature of much of the work, the diverse skills needed to perform the work, and the situational determination of much health care.

Support staff include both professionals and nonprofessionals whose work is necessary for management and the operating core to function smoothly. This component of the organization is organized as a mini-machine bureaucracy with highly standardized, predictable work. In a hospital this includes dietary, janitorial and physical plant maintenance, secretaries, security, laboratory, radiology, pharmacy, business office, and legal counsel. The majority are not professionals. Some support the strategic apex, such as legal counsel, some middle management, such as accounting, and others the operating core such as pharmacy.

The neck of the model is *middle line management,* also referred to as tactical management. Here are the functional vice presidents and administrators who are not a part of the executive team. Their primary function is to design systems and monitor progress of the implementation of strategic plans, mission, and objectives chosen by the executive apex. Within the operating core are managers who focus on daily operations that actually implement strategic plans and the organizational mission. Some smaller hospitals combine middle and operational management into the same role. Middle and operational managers are a relatively small group in professional bureaucracies due to the professional autonomy of the operating core.

The fifth, last and largest group in a professional bureaucracy is the *operating core*. They provide the services offered by the organization. For hospitals they secure the patients, provide health care services, and discharge patients. Mintzberg describes the operating core as the group with the most pull, thereby shaping this type of organization. Thus, it is the largest element in the diagram. Work is coordinated through professional training, which standardizes skills and knowledge creating mutual expectations of performance among colleagues. Each colleague carries out work using considerable discretion within mutually accepted parameters of standards of care.

Diversity of actions is loosely standardized through a diagnostic process of pigeonholing. Patients are admitted to departments with product or service lines that are logically similar functional services serving the same market segment. Thus, women in labor are admitted to women's services; a person with appendicitis is admitted to general surgery. Within these departments patients with similar categories of medical diagnoses receive similar services within the parameters of standards of care. Each professional has several sets of specialized skills that are employed based on their assessment of the patient and clinical judgment resulting in a diagnosis. For instance, a physician assesses a patient and then writes the diagnoses and list of orders. Each order is a preprogrammed routine work activity. The nurse also assesses a patient and generates another list of preprogrammed activities. Through this pigeonholing process patients with their unique life history, self-care practices, and reasons for seeking care are assessed, categorized, referred to appropriate professionals, and receive appropriate services. In this way individualized care is standardized and thereby increases organizational efficiency.

As you can surmise, the professional bureaucracy structure is designed to accommodate the professional autonomy necessary for health care practice. Coordination is by standardization of skills through lengthy training and socialization into the community of professionals rather than direct supervision or even mutual adjustment and review. To some degree each professional bureaucracy has two parallel structures that are organized quite differently: a decentralized professional structure and a centralized administration and support staff. Decision making in the decentralized professional structure is primarily through political negotiation and coalition building; decision making in the administration and support staff is more bureaucratic and rule based. As the environment becomes less stable for health care organizations, however, administrative and support decision making is now becoming, less bureaucratic and more political.

Age and size are less important factors in determining structure in a professional bureaucracy than in some other types of organizations. As we pointed out, the two dominant qualities are autonomy and democractic involvement of the professionals in governance through committees. These qualities are both its greatest strength, a mechanism to carry out professional work on a large scale, and its greatest weakness, little control by administration over work quality and extreme resistance to systematic innovation.

Rapid technological change, an information-based society, and rising costs of providing services have lead administrators to look for new ways to structure their businesses and management practices to foster innovation, increase integration of services, and restructure service lines rapidly to accommodate new technology and information (Toffler, 1980; Naisbett, 1982). Restructuring, however, requires dramatic change in the philosophy and internal processes of health care organizations. Thus, changes have been slow and often fragmented. OD consultants are increasingly used to assist administrators struggling to design and implement more responsive organizations.

CONTINGENCY MODEL

Contingency models emphasize environmental exchanges that drive organizational decision making, mission, and structure. Charns and Schaefer (1983) described a contingency model for health care organizations (Fig. 8–5). The triangles represent the two types of work in the organization, direct and managerial. Both are separated into three elements, structure, coordination, and people. The purposes and goals of the organization define the necessary direct work and managerial work describes the strategies by which the direct work is accomplished. The environment is seen as the most important element in the contingency model. It influences both the purposes and goals and the managerial work.

The first element of both direct and managerial work considered is structure, which is the grouping of individuals, tasks, and responsibilities. Structure creates interconnections and interdependencies that vary in intensity and type. Structure also creates the formal communication system and the legitimate power structure. Direct work structure is collegial; managerial work structure is bureaucratic. This is consistent with Mintzberg's description of the differences in the operating core and the management and support services.

The second element of work is coordination, which deals with processing information among structural elements. The degree and type of coordination needed varies with size, standardization of work, skills, output, interdependence of work, amount of slack resources, and expertise of workers. Coordination also encompasses mechanisms for handling conflict. The primary processes of coordination used in direct work and management work differ; the latter is bureaucratic and the former is political.

The third and last element of work is people, both as individuals and as work group members. People's abilities, skills, perceptions, motivation, produc-

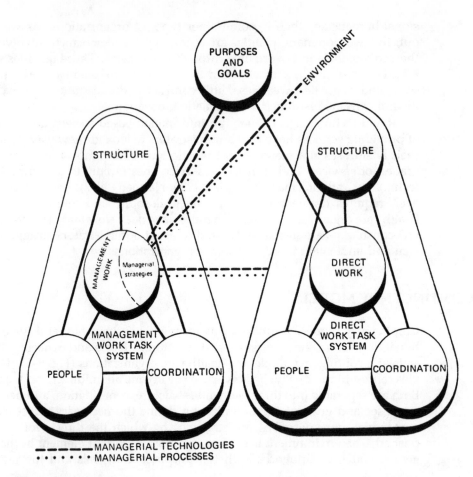

Figure 8-5. Contingency model. *(Source: Charns, M., & Schaefer, M., Health Care Organizations: A Model for Management. © 1983, p. 238. Reprinted by permission of Prentice-Hall, Inc., Englewood Cliffs, N.J.)*

tivity, and job satisfaction are the determinants of their contributions to the organization. Small group dynamics and other social processes are also included.

Direct work in health care organizations is the provision of services to patients and clients and the governance activities of providers. Management work is analytically divided into strategies and technologies. Strategies refer to decisions about relations with the environment, organizational design, internal managerial approaches, and strategic planning of organizational purposes and goals. Management technologies include: internal and external information gathering, planning and goal setting systems, scheduling systems, job descriptions, policies and procedures, protocols, allocation of scarce resources through budgeting and exceptions, evaluation and reward systems, and personnel systems. Implementation of both strategies and technologies occurs through the social processes of power and influence, interpersonal relationships, leadership style, personality type, conflict and cooperation, norms, and culture.

Although it is depicted as a small arrowhead outside the organization, the authors strongly emphasize the role of the environment in the contingency model. It is the source of all inputs and recipient of all outputs. The environment is defined as all individuals, groups, institutions, and forces that influence managerial decision making. Freeman (1984) refers to these interest groups as all stakeholders in the organization. The four major environmental characteristics influencing all organizations are stability, complexity, market diversity, and hostility. In addition, health care organizations need to assess legitimacy of possible providers, causal relationships among factors, spatial and cultural factors of a locale, and population changes in the marketplace.

The contingency model does not show the flow of inputs, transformation, outputs, and feedback, but assumes that they occur across all boundaries of the organization. Its emphasis is on the environment and delineation of managerial and direct work technologies and processes.

LIFE CYCLE STAGES OF ORGANIZATIONS

An organization's life cycle stage shapes the managerial challenges facing administrators and affects the selection and application of an open systems model for analysis and planned change. Structures, policies, and practices need to reflect not only characteristics of the work being performed and the workers, but also the life cycle stage of the organization. Galbraith and Nathanson (1978) refer to these stages as recurring metamorphoses driven by increasing complexity, age, and size. Griener (1972) describes the accompanying management approaches appropriate for each metamorphosis. The most common pattern of organizational evolution is shown in Figure 8-6 by the heavy line moving from top to bottom.

The young or entrepreneurial organization has a *simple structure*. All employees and the owner interact face to face more or less as equals performing the work. Financial rewards are low, but intangible rewards of participation in creating a new enterprise are high. The first crisis leading to a metamorphosis is when the organization grows to the point where informal interaction is no longer intense or frequent enough to sufficiently coordinate work. Volume of work dictates a need for increasing division and specialization of labor. Management emerges as a separate position from direct work.

If management meets this leadership crisis by restructuring with a hierarchy and formal control systems, then the organization may effectively deal with new challenges and grow. Accompanying changes include formalization of the reward system with development of job descriptions, standards of organizational expectations, and associated rewards and recognition through financial rewards and participation. Figure 8-6 shows that several different types of structures may be chosen at this stage depending on the technology of the organization

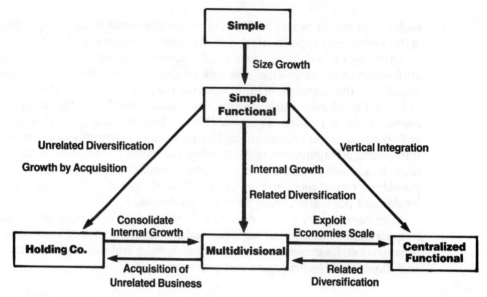

Figure 8-6. Structural patterns of organizational evaluation. *(Source: Reprinted by permission from Strategy Implementation: The Role of Structure and Process, by Galbraith, J., & Nathanson, D. Copyright © 1978 by West Publishing Company, p. 115. All rights reserved.)*

and the environmental contingencies it faces. Hospitals traditionally use the most common *simple, functional* structure.

Eventually, as the organization grows beyond 500 employees it diversifies its products, services, or sites within a local region. At this point, new managerial practices are again needed. Often the organization more clearly delineates levels of management and begins to expand into a wider variety of products and services within their usual product and service lines.

The new crisis leading to another major change is autonomy (Griener, 1972). Administrators responsible for different sites and product or service lines begin to assert that they lack the authority commensurate with their responsibilities. They are more aware of the changing needs of their local market and need the autonomy to respond rapidly to opportunities and contraints that often change as they wait for information to move up to top management and decisions to filter down to them.

The most common response to this growth is not another dramatic structural change but an elaboration of the functional structure into a *centralized functional structure.* Here, management is divided into executive, middle, and operational levels with an elaboration of staff support roles and increasing decentralization of authority and responsibility. Over time, the organization begins to be unwieldy, requiring increased formalization of reporting systems. New layers of management are added and more specialized functions become full-time positions. Within nursing, the top administrator becomes fully occupied with executive, strategic functions and delegates the tactical and operational management functions to others. Specialty staff positions emerge such as director of quality assurance, financial systems coordinator, and coordinator of recruitment and retention. First-line operational managers must now be trained to assume new functions such as preparing and monitoring budgets and manpower needs, marketing services, and monitoring quality of care.

The resultant growth through delegation is either by acquisition of other organizations or by horizontal or vertical integration (Griener, 1972). For instance, a hospital may expand vertically by restructuring into subunits offering different services such as skilled nursing facilities, hospice, home health care, work site health screening, rental offices for physicians, and sales of medical devices. Another pattern is horizontal growth or the addition of similar subunits as when a nursing home grows by opening similar facilities throughout a geographic region. A third mode of growth is by contracts, mergers, acquisitions, as when a health care agency purchases other service lines or facilities rather than developing new ones. Most organizations grow through a mixture of these approaches.

The reward system for managers changes to more impersonal measures such as return on investment (ROI) and profit contributions. Decisions to expand, terminate, or initiate sites and product or service lines are made impersonally using financial data. Again the organization grows and existing practices do not allow for directing multiple diverse units while maintaining control over entry and exit of new product or service lines and allocation of scarce resources such as capital funds between units. Lack of control leads to a major crisis, producing a metamorphosis into a *multiple division structure* to allow simultaneous autonomy and control. This type of organization in health care is often found in regional, statewide or national corporations. Growth is coordinated by corporate headquarters, which is usually separate from the operational divisions. Different types of management practices are now in place at differing levels within the organization. Participants may experience an entire career within one unit or organizational level, most are not familiar with or know participants from other units of the organization. Units vary widely in size, technology, age, complexity, and autonomy from the corporate headquarters.

This complexity eventually leads to a crisis of red tape as the headquarters, regional division, and local units each require different reporting and control information at various intervals (Griener, 1972). The organization begins to suffer from being "top heavy" and unable to coordinate its diverse, geographically dispersed enterprises with acumen. This crisis is resolved if the organization can begin to free itself of centralized responsibility at the corporate level for all major allocation and new venture decisions through collaboration of major divisions acting in parallel, rather than subservient to a central hierarchy. Management becomes more flexible and uses more behavioral approaches such as values confrontation, quality circles, interdisciplinary teams, conferences, and educational programs. The reward system shifts its focus from individual to team rewards. This collaborative structure often exists in multinational corporations with diverse holdings and product or service lines. Few, if any health care agencies have reached this stage, although some appear to be reaching the crisis of red tape. Galbraith and Nathanson (1978) also point out that all organizations do not need to continue to grow and follow these patterns to survive. In fact, many may decide to stabilize at some size and complexity level and maintain their vitality through environmental scanning and adaptation to their changing markets.

USING OPEN SYSTEMS MODELS

The nurse administrator may use the open systems models to assess organizational problems, guide organizational changes, and evaluate outcomes. The first step in applying open systems models is to select a model that reflects your organization's life stage and situation. For instance, if the organization is relatively young and rapidly growing, which crisis in the life stage model seems appropriate? Which open systems model would seem to best address this crisis? Even a cursory examination shows that each open systems model emphasizes certain elements and processes. After tentatively choosing a model, the administrator should go to the primary source describing the model for an in-depth description of both the model and how to use it to diagnose organizational problems.

The selected model directs the nurse administrator in choosing what information to focus on to diagnose the organizational problem and grasp its overall impact on the organization. Many administrators choose to hire an OD consultant to assess their organization rather than using a task force, standing committee, or the management team. A consultant offers an external perspective that many executives find enhances communication concerning sensitive problems.

After diagnosing an organizational problem the selected open systems model suggests how the problem is connected to critical elements throughout the organization and its environment. It is also useful in building scenarios to consider alternative strategies for problem resolution. Finally a model is useful when constructing criteria to evaluate the outcome of a planned change for problem resolution. Writings about OD usually include suggested actions frequently used in the resolution of common organizational problems.

In practice, the evaluation of organizational changes is complex and often problematic to assess. Organizations are infamous for appearing to absorb attempts at change to improve overall outcomes. For instance, the effect of a worthwhile change in one area may be offset by adaptation in another with the result of no overall improvement in organizational productivity.

Cameron (1982), synthesizing research on organizational change, has identified the four most frequently used criteria. They are: goal achievement, ability to acquire needed resources, optimization of internal processes, and extent of satisfaction of all stakeholders involved in the organization. Managers usually use a combination of these criteria.

Measurement of change is also problematic because each criteria has conflicting dimensions. Goals are multiple and sometimes conflict; priorities of different stakeholders result in varying definitions of needed resources; internal processes also conflict as managers attempt to satisfy different stakeholders. Actions effective to achieve one goal, block another, such as adding amenities increases patient comfort, a goal of patient care, but also increases costs, thereby decreasing achievement of the goal of cost containment. Data collected to measure goal attainment may indicate success, but interviews with those involved may indicate failure as they focus on a different aspect of work life. Conclusions comparing the organization with its goals, competitors, itself over time, or "ideal" models yield very different measures of success. Based on these conflicts Cameron (1982) suggests the evaluator take into account goals, constituencies, subgroup level of analysis, temporal frame, bias of data sources, and referent comparisons when designing an evaluation plan. Evaluation is for the purpose of decision making, therefore, data needs to be collected using feasible, valid, and reliable methods.

Health care organizations are increasingly employing OD consultants to develop and evaluate managerial changes and change employee behavior to accept and support rapid innovation, as they become interested in managerial changes to support innovation and marketing of services. No longer can work be designed primarily with efficient use of technology in mind. Work design must also include the interests and skills of providers and the perceptions and expectations of consumers receiving services. This major change in focus is necessitated by the move from a not-for-profit community service agency in a relatively certain environment to a profit-oriented business in a competitive uncertain environment (Burke, 1987). Organizational development interventions have been used for over 20 years to develop and support participative management practices in traditional businesses. They are now a popular choice to institute such changes in health care organizations. Nurse administrators will find open systems models and consultation from OD experts useful tools to increase the responsiveness and adaptability of the health care organizations they participate in administering.

BIOGRAPHICAL SKETCH

Jackie Dienemann is currently Associate Professor and Coordinator of the masters program in Nursing Administration at George Mason University where she has worked since 1983. Curriculum changes under her direction have focused on development of courses in financial management, nursing informatics, and, most recently, case management. She received the outstanding graduate nursing faculty award from students in 1988. Her publications and research have focused on development and evaluation of organizational power, research programs, collaboration between service and educational nursing departments, and nurse performance. She consults with divisions of nursing on automation of nursing information, performance evaluation, and research program development. Her background includes a BS from Mount St. Mary's College in nursing; practice as a community health nurse and home health nurse; an MSN degree in psychiatric-mental health nursing from Catholic University of America; teaching nursing at Columbia Union College; and a PhD in Sociology from Catholic University of America. She is active in Sigma Theta Tau, Maryland Nurses Association, Academy of Management, and American Organization of Nurse Executives where she has held numerous leadership positions.

SUGGESTED READINGS

Systems Theory

Bertalanffy, L. von. (1967). *Robots, Men and Minds.* New York: G. Braziller.

Luthans, F. (1981). *Organizational Behavior.* New York: McGraw Hill.

Rackich, J., Longest, B. Jr., & Darr, K. (1985). *Managing Health Services Organizations.* Philadelphia: W.B. Saunders.

Shortell, S., & Kaluzny, A. (1988). *Organization Theory and Health Care Management in Health Care Management,* 2nd ed. Shortell, S., & Kaluzny, A. (eds.). New York: John Wiley & Sons.

Organizational Development

Harrison, M. (1987). *Diagnosing Organizations.* Beverly Hills, CA: Sage Publications.

Kotter, J. (1978). *Organizational Dynamics.* Reading, MA: Addison-Wesley.

Weisbord, M. (1978). *Organizational Diagnosis: A Workbook of Theory and Practice.* Reading, MA: Addison Wesley.

REFERENCES

Burke, W.W. (1987). *Organization Development.* Reading, MA: Addison Wesley.

Cameron, K. (1982). *Organizational Effectiveness: A Comparison of Multiple Models.* New York: Academic Press.

Charns, M., & Schaefer, M. (1983). *Health Care Organizations.* Englewood Cliffs, NJ: Prentice Hall.

Droste, T. (1988, July). Product-line management: Misunderstood, feared. *Hospitals,* pp. 30–33.

Freeman, R.E. (1984). *Strategic Management.* Boston: Pitman Publishing Co.

Galbraith, J., & Nathanson, D. (1978). *Strategy Implementation: The role of structure and process.* St. Paul: West Publishing Company.

Griener, L. (1972). Evolution and revolution as organizations grow. *Harvard Business Review, 51*(4), 37–46.

Hackman, J.R., & Oldham, G.R. (1975). Development of the job diagnostic survey. *Journal of Applied Psychology, 60*(1), 159–170.

Mintzberg, H. (1979). *Structuring of organizations.* Englewood Cliffs, NJ: Prentice Hall.

Morgan, G. (1987). *Images of organization.* Beverly Hills, CA: Sage Publications.

Nadler, D., & Tushman, M. (1982). A model for diagnosing organizational behavior: Applying a congruence perspective. In Nadler, D., Tushman, M., & Hatvany, N. (eds.): *Managing organizations.* Boston: Little Brown & Company.

Naisbett, J. (1982). *Megatrends.* New York: Warner Books.

Scott, W.R. (1987). *Organizations,* 2nd ed. Englewood Cliffs, NJ: Prentice-Hall Inc.

Tichy, N., & Beckhard, R. (1982). Organization development for health care organizations. In Marguilies, N., & Adams, J.D. (eds.) *Health care organizations.* Reading, MA: Addison Wesley.

Toffler, A. (1980). *The third wave.* New York: Morrow.

APPLICATION 8-1

Management Consultation
Kitty S. Smith

Need for change is the reason why many nursing administrators hire consultants whether related to nursing practice, staff, management, or new services. Change is inevitable but an administrator may assume some control through planning. The problem is how to establish a plan that is as rational as possible and at the same time produce a minimum of side effects and a maximum of satisfaction for all involved.

The current extensive changes in health care delivery systems make it imperative that administrators consider restructuring and job design to assist nursing personnel in achieving a level of desired productivity. A decision for attacking each specific area of concern is more likely to be successful if based on a well-thought through plan. Valuable time and money are often expended with minimal positive impact when hasty decisions are made without appropriate planning. Let us assume you have a need to change the organizational structure of the nursing department. The best solution appears to be the combining of several units under one manager. What changes are needed to implement this decision?

Consultation is being used more frequently by nurse executives to achieve organizational goals. They are seeking guidance and counseling from educationally prepared, experienced consultants to bringing about changes such as adding new services, changing nursing care modalities, redefining manpower needs and utilization, evaluating patient care, and developing management skills.

THE CONSULTANT

Choosing the right consultant is a crucial step to be taken by the nurse administrator. The consultative process is a personal relationship between the consultant and the persons involved in solving a problem or developing a plan. Accepting this basic premise, it can be agreed that two aspects of any consultation relationship are (1) work carried out on a problem and its solution and (2) the relationship between consultant (the helper) and client (persons being helped).

Conversely, acceptance of a consultative role is a critical decision for the person being asked to help. The consultant recognizes the client as involving persons with authority achieved through possession of specialized kowledge, position, and experience. The nature of this power must be understood and skills developed and used in a manner that will be viewed as being helpful. A nurse consultant entering this relationship must be able to assess the situation and have the ability to diagnose the client's problem. Paramount to the relationship is the recognition and understanding of the strengths and limitations of one's own resources and one's motivation for providing consultation. It is unethical to accept a consultative offer when one does not have the expertise or credentials.

THE CONSULTATIVE PROCESS

Relationship Conditions
The consultant recognizes that the persons seeking help may reveal a number of feelings or attitudes during a consultative relationship. Typically, these include uncertainty, resistance to change, and overly optimistic time expectations.

Uncertainty. There may be suspicion or a tendency to proceed cautiously when the client coming to the consultant for help is uncertain as to the amount of authority the consultant has or will attempt to use. In asking for help the client may be unclear about what organizational relationship to establish with the consultant. There may be concern that the consultant will assume too much authority and take over certain areas of problem solving causing the client to be looked upon by their superiors or subordinates as ineffective.

Resistance To Change. When change is contemplated, the natural reaction is resistance, especially if status quo has been comfortable. Fear and uncertainty of the unknown and concern for potential impact on the client's position if failure results from change or organizational inertia blocks change. Feelings balancing this resistance, however, are curiosity, interest, and desire to explore the unknown.

Time Schedule. The client may expect quicker solutions to a problem situation by having a consultant. For the consultation process to be effective, however, time must be spent in establishing of relationships, developing of roles determining responsibility/authority distribution, learning how to work together, and working on the problem. None of these steps should be bypassed or short changed.

Establishing Consultant–Client Relationship

Establishment of an effective consultative relationship may be hampered by the problem of dependency associated with receiving help. On one hand, a client may have the tendency to be over-dependent on the consultant. Rather than participating in thinking through the problem, those being helped may want to be told what to do. On the other hand, a client may resent dependency and tend to resist assistance or make the consultant prove him or herself. The effective consultant recognizes these problems and works toward solving the client's reaction to dependency first rather than immediately proceeding to solving the organization problem under consideration. The consultant facilitates a trusting relationship and joint exploration of the actual problem at a pace comfortable to both parties within the established timetable. Efforts should be made to be nonjudgmental and reduce any threat the consultant may be to other persons. Remember, listening is as important as giving information. Relationships must be developed and understood before other problems can be resolved.

Problem Solving Phases

To attack the problem, it is essential that the consultant and the client be conversant with the several phases of the problem solving process—defining the problem, working on the problem, implementing an action plan, and evaluating and replanning.

Definition. The client's statement of the problem is presented and through joint exploration, a working definition of the problem is developed. Diagnosis of the real problem is the crux of the process. Frequently a situational symptom is presented as the problem.

A systematic diagnosis of the status quo that is to be changed must be carried out. To assist in the identification of those forces pushing for change or impeding the change process I have developed a general systems model for use in consultative work. This model provides order to a comprehensive assessment of a specific nursing unit or situation (Fig. 8–7). Other systems, models, described in the preceding chapter, could also be used for organizational diagnosis.

The model can be used either in its totality or in part. Regardless of the unit size (whether a home health care agency, clinic, nursing unit, or nursing service department) and regardless of the primary problem, the model assists the consultant and the client in the recognition of internal and external forces impacting the agency and the problem area. Identification of system components helps in explaining appropriate and realistic use of management processes. Application of a model assists in the differentiation of "what is from what ought to be."

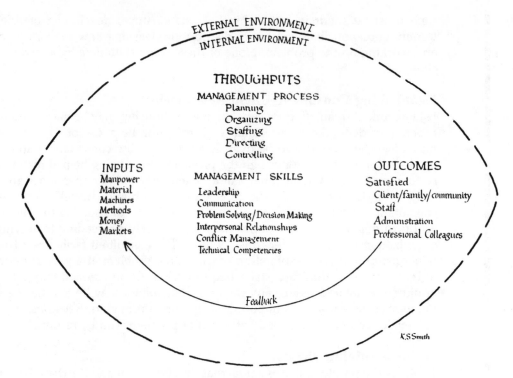

Figure 8–7. Assessment model: management development programs.

Environment. The many and varied external forces in the community impacting on decision making and planning include political climate, economic status of citizens, legislation, physical environment, health and science advancement, health-related knowledge, culture, major health problems, availability of services, sources of payment for services, and educational level of population. Careful analysis of these forces provides a greater understanding of the community and the individuals being served, whether they be patients or employees.

Internal environmental forces having impact on the problem situation are the organization's statements of mission, philosophy, goals, and organizational and physical structures. It is important to determine the compatibility of the nursing service department and its units with these elements.

Inputs. Resources determine how goals can be accomplished, thus making it essential for the consultant and the client to know what is available to them. What is the manpower supply and demand? What types and numbers of nursing personnel are needed to implement anticipated change? Are they available in the marketplace for hire? What types of expendable supplies are available? Is the available equipment and technology appropriate and adequate for achieving goals? What rules, procedures, and regulations govern the management of the employees and how they perform while at work? Are there unions? What monies are available? How are the changes to be promoted?

Assessing the readiness of the situation for change poses two questions for consideration by the consultant. Given the existing conditions, to what degree is it realistic to hope one can affect the situation? How strong are the forces for or against change?

Working on the Problem. Diagnosis of the problem situation having been made, the consultant and the client embark on developing a plan of action with alternatives. Goals are agreed upon and objectives established for their achievement. Goals should be based on readiness and potential for change. Should a complete solution of the problem be sought (e.g., total reorganization of nursing service) or would it be more realistic and appropriate to approach one aspect of the problem (e.g., reorganization of one pilot unit)? Objectives developed to achieve goals should be stated in terms that are measurable, realistic, necessary, understandable, consistent, and challenging.

Forecasting in light of the objectives is essential to the development of strategies. A timetable for long-range and short-range planning must be established. Determination of manpower and material needs and the establishment of capital costs are the next step. Strategies are set to reflect an operating plan with clear and prioritized objectives. Policies or directives with a support system of procedures and methods must be professionally, financially, and politically effective. When priorities are set, adhere to them.

Decisions are now in order as to what positions will be changed or created with what responsibilities. What associated authority is needed by each person to accomplish assigned responsibilities? The client with consultant input decides the appropriate way to divide the total task into its managerial and clinical components. Well-developed position descriptions provide a structure for delegation.

The ability to accomplish the task depends on the complexity of the work, similarity of tasks, degree of interdependence among the workers or degree of physical dispersion, degree of standardization, education of workers, training and general capabilities of workers, level of initiative, competence of the administrator/manager, degree of interaction required in the setting, and the time the client must give to accomplish a task. Involving staff who are interested in the planned change makes assignments easier and provides for commitment to the project. The time spent by staff on the project should be commensurate within their regular workload and associated rewards.

Acceptance of a task by an employee carries both the responsibility and accountability for satisfactory performance of assigned duties. Delegating the responsibility for a particular function to an employee in no way diminishes the person's responsibility for that function. Authority to take or initiate action should be delegated as close to the scene of action as possible. The number of levels of authority should be kept at a minimum. Taking time to know the organization, lines of authority, and the agency as a social system provides the client and the consultant with an informed basis for assigning tasks.

Implementing Action Plan. Putting the organized plan into action through deployment of resources and translation of strategy into tactics follows the planning and organizing activities for changing the system. Delegation, supervision, coordination, and control are the essential elements for actuating the plan. Delegation, if handled well, assures each involved employee fair and equal treatment during the implementation of the plan.

Directing activities to fit interests and values of staff is the task of supervision. Supervision undertakes the direct oversight of tasks assigned to individuals or small groups to assure appropriate performance. Supervision poses many challenges to the individual responsible. How does one create a climate in which spontaneous team work is possible? How does one bring together the goals of the individual with those of the group? How does one motivate individuals to fulfill their potential of professional functioning? If supervision of the project and administration are effective, then coordination becomes effective.

Coordination is the orderly bringing together of individual efforts on the project with respect to their number, time, and direction so that a common frame of reference is implemented for achievement of the stated goals. Coordination prevents fragmentation of individual effort and maintains the control system for assessing the project's process.

The manager need not lose control in decentralization but must learn to use safeguards, such as regular feedback, to identify impending difficulties. Self-control on the part of all workers is essential.

In implementing the action plan roles are worked out between the consultant and the client on individual responsibilities concerning a solution of the problem. What assistance does the client need in implementing an action plan? What should the consultant do during this first action phase? When should the consultant withdraw? In most cases the client should have the action role and the consultant withdraw, at least temporarily.

There are a number of ways the consultant can assist the problem solution. Careful consideration should be given to what is deemed appropriate by the client rather than what the consultant would ideally like to do. Consultants can implement their role as helper by

1. Remaining on the outside of the problem and confining the role to suggesting new ways or changes in the work situation, relationships, procedures, and methods. Challenging traditions is often a valuable service.
2. Collecting information within the organization and making it available to the client and other appropriate persons.
3. Providing methodological assistance for the assessment of the problem situation.

4. Suggesting use of outside methods, experiences, experts for working on the problem.
5. Providing seminars and workshops around identified learning needs.
6. Meeting with strategic organizational people and offering interpretation of the consequences of the status quo and suggestions for change.

Evaluation and Replanning. The ultimate outcome is hopefully a satisfied client, administration, staff, and professional colleagues. Outcomes should reflect achievement of stated goals and objectives in terms of effectiveness and efficiency in time, money, and energy. The planned level of goal achievement and degree of predicted change dictates feedback for modification of the plan. This modification of the original plan may take place at any step in the process.

In an effective relationship, the consultant will repeatedly evaluate progress and assist the client in planning the next step in the action plan. Support should be readily available to the client as obstacles occur and delays are encountered. In many instances it is the consultant who holds the project together when barriers and emotions interfere with action plan achievement.

PLANNING FOR MANAGEMENT DEVELOPMENT PROGRAMS

A study of problem situations through the consultative process model provides detailed input for planning management development programs.

In increasing numbers, large agencies with a goal of effective handling of the entire organizational operation have developed extensive human resource development programs. These programs provide an ongoing objective assessment of the needs of the agency in recruiting, maintaining, and promoting qualified administrators. The agency's master program in management development includes clinical/technical and administration phases and is generally composed of basic, intermediate, and advanced courses. The basic courses provide for the acquisition of fundamental concepts to be used by first-level managers. The intermediate phase covers application and adaption of techniques such as marketing and quantitative methods for middle management personnel. The third phase comprising policy formulation, organization change and trend analyses is for development of the executive. Over and above the institution master program for management development, nursing service adds courses that are specific to nursing (e.g., staffing, scheduling, professional staff development, nursing care plans, and quality assurance).

Management development programs in most institutions are less comprehensive. Often they include only orientation for new employees with an occasional employee training program to meet a specific agency need. Planned programs for development of head nurses is becoming common place; however, little planning is done for continued growth and upward mobility of these individuals. Additional courses may be provided by a consultant as described as part of an organizational change. Also many agencies are now sending their employees to external educational programs in management or contracting with educational institutions to provide a wide range of offerings.

BIOGRAPHICAL SKETCH

Kitty S. Smith, MSN, RN, Associate Professor, George Mason University, Fairfax, Virginia, provided leadership in the development of a master's program in nursing administration and served as coordinator of the program for 10 years. She serves as a management consultant to health care-related agencies and curriculum consultant in program development and administration to schools of nursing. Consultancies have extended to hospitals and nursing schools in Taiwan and Beijing, China. Her professional career includes staff, supervisory, and managerial positions in community health nursing in local and state health departments and the U.S. Public Health Service, faculty and administrative positions at the Catholic University of American University and Radford University, and elected offices in several nursing organizations.

CASE 8-1

Changes in Medicare Reporting: Its Impact on a Home Health Agency
Emilie M. Deady

General systems theory assumes that there is a continuous relationship between the environment and the organization. The main points of most definitions by systems theorists are that systems are composed of interdependent parts (components) that are separated by a boundary from their surrounding environment, (Farace, Mange, & Hamish, 1977). Systems analysis is the breakdown of a system in a logical fashion into its constituent parts, the detection of the relationships of the parts and the way they are organized. Its use is twofold: (1) for descriptive purposes and (2) for analysis of a problem. Important characteristics of general systems theory are an emphasis on multiple organizational goals and the closely interrelated functioning of subunits within the system (Anthony, Dearde, & Norton, 1984). It emphasizes the use of groups of people to interdependently deal with management problems and decisions. This case application uses general systems theory to describe the interaction and interdependence between the Visiting Nurse Association of Northern Virginia and the Medicare health insurance program of the federal government.

The Visiting Nurse Association of Northern Virginia (V.N.A.) is a private, nonprofit voluntary home health agency that serves the residents of northern Virginia within a 120-square-mile area. From its founding in 1937, the main purpose of the agency has been to provide quality in-home health services to the sick and disabled of northern Virginia regardless of the individual's ability to pay for service. The V.N.A., in fiscal year 1987, had a budget of over 4 million dollars. About 70 percent of V.N.A. patients are elderly and the largest source of revenue has been from Medicare. Revenues also come from private insurance payment and patient paid fees. An additional 4 percent of our budget is provided by the local United Way charity campaign to cover uncompensated care. The V.N.A. is the largest nonofficial home health care provider in the state and is accredited by the National League for Nursing.

The agency is governed by a volunteer Board of Directors who hire an Executive Director to carry out day-to-day operations. Currently the agency provides service through a multidisciplinary staff of nurses, physical, occupational, and speech therapists, home health aides, and medical social workers. The V.N.A. has recently added clinical specialists to its staff to meet the needs of its increasingly acutely ill patients and to complement its other staff. Because of shorter average hospital stay, V.N.A. staff now care for patients with a high acuity level of illness who are in need of more specialized, intensive care, such as intravenous therapy. In conjunction with this increased need for specialized care, staff are also available 24 hours a day.

The V.N.A. has changed over the past 50 years in response to the environment in which it interacts. The agency may be seen as a system that responds to other systems and the suprasystems in which it functions. Many internal changes have occurred as responses to changes in community needs and demands from Medicare, other third-party payors, and regulatory agencies.

Because the V.N.A. is approximately 70 percent Medicare funded the regulations and requirements for participation in that program heavily influence the operations of the agency. Medicare and its requirements is perceived as the primary system that interacts with and significantly impacts on the V.N.A. system (Fig. 8-8).

In September of 1985, the Medicare system introduced a new form to obtain written physician's orders. These forms were mandated as a requirement for participation in that program. Previous regulations had required signed physician's orders every 60 days on all Medicare patients using a form available from the federal government or its own form providing certain issues were addressed. The new mandated forms titled 485, 486, and 487 eliminated that option. The 485 form is the primary physician form and the other forms are addendums to it. All providers of services must complete the information using these forms and combine this into one order per patient. In addition, this physician signed form must accompany monthly invoices for service.

The introduction of these forms into the V.N.A. clearly illustrates the interdependence of each system or component within the total system. The guidelines for completing these forms arrived at the V.N.A. in the latter part of July with an implementation date throughout the country of September 1. Careful scrutiny of the forms revealed that an excessive amount of field staff time would be spent on completing them. Similar information was asked in several different areas. The underlying theme was to detect if the caretaker could provide the

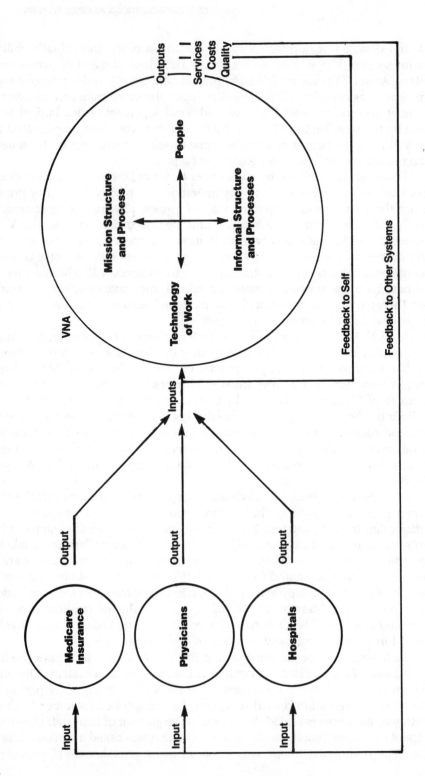

Figure 8–8. Systems involved in the introduction of 486 forms to VNA.

services done by the home health aide and, therefore, indicate that home health aid service was not needed. The management staff studied the guidelines and determined that the processing of this form with the correct information would impact on the total agency staff in some manner. All disciplines that would be providing service to a patient had to combine orders and observations onto one 485 form and the necessary addendums. Because of the high acuity level of patients there is frequently more than one discipline involved in providing care. The seemingly simple task of having a nurse, a physical therapist, and a social worker complete one form is challenging, as the staff are not all in the office at the same time.

A small multidisciplinary task group, including secretarial and billing staff, was delegated the task of developing a mechanism for implementation. To accomplish this goal the group was given a 2-week block of time to work together on developing a checklist for the forms and then the paperflow through the agency. For this task group to produce this in 2 weeks other members of the management team had to cover and perform their daily work.

A checklist for physician's orders had been previously used by field staff who would complete the form and turn it in for typing by the secretarial staff. This checklist gave several options from which staff could choose the desired order or outcome. The original checklist reduced the amount of time that the nurses and the therapist spent in completing paperwork. It was anticipated that a checklist for these forms would do the same for field staff.

Assessment of the capabilities of our computer at that time was that additional hardware was needed for storage and retrieval of the forms. The staff planned for a time lag in ordering the equipment and a November deadline for implementing the computer automation. The additional expense had been anticipated in planning the operational budget so the hardware was ordered. Delivery of the equipment was late, which then caused a delay in programming the software. Actually the implementation of the computerized 485s did not take place until April of the following year. We had anticipated that the programming could be done within 3 months; in reality it took much longer because of the size of the design and its impact on other software programs already in use. All the while, despite these problems the 485 forms were flowing through the agency, out to the physician, back into the V.N.A. and to Medicare in a timely manner.

The task force decided that much of the identifying information required by the forms could be captured from the referral source at the time of the initial intake process. This changed the amount and kind of information that was requested by the intake department from hospital liaison staff. One of the few initial changes that these forms caused was on the tracking system that the secretarial staff used in monitoring the flow of the form from referral to nurse/ therapist to physicians to patient record. The greatest impact within the V.N.A. was on secretarial staff in typing from the checklist to the appropriate forms. To cope with this added typing, additional secretarial staff were employed and added to each team. This addition of extra secretarial staff caused problems as to where to locate them in an already crowded noisy office.

One of the greatest concerns to management was to maintain field staff productivity during the change over. We anticipated that there would be some down time as staff learned how to use the new forms but we hoped that this would not continue for a long time. Because this form was mandated for all home health agencies throughout the country, we were able to confer with other agencies to determine its impact. The V.N.A. considered itself fortunate in that the average visits per day for staff were not adversely affected. Other agencies told of actual decreases of one visit per day. We hired additional staff and determined that this increase and processing of paper added at least $2.50 to our per visit cost.

Thus, a seemingly simple change to a new set of forms by Medicare impacted the hospital referring patients, the computer system at the V.N.A., the work and working conditions of secretaries, and the cost per home visit. The interdependence of the system components was obvious. The task force's attempt to plan the change and monitor system impacts benefited from a general systems viewpoint.

The V.N.A. as a system interacts with other systems and its environment. The physician system is a key element in home health as orders and consultation about care plans must be obtained and documented for payment. Most of the physicians that work with the V.N.A. are accustomed to signing orders and returning them to the agency with corrections or additional comments if needed. The new forms left little, if any, room for physician comments. Now instead of a one-page form there were two or three with the physician's signature needed on the 485 form and not the addendums. Plans for the change included a letter sent with every new 485 form to the physician explaining the reason for the new form and the need to have it returned as early as possible. We found that these forms required more than the usual postage, which added to the overhead expenses of the V.N.A. for metering and secretarial time. The task force suggested envelopes with postage paid to ensure that the physician would return the forms promptly and the V.N.A. would avoid postage due problems. The secretarial staff monitor closely the date the form is mailed and returned. If orders are not returned in a timely manner, the secretary telephones and/or visits the physician's office to pick up forms. Because of these built-in controls and monitoring, the new forms have been sent into the Medicare fiscal intermediary without major problems.

Once the forms are returned to the V.N.A., the secretary processes it through to the billing department. In this department the forms are attached to the individual patient bill with another verification before being sent to the fiscal intermediary. Billing department staff validate the forms with the bill to determine if the appropriate visit count and disciplines ordered match.

Using general systems theory, the V.N.A.'s output is the fiscal intermediary's (FI) input and its feedback to the V.N.A. is an input. The 485 forms request more in-depth information on all levels of the patient's and family's functioning than had previously been given. This information is reviewed on all claims by the fiscal intermediary who either judges services appropriate or questions the care plan. If the care plan is questioned the FI asks for more information from the agency, such as why were three visits charged for a monthly catheter change when only one was on the 485 form. This causes a response in the V.N.A.'s system with more information and photocopying returned to the FI.

The flow for monitoring additional requests had been an established system before the 485 forms and, therefore, did not have to be developed. What we did not anticipate was the FI interpreting guidelines more stringently resulting in raising the volume of requests not only on current patients but often on patients who had been served as much as a year before. In the review process the FI may determine that services were inappropriate and deny payment for such care. All denials activate a review of the documentation of patient care and frequently initiated a challenge within a defined time frame. This increased frequency of requests and denials has had an effect on staff who are providing care. Staff are concerned that payment for services will be questioned and ultimately denied. They have become very careful about documentation of care plans and the estimate on the number of visits, in fact, care is rationed. The staff subsystem within the V.N.A. system responded to change in the denial rate by an outside system with informally enforced reduction in patient care. To offset this informal service reduction, coordinators and senior staff work closely with nurses, therapists, and social workers to interpret the Medicare guidelines so that patient care will not be adversely affected.

The V.N.A. services emanate from two offices. The satellite office houses a district or a team composed of a coordinator, nurses, and secretarial staff with therapists occasionally reporting to that office. Other teams along with administration and billing are located in the main office. The management staff did foresee problems in the satellite office with using the 485 forms because the therapist team was located at the main office and all disciplines were to write on the same form.

To enhance communication and reduce the coordination necessary for the new forms the therapists were decentralized and a team physically located in the satellite office. The plan was to pilot the program for 3 months and to monitor carefully the issues of demand, paper flow, and supervision of care. These results were all positive. Staff enjoyed the multidisciplinary team work that developed from being physically located in the same area and all working with the same patients. The only problem was that now the office, which had been designed for a staff of 8 to 10 people, had to accommodate up to 16. This created a need for finding larger offices. Because the pilot was so successful, the other nursing teams in the central offices also wanted to have the therapists assigned to share the same patients.

Each discipline at that time had their own patient record that was taken into the home at the time of the visit and only combined into one record at the time of discharge. This was a practice for many years, not only in the V.N.A., but also at other agencies. The Record Committee was in the process of developing a patient record that would allow for centralization of the record for all disciplines with a traveling file for home visits. We all perceived that the decentralization of staff would be easier to accomplish after implementation of the new central record. Thus implementation of the new forms also hastened decentralization of multidisciplinary staff and major changes in our patient records.

Field staff and the billing department were both affected by the new forms. The billing department became over-crowded due to the additional staff, more paperwork, and the expansion and reprogramming of the agency's main computer. As has been explained earlier, additional computer hardware and software was needed to implement the automation of the new forms onto the system. After 6 months the software for implementing a new intake information process was ready. The plan was to have as much information as possible gathered at the time of intake, which could then be entered on the 485 forms by the computer before home visits began. Nurses and therapists going on home visits would have a printout of the intake information to take into the field.

The implementation of a new form was causing changes in a domino effect throughout the V.N.A. We are finally into the final phase of "bringing up" the new forms on the computer. The forms have been entered by secretarial staff and flowed through the agency as we had planned. The implementation of the forms on the computer is anticipated to bring about less change than the initial introduction. This will be the end result of planning started over a year ago. Over the year plans have been evaluated and revised in relationship to unanticipated consequences of the new forms. The process has required work by groups at all levels of the agency's system and in all departments.

The implementation of the 485 forms would have been more stressful if the concepts of general systems theory had not been used as a framework to plan the changes. Every change in one part of the system brought about or supported a change in another. Some of the changes within our system we were able to plan for and anticipate; others we were not. Systems outside of the V.N.A. were not within our control but we attempted to collaborate with both hospital discharge planners and physicians to manage problems. The system that the V.N.A. presently has is more complex, involves two decentralized multidisciplinary teams that offer better coordinated services, and a more sophisticated automated intake and billing system.

BIOGRAPHICAL SKETCH

Emilie Deady is Executive Director of the Visiting Nurse Association of Northern Virginia. She has been in the home health field since 1966 and has worked in positions of staff nurse, supervisor, and now director. Previous positions include clinical specialist in community ambulatory care at Childrens Hospital National Medical Center and consultant for Nurses Coalition for Action in Politics (NCAP), American Nurse Association. In addition to serving on local committees, she serves on the Board of Directors of Virginia Association for

Home Care. She has master's degrees in Community Health Nursing from Catholic University of America and General Administration from the University of Maryland.

REFERENCES

Anthony, R.N., Dearde, J., & Bedford, N. (1984). *Management Control System.* Homewood, IL: Richard D. Irwin, Inc.

Farace, R.V., Mange, P.R., & Russell, H. (1977). *Communicating and Organizing.* London: Addison-Wesley Publishing Company.

9

Organizations as Financial Systems
Lloyd M. DeBoer

This chapter describes how a unit contributes to the entire organization's financial well-being and some ways all levels of nursing administrators may better understand the financial management of their facilities. Specific references are made to the financial management responsibilities of both nurse executives and nurse middle managers.

INTERPRETING FINANCIAL STATEMENTS

The overall financial condition of any health care organization is primarily portrayed by two financial statements: the balance sheet and the statement of revenues and expenses.* The budget that nursing unit directors submit and how well these directors managed their budget this year have a direct impact on the expense portion of the organization's statement of revenues and expenses and an indirect influence on other parts of the balance sheet. Initially, we focus on these two statements that are of primary interest to nurse executives and then introduce other statements that managers use in the financial management of units within their organizations.

The Balance Sheet and Statement of Revenues and Expenses
Tables 9–1 and 9–2 are a balance sheet and statement of revenues and expenses. To understand these statements the nurse executive needs to know these seven

---

The discussion in this chapter is for a not-for-profit organization as this accurately describes the majority of health care organizations. There are some differences in the financial statements prepared for a not-for-profit organization as compared with those prepared for a for-profit organization. The more significant differences are noted.

*For a for-profit organization this statement is called an income statement or a profit-and-loss statement.

TABLE 9-1. GOODHEALTH HOSPITAL BALANCE SHEET AS OF DECEMBER 31, 19XX (AMOUNTS IN THOUSANDS)

Assets			Total Liabilities and Fund Balance	
Current Assets		Totals	**Current Liabilities**	Totals
Cash		$ 2,146	Accounts payable	$ 1,286
Short-term investments		3,000	Short-term notes payable	1,470
Accounts Receivable	$18,701		Long-term bonds payable within one year	1,343
Less: Provision for allowances	3,740	14,961	Accrued salaries	3,005
Supply Inventory		1,144	Accrued wages	790
Other current assets		2,477	Accrued other liabilities	890
			Deferred revenues	3,890
Total current assets		$23,728	Total current liabilities	$12,674
Fixed Assets (Property, plant, & equipment)				
Land	$ 794		Long-term bonds payable	34,306
Building	45,485		Other liabilities	2,001
Medical equipment	33,756			
Office equipment	4,744		Fund balance	46,313
Total fixed assets	84,779			
Less: Accumulated depreciation	35,607			
Total fixed assets		49,172	Total Liabilities and Fund Balance	$95,294
Long-term investments		12,865		
Other Assets		9,529		
Total Assets		$95,294		

TABLE 9-2. GOODHEALTH HOSPITAL STATEMENT OF REVENUES AND EXPENSES FOR THE PERIOD ENDING DECEMBER 31, 19XX (AMOUNTS IN THOUSANDS)

Revenues		Totals
In-patient revenues		$135,040
Out-patient revenues		19,422
Emergency room revenues		8,176
Total gross patient revenues		$162,638
Less: Deductibles (uncollectible accounts, contractual allowances, Medicare, Medicaid, indigent care)		34,154
Net patient revenues		$128,484
Other operating revenues		4,673
Total operating revenues		$133,157
Operating Expenses		
Salaries	$ 61,450	
Wages	18,940	
Employee benefits	10,762	
Employed physicians	10,684	
Interest expense	3,186	
Utilities	9,168	
Supplies	5,632	
Depreciation	8,944	
Total operating expenses		$128,766
Net operating income		4,391
Nonoperating revenues		2,277
Excess of Revenues Over Expenses		$ 6,668

concepts: basic accounting equations, major classes of accounts, double entry bookkeeping, fiscal period, profit, not-for-profit, and accrual accounting.

All organizations must know their financial status, both for operational decisions and to report to external interested parties such as shareholders, investors, Board of Trustees, lending institutions, and federal Internal Revenue Service. The accounting department records all transactions and creates reports for administrators and trustees to use for decision making.

Basic Accounting Equations

To decipher what these reports mean, one must understand the basic accounting equations used by all organizations. The first is:

$$\text{assets} = \text{equity}$$

An organization's *assets* are expressed as the economic value of all resources. These may be broken down into (1) current assets, which include cash and that which will become cash in 1 year or less, e.g., short-term investments, accounts receivable, and inventory of supplies; (2) fixed or long-term assets, which include land, depreciable assets of buildings and equipment, long-term investments; and (3) contra assets, which may be current or long-term, expressed as reserve accounts for which funds may be set apart and restricted in use for specified purposes, e.g., uncollectible accounts, depreciation of building or equipment.

For accounting purposes, assets must always equal *equity*. Equity is a broad term that is commonly broken down into:

liabilities + organization's equity + retained earnings

An organization's *liabilities* are basically monies owed. These are usually divided into short-term and long-term amounts with the division based on whether they are to be paid within 1 year or over a longer period.

The second component is the *organization's equity*, which is the value of the assets provided when the business was established or expanded. The third and last component, *retained earnings*, is the net cumulative result of operations, that is, revenues minus expenses. These two components, organization's equity and retained earnings are usually combined into a single item called *fund balance* for a not-for-profit organization.

Therefore, the basic accounting equation can also be written as:

assets = liabilities + organization's equity + revenues − expenses

Revenues are amounts owed by persons or businesses for purchased services or goods, or both. *Expenses* are monies paid for operations—these include wages, rent, electricity, telephone, other utilities, and other regular costs of operating the business.

Major Classes of Accounts

The last accounting equation given (Table 9-3) contains the five major classes of accounts used in both financial statements in Tables 9-1 and 9-2. The definition of each major account class and illustrative subaccounts included within each are:

- *Assets*: are resources with economic value for productive operations or with exchange value. Illustrative subaccounts are *current assets—cash, accounts receivable, inventories, short-term investments* (less than 1 year); *fixed or noncurrent assets* (longer than 1 year), i.e., land; building; equipment, long-term investments.

TABLE 9-3. BASIC ACCOUNTING EQUATIONS

Assets = Equity
where
Equity = Liabilities + Organizational Equity + Retained Earnings

Assets = Liabilities + Organizational Equity + Retained Earnings
where
Retained Earnings = Cumulative (Revenues − Expenses)

Assets = Liabilities + Organizational Equity + Revenues − Expenses

- *Liabilities:* are the amounts that the organization owes for services provided, materials purchased, repayments of funds borrowed, and/or operating expenses incurred but not yet paid.
- *Short-term liabilities:* are liabilities due to be paid within 1 year. Long-term liabilities are usually for funds obtained from the sale of bonds or from a bank and represent amounts to be paid within a time period more than 1 year from the date of the balance sheet.
- *Organization's equity:* represents the value of cash, building, and/or equipment provided when the business was established or when the business was expanded.
- *Revenues:* represent the amounts owed by persons and/or businesses that purchased services and/or goods from the organization. A not-for-profit organization distinguishes three types of revenues: *operating,* revenues received for services provided to patients; *other operating,* revenues received from programs that support patient care but are not directly involved in it, such as a gift shop; *nonoperating,* revenues received from sources other than current operations, such as nonrestricted donations, net sales of fixed assets. Illustrative patient revenue accounts are *inpatient, outpatient,* and *emergency room.*
- *Expenses:* are the costs paid and/or incurred for operating the business. Illustrative subaccounts are *wages, salaries, rent, heat, light, and power, and telephone.*

Double Entry Bookkeeping

The accounting department in recording all financial transactions, revenues earned and expenses paid, uses a system called double entry bookkeeping based on a chart of accounts. Every financial transaction is recorded in a journal under a specific account for a specific cost center, revenue center, or investment center. For example, the hospital purchases 60,000 aspirin tablets from a pharmaceutical company. The payment is recorded in the journal "drugs" account for the "pharmacy" cost center. Each organization may have a different chart of accounts and different cost, revenue, and investment centers.

Periodically, all journal entries are summarized into ledger accounts. Values for ledger accounts are used to prepare the balance sheet and the statement of revenues and expenses.

Double entry bookkeeping means *every* transaction is recorded in a *journal entry* affecting two or more accounts. The rationale is to create a checks and balances monetary system for financial recording. Notice the *two sides* of the balance sheet in Table 9-1 *total to the same amount.* Using double entry bookkeeping each major account in the financial statements is defined as being a debit (asset, expense) or credit (liability, equity, revenue) according to generally accepted accounting practices (GAAP). What is important is consistency and that every transaction is entered as a debit into one or more accounts and as a credit into one or more accounts so that the net effect is a balance. If all transactions are recorded properly, then the totals of the debit balances and the credit balances in the accounts will balance. Otherwise, a review of the transaction entries must be made to identify the error.

Table 9–4 presents a summary of the sequence of accounting activities that result in the financial statements of balance sheet and statement of revenues and expenses.

Nurse Administrators and the Chart of Accounts. The nurse executive wants to know—does the listing in the chart of accounts result in meaningful categories? A "good" chart of accounts assists an administrator in identifying financial problems in each department. The chart of accounts listing is the basis for "line items" in budgets. Thus, categories chosen are crucial for financial planning.

The middle and first line managers need training to use the chart of accounts in budgeting, reporting expenditures, and interpreting budget variances. They do not need to know double entry bookkeeping but they do need to know its basic ideas and when to call the accountant and what to ask for clarification.

Fiscal Period

One important concept in reading balance sheets and statement of revenues and expense is *fiscal period.* They are both historical documents and the dates used on each are important in understanding the information being conveyed in each statement. Note the date on the balance sheet is as of a specific date and on the statement of revenues and expenses for a specified time period (called fiscal or reporting period), usually 1 year (see Tables 9–1 and 9–2). Different reporting periods are used by different organizations and within organizations for different purposes. For many the fiscal year is not January to December. This is important to note if the time periods are the same when comparing financial statements for different organizations.

TABLE 9-4. SEQUENCE OF ACCOUNTING ACTIVITIES

Transaction

(↓)

Journal Entry

(↓)

Ledger Account

(↓)

Statement of Revenues and Expenses

(↓)

Balance Sheet

The *balance sheet* reports assets owned and the sources of funds to acquire these assets. It is used primarily for reporting the ownership status of the business. It is normally included in reports to external agencies and in any reports provided to community members that support the hospital through volunteer work or membership in a professional organization.

The *statement of revenues and expenses* is prepared whenever a balance sheet is prepared. It differs from the balance sheet in that it reports the results of operations in terms of revenues produced and expenses incurred. It is used primarily to establish the profitability of the activities in which the organization is engaged. It is normally included in the same reports as the balance sheet as these statements together provide the picture of how well the organization is doing in a financial sense.

Nurse executives are primarily interested in the statement of revenues and expenses as they are involved in activities that produce revenues and require the expenditure of funds that make it possible to obtain those revenues.

For Profit and Not-For-Profit Financial Statements

Increasingly health care agencies may be *for profit*, *not-for-profit*, or include both types of agencies within one corporate structure. These two types of organizations differ in several important ways.

The major accounts and subaccounts in the financial statements reflect how these two types of organizations differ in their sources of equity, sources of funds, and recording of revenues and deductions. These differences are shown in Table 9–5.

Not-for-profit organizations use fund accounting rather than corporate accounting. This is to recognize that these organizations are financed by funds that come from several sources but the providers of these funds do not obtain an ownership interest in the organization such as occurs when one buys stock in a profit organization.

Cash Versus Accrual Accounting

Small organizations may use cash accounting, that is, the organization records transactions that recognize revenues and expenses only when cash is received or paid. Most individuals handle their personal finances this way. It is less complex but does not record outstanding debts to be paid or monies due to be received.

Hospitals, as all larger organizations, use accrual accounting, which is more accurate for the fiscal period being reported. Under accrual accounting revenues are recorded as a transaction when earned without regard to when cash is received, and expenses are recorded as a transaction when incurred without regard to when cash payment is made. This carries out the "matching principle" for double entry bookkeeping, which is that all costs and expenses incurred in generating revenues must be recorded in the same reporting period (fiscal period) as the related revenues.

Accrual accounting requires a set of adjusting entries to be made at the end

TABLE 9-5. KEY DIFFERENCES BETWEEN PROFIT AND NOT-FOR-PROFIT ORGANIZATIONS

	Not-For-Profit	Profit
Source of equity	Community investment and Government investment and Endowments and Gifts	Single proprietorship: personal investment or partnership: personal investment or corporation: common or preferred stocks
Source of funds	Charges for products/services Private bonds Bank loans Gifts or endownment earnings Public financing in the form of industrial revenue bonds, general obligation bonds, etc.	Charges for products/services; private bonds; bank loans; gifts or endownment earnings,[a] common or preferred stock
Recording of revenues & deductions[b]	Revenues recorded at full value of charges even though some are never expected to be paid at that amount	Revenues recorded at the value of the sale made even though some will not be collected
	Deductibles include discounts for less than full charges paid by third payors; Medicare; Medicaid; uncollectible accounts (bad debts); indigent care patients; contractual allowances granted HMOs, PPOs, and other organizations	No deductibles are defined or recorded on the statement

[a]If the profit organization has a foundation that is recognized by the IRS as a 501 (C) 3 tax exempt foundation to receive these gifts or endowments they would be tax exempt to the contributor but earnings from their investment may be restricted to use for specified purposes that are acceptable under tax law.

[b]These revenues and deductibles are recorded on the income statement only but influence the organization's financial health through their impact on net income or excess of revenues over expenses, that is, the retained earnings for the organization as reported on the balance sheet.

of the fiscal period to reflect all revenues earned and expenses to be incurred. For example, wages due persons who have worked a period of time but their actual payday is after the end of the fiscal period are recorded for up to the last day of the fiscal period.

Cash Flow

It is important to know if your organization uses cash or accrual accounting when you interpret the financial statements. This is especially important when an accountant reports that the organization has a "cash flow" problem and certain expenditures need to be postponed temporarily.

For an organization using accrual accounting nurse executives need to keep in mind the difference between the flows of revenue and of cash. The flow of revenues is the amount of charges or sales over time that represents the flow of potential cash to be received from providing services or goods to a purchaser. On the other hand, cash flow represents the actual cash available for an organization to pay its bills.

An organization's statement of revenues and expenses may reflect an excess of income from revenues, and its balance sheet substantial potential cash owed to the organization by purchasers but simultaneously be experiencing cash flow problems and unable to pay its bills. In developing a business plan the nurse executive needs to include not only a proposed budget but also determine cash flow to assess the fiscal soundness of the proposal being made.

Talking With Financial Managers

By using these concepts and familiarizing themselves with financial management terms, nurse managers are better able to understand the connection between unit variances and the hospital's financial condition. Also they could seek with confidence the assistance of the hospital's accountant due to familiarity with basic accounting terms and procedures.

Nurse executives should use these concepts and terms in discussions with the hospital's financial officer, accounting department, and unit managers to plan innovations, decide when to reduce certain activities, and to contribute to formulating the executive team's strategic plan. In addition to these basic concepts and terms, executives also need to know common indicators used in financial analysis to justify fiscal decisions.

FINANCIAL ANALYSES

Ratios for Strategic Planning

The financial statements report what has happened financially to the organization for the fiscal period covered but give only limited insight into how well the organization is doing over time or in comparison with other health care organizations. These measures of financial performance are done through the use of financial ratio analysis.

The ratios that are computed in doing this analysis can be divided into five groups. The formula for each ratio is shown in Table 9–6. The information provided by each set and the ratios* included in each are:

- *Liquidity:* These indicate the extent to which short-term obligations can be met. The ratios include the current ratio, acid test ratio, days in accounts

---

*The ratios identified and the grouping into which each is placed is according to the Health Care Financial Management Association, as reported in their annual report of ratio values obtained from its analysis of financial statements from more than 1300 health care organizations.

TABLE 9-6. FORMULAS FOR FINANCIAL RATIOS

Liquidity Ratios

1. Current ratio = current assets/current liabilities
2. Acid test = cash + marketable securities/current liabilities
3. Days in accounts receivable = net patient accounts receivable × 365/net patient service revenues
4. Average payment period = current liabilities × 365/operating expenses – depreciation
5. Days cash on hand = (cash + marketable securities) × 365/operating expenses – depreciation
6. Quick ratio = cash + marketable securities + accounts receivable/current liabilities

Profitability Ratios

7. Return on equity = excess of revenues over expenses/fund balance
8. Return on total assets = excess of revenues over expenses/total assets
9. Operating margin = total operating revenues – operating expenses/total operating revenues
10. Nonoperating revenues = nonoperating revenues/excess of revenues over expenses
11. Discounts and allowances = deductions/gross patient services revenues
12. Mark-up = gross patient revenues + other operating revenues/operating expenses
13. Reported income index = excess of revenues over expenses/change in fund balance

Activity Ratios

14. Total asset turnover = total operating revenues/total assets
15. Current asset turnover = total operating revenues/current assets
16. Fixed asset turnover = total operating revenues/net fixed assets
17. Inventory turnover = total operating revenues/inventory

Leverage Ratios

18. Long-term debt to equity = long-term liabilities/fund balance
19. Equity financing ratio = fund balance/total assets
20. Cash flow to total debt = excess of revenues over expenses + depreciation/current liabilities + long-term debt
21. Fixed debt financing = long-term liabilities/net fixed assets
22. Times interest earned = excess of revenues over expenses + interest expense/interest expense
23. Debt service coverage = excess of revenues over expenses + depreciation + principal payment + interest expense/principal payment + interest expense

From Cleverley, WO., 1986, pp. 70, 71.

receivable, average payment period, days of cash on hand, and quick ratio.

- *Profitability:* These define the extent of net revenue and usually compares it with a given level of equity. The ratios include the return on equity (fund balance), return on total assets, operating margin, nonoperating revenue ratio, discounts and allowances ratio, mark-up, and reported income index.
- *Activity:* These measure the efficiency of an organization in using its assets. The ratios include the total asset turnover, current asset turnover, fixed asset turnover, and inventory turnover.
- *Leverage:* These describe the amount of financing from debt as compared

with that from equity. The ratios include long-term debt to equity, equity financing ratio, cash flow to total debt, fixed debt financing, times interest earned, and debt service coverage.

- *Other:* Each organization undoubtedly will compute certain ratios that have particular meaning for it which do not fit into one of the major groups described previously. Illustrative other ratios include the average age of plant, price-level adjusted depreciation, operating margin (price-level adjusted), and restricted equity.

To ascertain the financial health of an organization the ratio values for this year are compared with those of previous years to identify any trend changes in values and to a set of industry data such as provided in the annual reports from the *Health Care Financial Management Association* to compare their performance with their competitors. These comparisons should be done for each group of ratios, as a single ratio does not provide a complete picture of what is happening with respect to any given focus. From these comparisons conclusions about how the organization is doing financially can be developed. Keep in mind the chances for error in multiple calculations and the need for expert judgment in interpreting comparative data. Based on these conclusions the executive team then develops a set of recommendations as to what actions should be undertaken to preserve or improve the financial health of the organization.

Expanding or Adding New Services

When the nurse executive is planning to add a new service that will be revenue producing a set of *pro forma statements* for each of the first 3 to 5 years of operations should be developed. Pro forma statements are projected financial statements prepared using as their basis a set of assumptions about the operations of the new service as to levels of activity, capital and expense costs incurred for the service, anticipated revenues, planned growth, and any other items needed to describe the internal and external environment for that service. Sometimes three sets of assumptions are prepared—worst case, most optimistic case, and most probable case—with a set of pro forma statements developed for each set of assumptions. Some authors refer to this as scenario analysis.

The nurse executive should work closely with the chief financial officer in preparing these assumptions and their translation into the pro forma statements. The nurse executive probably has the best knowledge and judgment about the operating environment for the new service, whereas the chief financial officer understands better the translation of the assumptions into financial terms and how this new service fits into the present and future financial operations of the organization. Working together they should develop a set of pro forma statements that will represent an accurate forecast of the financial results if the new service is added.

These statements let the nurse executive know if the proposed new service will produce financial results that support its addition by meeting the financial performance standards used by that organization. Comparison of the best, worst, and probable sets of pro forma statements lets the nurse executive identify which assumption(s) appears to be most critical in determining the financial results. Thus, if the new service is offered, the activities represented by these critical assumptions should be carefully monitored as it is obvious their behavior will determine the operational success of the new service.

Cash Flow Analysis

The old saying, "money makes the world go round" applies to all health care organizations. In doing cash flow analysis one estimates for a defined future time period, usually in intervals of 1 month each, what cash will be coming into the organization from cash revenues, collections of accounts receivables, earnings from investments, and additional cash investment from one or more sources of funds for this organization, and what cash will be flowing out to pay expenses, repay borrowed funds, be used for investments, and be transferred into a restricted fund for a specified purpose. The analysis starts with a cash balance at the beginning of the month and after the transactions for the receipts and payments of cash for that month are detailed, a cash balance as of the end of the month is obtained. Assumptions as to time lag in collections of accounts receivables, payment of payables, returns on investments, and so on are made based on past experiences or on any changes made in operating procedures that will affect these activities. The accounting department usually prepares the cash flow analysis for use by the nurse executive.

From this analysis the nurse executive can learn when additional cash will be needed. Most organizations establish a minimum cash balance they wish to keep on hand at the end of each month to handle variations in the flows of receipts and payments. If the need for additional cash is seasonal or is of short duration an organization usually establishes a line of credit with its bank that will let it borrow the cash whenever needed up to the limit set by the line of credit. There is a small charge for having the protection of a line of credit and the interest charge for the amount and period of time for which the cash is borrowed.

This analysis may also help the nurse executive identify opportunities for changes in policies and practices that would reduce the need to borrow cash, or require a smaller amount to be kept on hand. Cash kept as cash produces no earnings for the organization. Thus, the chief financial officer will often use investments in government securities, such as treasury bills, to produce some earnings and also provide an immediate source of cash, because they can be sold within minutes whenever a need for cash should develop.

Working Capital Analyses

A major short-term concern for administrators and the Board of Trustees is to have sufficient working capital to pay operating expenses and make purchases to implement strategic plans. Net working capital is defined using this equation:

$$\text{Net working capital} = \text{Current assets} - \text{Current liabilities}$$

This represents the *net* funds you have available to handle the day-to-day operations of the business.* This is calculated as part of the statement of changes in fund balances, which is prepared simultaneously with the statement of revenues and expenses and balance sheet for each fiscal period.

What are the questions to be asked or the analyses to be made for each current asset and current liability account to analyze net working capital?

Current Assets

- Cash: *What is the flow of cash into and out of the business*? This is answered by doing a cash flow analysis as described previously. What is the minimum cash balance to be kept on hand and how is a temporary shortage or excess of cash handled? The choice includes consideration of the right combination of risk incurred, rate of return payment on investments, and readiness of access to the invested funds.
- Marketable securities: *Were the temporary cash excesses relative to cash needs invested and in what securities*? In selecting among the several alternative investments, management will need to balance the risk of possible loss of the amount invested in the security instrument, the yield earned, and the quickness by which the investment can be converted into cash. Alternative instruments include U.S. Treasury bills, certificates, notes (T-bills); prime commercial paper; negotiable certificates of deposit that have varying maturity dates; governmental notes; savings accounts; corporation stocks, notes, bonds, and certificates of deposits (CDs).
- Accounts receivables: *Are all bills prompt and accurate*? Monitor if all charges are recorded accurately in the bill provided to the patient, if bills are ready for the patients when the delivery of services is completed, and if bills to be paid by a third-party payor are rendered promptly. The results from monitoring these activities should establish if the first step in good management of accounts receivable is occurring.
  Do credit terms facilitate and enourage full payment? Identify credit terms for payment extended to patients or third-party payors. Monitor how promptly each class of payors pays. It makes little sense to extend credit terms that are very inconsistent with how payments are actually being made. Two analyses are to: (1) examine the cash flow analysis for the flow of cash from payment of accounts receivable and (2) age the accounts in terms of how long they have been carried on the books. These analyses should be done for each class of payor as differences could be important in understanding what is happening in terms of payment and in guiding management as to what corrective actions, if any, should be implemented.

---

*Current assets represent working capital as they are available for several uses in the organization, including payment of current liabilities. The term working capital, also, is frequently used to represent net working capital and to describe these analyses.

What collection procedures does the organization follow to assure collection of all accounts receivable? This involves examination of the several steps in the process—How frequently is contact made with the account payor? What statements are being made as to the potential penalty of continued delinquency? When is the account turned over to a collection agency? and What legal steps, if any, will be implemented, and when, to obtain collection of the account? The financial ratio for the number of days of accounts receivables are on the books indicates the relationship between the flow of revenues into the organization and their average conversion into cash.

- Inventories: *Are inventories current and sufficient?* For health care organizations the major concern in the management of inventories is to have the right supplies on hand when needed and in amounts that, when compared with their frequency of use, assure that the supplies are fresh. Analysis of special orders for specific supply items and of reports of supplies discarded because they are outdated or otherwise unusable help establish the adequacy and freshness of the inventory items. For nonperishable items management will also be interested in the relationship of the quantity on hand, the rate of usage, the quantities ordered, and any discounts in purchase price available if certain quantities are purchased.

Current Liabilities

- Accounts payable: *What credit terms are suppliers providing to us? Are we taking advantage of all discounts provided?* An organization should delay paying any bill until its due date so as to use its cash for its own operations. The only exception is to meet the requirements for any discount for prompt payment or purchase of a large quantity. Taking advantage of discounts usually give a rate of return on the money involved in the transaction that far exceeds the cost of borrowing an equal sum of money. For example, a cash discount of 2 percent if a bill is paid within 10 days represents an annual return of 35 percent.
- Accrued liabilities: *Are there any expenses for operations for which the organization has incurred a liability but has not paid it? Has the organization received payment for services it has not yet rendered?* As described earlier, by use of adjusting entries accounting records a liability, that is, a claim against the assets, in both of these situations.
- Short-term liabilities: *Is the organization required by terms of the borrowing agreement to pay off within 1 year some or all of the amount borrowed?* If such a repayment requirement as to time period exists it is a short-term liability. An organization's failure to meet this repayment requirement when due jeopardizes its credit standing, which can affect its ability to borrow additional funds in the future *and* the rate of interest to be paid for those borrowed funds. In the extreme case, creditors could take legal action that could force the organization into bankruptcy.

After examining each current asset and current liability account and analyzing why it has changed, the administrator can institute changes to correct the identified problems.

The next step is to examine changes in net working capital and the amounts of current assets and liabilities. An increase in net working capital from one fiscal period to the next alerts the administrator to see how the balance and amounts of current assets and liabilities have changed. Current assets may increase due to an excess of revenues over expenses for that period, reporting of a depreciation expense for the period (appearing as a source of new funds because it requires no actual expenditure of cash funds), sale of bonds, direct receipt of unrestricted funds, earnings from endowments, or a transfer of funds from restricted funds (restricted funds are not current assets because how they can be spent is delimited).

A decrease in current assets may be due to purchase of additional fixed assets with current funds, renovation of buildings or major equipment, establishment of and transfer of current assets into new restricted funds for specific purposes such as a future replacement of existing buildings or equipment, a reduction in revenues or an increase in expenses.

Similar changes may occur in current liabilities changing the balance between the two or offsetting the changes in current *assets*.

COST CONCEPTS AND CONTROLS

Within the last few years cost control has become much more important for health care organizations as the competitive environment within which they operate has undergone significant changes. Four key changes are: a change in reimbursement basis for Medicare from a cost-based reimbursement to a prospective payment system (PPS) based on diagnosis-related groups (DRGs); private industry directly negotiating with health care organizations for volume discounts; the entry of entrepreneurs into the health care market who frequently target the more profitable activities for their ventures; and the possible disappearance of certificate of need (CON) laws or their significant modification, which will remove the franchise protection an organization received when granted permission to add a service.

To respond to this need for better cost controls administrators must develop policies and procedures that do indeed keep costs in line with operating revenues. There are two parts to a cost control program. One is the budgeting process and the use of the annual budgets to set standards for individual costs for each budgeted activity. These topics are discussed in a later section of this chapter. Another is for the administrators to understand and use properly the concepts that describe different types of cost behavior.

A nurse executive and a unit manager occupy important roles in both parts of a cost control program because they have primary responsibility for one area of major costs in any health care organization—nursing salaries. Unit managers discharge their responsibility in managing the day-to-day operations of their units and nurse executives discharge theirs by participating in top management decisions of adding, deleting, contracting, or expanding particular service activities.

Table 9–7 groups the different cost concepts into four categories: asset valuation, managerial control, decision making, and volume. The concepts in each category focus on a particular set of problems with which management must deal.

Asset Valuation

Management needs an accurate valuation of the organization's assets to know if the results of operations are increasing the value of the assets and to have a basis for persuading investors to provide additional capital when needed.

Historical/Replacement. These concepts are concerned with the valuation of the fixed assets on the balance sheet. Use of a historical basis means the fixed assets are valued at their purchase price and this value is used when computing the depreciation expense incurred from operations. Through the process of charging depreciation expense against operations and accumulating a depreciation reserve an organization retains asset values in the business that can be used for future replacement of a fixed asset. When the cost of a new fixed asset is increasing due to inflation, depreciation will not offset replacement cost. When this occurs the additional funds needed for the actual replacement of the fixed asset

TABLE 9–7. CATEGORIES OF COST CONCEPTS

Asset Valuation
    Historical/replacement
    Cash/accrual

Managerial Control
    Controllable/noncontrollable
    Direct/indirect
    Committed/noncommitted
    Budget/actual

Decision Making
    Sunk costs
    Incremental costs
    Opportunity costs
    Avoidable or escapable costs

Volume
    Fixed costs
    Variable costs
    Semifixed or semivariable costs
    Step costs

Adapted from Neumann, Suver, and Zelman, 1984, p. 170.

must be obtained from the excess of revenues over expenses kept as retained earnings and/or an infusion of additional capital.

Cash/Accrucal. These concepts affect when the cost of using a fixed asset is recognized on the statement of revenues and expenses. With cash accounting its cost is recorded when the expediture is made. With accrual accounting its cost is recognized as the asset used up in producing goods or services. The latter basis is used more frequently because it records on the balance sheets within the same fiscal period both the cost of producing revenues and the revenues earned.

Managerial Control

These cost concepts are used by administrators in their management of costs associated with operations.

Controllable/Noncontrollable. When evaluating the performance of a unit manager as to how well the operating costs for that unit were managed during the fiscal period the nurse executive must consider which costs the unit manager can control and which ones are outside of the manager's control. For example, if the unit manager determines the scheduling of nursing coverage and the use of agency nurses that cost is considered to be controllable. On the other hand, the unit manager does not determine raises in nursing salaries; therefore, this would be a noncontrollable cost.

Direct/Indirect. Direct costs are those costs that can be traced to a specific unit or activity that incurred the cost, whereas indirect costs are shared by or common to two or more units or activities. These concepts are used when administrators are determining if the revenues generated by a given unit or activity are sufficient to cover its costs. A particular cost may be a direct cost for one analysis and an indirect cost for another. For example, the operating cost of the MRI machine is a direct cost of the radiology department, but an indirect cost for each of the departments whose patients obtain a MRI scan. For these latter departments the administrators must use a basis for allocating the MRI costs to the using department, which is accepted as providing a good estimate.

Committed/Noncommitted Costs. These concepts are used in the budgeting process to define which costs have been committed to a particular activity (nurses salaries) or to the acquisition of certain assets (supplies; piece of equipment). Normally, certain funds will be left uncommitted to be available to cover fluctuations in operations, or an unanticipated acquisition or repair of fixed assets. These may also be referred to as discretionary funds.

Budgeted/Actual. These concepts are used as an integral part of the budgeting process. Budgeted costs are the operating costs planned for the next fiscal period given the assumptions of levels of activity whereas the actual costs are those actually incurred from the operations. A comparison of the actual costs to the budgeted costs is frequently used by administrators to determine the quality of performance at each level of the organization. Large variances from the budgeted amounts are a signal that the organization may be in serious trouble.

Decision Making

The cost concepts in the decision making category are used by administrators in making decisions about adding, deleting, or modifying a service. This involves a comparison of alternative uses of resources. A subgroup of these decisions are called make-or-buy decisions.

Sunk Costs. This recognizes that a cost incurred cannot be undone and should not be considered when deciding whether to delete a service. Frequently, these are costs associated with the replacement of a fixed asset. For example, a health care organization should not decide to continue to use its present computerized billing system solely because it owns it. Its purchase was a sunk cost that should not be "charged" in a replacement decision.

Incremental Costs. These are added costs that occur when a complementary service is added or represent the additional cost for one alternative as compared to another alternative. The use of the incremental costs concept in decisions recognizes only the additional costs the new service or alternative will incur and does not consider other costs that are already present in the organization, such as building costs, top management salaries, that will not increase with the addition of the new service. It is expected that the projected revenues for any new service minus the incremental costs will provide a contribution to the general overhead of the organization and to its excess of revenues over expenses.

Opportunity Costs. These costs are the value of the benefits foregone because the organization invested a set of resources in one new service and not in another. Thus, when one is evaluating what the new service will contribute to the organization both the operating costs and the opportunity costs will be deducted from the projected revenues to arrive at the contribution this use of resources will make to the organization. Then management can focus on the question—Is this contribution sufficiently large enough to support the risk associated with this investment of resources? Once the resources are invested they are not available for another use.

Avoidable or Escapable Costs. This cost concept is used in decisions to delete a service. It recognizes that not all costs will be reduced or saved if a given service is discontinued. If an organization needs to reduce its total costs it needs to identify those services that will in fact result in a reduction of costs when deleted. In such decisions management must also recognize that the contribution from that service to the general overhead and the excess of revenues over expenses for the organization will also be lost.

Volume

Volume concepts deal with the behavior of costs as the volume of operations changes. In examining cost behavior with respect to changes in volume the nurse executive must keep in mind that these observed behaviors only hold true for a relevant range of volumes and a specific period of time.

Fixed Costs. These are costs that do not change with a change in volume of operations.

Variable Costs. These are costs that do change in a definite relationship with a change in volume of operations.

Semifixed or Semivariable Costs. These are costs that are mixed as to how they react to changes in volume, partially fixed and partially variable. The labeling of these costs as semifixed or semivariable reflects which cost element is dominant.

Step Costs. These describe costs that are fixed to a certain volume level and then increase by a fixed amount when this volume level is exceeded. An example of a step cost is the increase in salary costs from the addition of another nurse to a unit as the patient load increases above a particular level.

These cost concepts for the category of volume are used in doing break-even analysis to answer the question—What volume in units or revenues is needed to equal the total costs of producing that volume? The break-even volume is the number of units where total revenues equals total costs (total fixed costs plus total variable costs). If the organization has established some level of expected dollar or rate of return for any new venture this amount is also included as part of the total costs. An example is provided in Table 9–8.

The real value of break-even analysis is that it forces the nurse executive to understand what costs are involved in providing the new service, their relationship to changes in volume, and what volume is needed to achieve a break-even volume. After doing the break-even analysis the management question then becomes—Will the organization achieve this volume? If management has done the break-even analysis carefully it can have confidence its answer to this question is accurate as to what would happen if the new service was indeed instituted.

An adaptation of break-even analysis can be used by nurse executives to see what volume changes are needed, that is, what new volume level, to maintain the same amount of excess of revenues over expenses if a contractual allowance is provided to a HMO or a PPO in exchange for your organization becoming a preferred provider to their members. Also, if an organization is not achieving a positive excess of revenues over expenses it may wish to do a break-even analysis to see what volume is needed to achieve break-even, or the specific dollar amount of excess of revenues over expenses above break-even desired.

TABLE 9-8. BREAK-EVEN ANALYSIS AT THE GOODHEALTH CLINIC

The Goodhealth clinic plans to provide clinical services in its clinic as well as an in-home visitation service. Staff for the clinic includes two physicians and two RNs. The one LPN does the in-home visitation service.

These are the operating assumptions management made to have a basis to determine the volume needed for a break-even operation and to earn an excess of revenues over expenses equal to 4% of gross revenues.

1. The expected revenue per visit is $45 for a clinic visit and $20 for an in-home visit.
2. The annual salaries are $30,000 for each RN, $65,000 for each employed physician, and $21,000, for the LPN.
3. The telephone charge is $23.50 per line per month. There are two lines for the clinic and one line for the in-home service.
4. The LPN is paid $0.21 per mile traveled and it is assumed each patient visit requires 8 miles of travel.
5. The rent is $2000 per month.
6. The cost for supplies is $200 per month plus $3.50 per patient visit for the clinic and $1.00 per in-home visit.
7. The laundry cost for the clinic is $3.00 per patient visit.
8. The custodian works 20 hours per week to clean the clinic and is paid $7.50 per hour.
9. Depreciation expense for medical and office equipment used in the clinic is computed by use of the straight-line method.

The steps for completing the break-even analysis demonstrated below are:

1. Determine the total costs for the time period for which you wish to determine the volume needed to achieve break-even or a volume that results in an established dollar amount of excess of revenues over expenses;
2. Identify each cost as fixed, variable, or semifixed or semivariable;
3. Determine the total fixed costs, the unit variable cost, and the revenue per unit;
4. Determine the break-even volume and/or the volume needed to achieve a given level of excess of revenues over expenses.

	In-home		Clinic	
	Fixed costs	Unit variable costs	Fixed costs	Unit variable costs
Employed physicians			$130,000	
RN-salaries			60,000	
LPN-salary	$ 21,000			
Telephone	282		564	
Rent			24,000	
Supplies		$ 1.00	2,400	$ 3.50
Laundry				3.00
Custodial services			7,800	
Mileage		1.68		
Depreciation			10,000	
Totals	$ 21,282	$ 2.68	$234,764	$ 6.50

A. Break-even volumes

In-home:

$$\$20x = \$21,282 + \$2.68x$$
$$(\$20 - 2.68)x = \$21,282$$
$$\$17.32x = \$21,282$$
$$x = 1229 \text{ visits}$$

Clinic:

$$\$45x = \$234,764 + \$6.50x$$
$$(45 - 6.50x = \$234,764$$
$$\$38.50x = \$234,764$$
$$x = 6098 \text{ visits}$$

B. Volume needed to achieve an excess of revenues over expenses = 4% of gross revenues

In-home:

$$\$20x = (21,282 + \$2.68x) + (.04)(\$20x)$$
$$\$20 = \$21,282 + \$2.68x + \$.80x$$
$$(\$20 - \$3.48)x = \$21,282$$
$$\$16.52x = \$21,282$$
$$x = 1288 \text{ visits}$$

Clinic:

$$\$45x = (\$234,764 + \$6.50x) + (.04)(\$45x)$$
$$\$45x = \$234,764 + \$6.50x + \$1.80x$$
$$(\$45 - \$8.30)x = \$234,764$$
$$\$36.70x = \$234,764$$
$$x = 6397 \text{ visits}$$

C. This may be graphically displayed

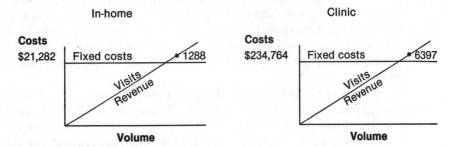

Revenues and costs intersect where revenues = expenses. Point shown is 4% excess.

BUDGETING

Purposes and Types

The activity of budgeting for the next fiscal year contributes significantly to two functions for an organization: planning and control. For planning it represents the financial definition of an organization's plans and the articulation of specific resource allocations. For control it establishes the financial expectations of the organization to which actual performance is compared. Control is accomplished at the start of the fiscal period when management determines if achievement of the financial expectations set forth in the budget will enable the organization to accomplish the goals and objectives established by its planning process. It is also accomplished during and at the end of the fiscal period when actual perform-ance is compared with the expectations set forth in the budget, which are treated as standards.

Three different budgets are prepared for each fiscal period: operating, capi-tal, and cash. The *operating budget* forecasts revenues, expenses, and excess of revenues over expenses. The *capital budget* establishes what expenditures will be made for plant and equipment. It usually covers a period of several years so that the organization will know what total funds it will need to finance these capital expenditures and the expected sources of these funds (see Table 9–5). When doing the capital budget for the next fiscal period the appropriate elements of the long-term capital budget are used. The *cash budget* forecasts cash receipts and cash payments for the fiscal period. In preparing these three budgets many of the concepts discussed previously are used.

Process

The preparation of these budgets requires management to provide detailed op-erating guidelines, participation by many individuals, and an iterative process of submission, review, and adjustments. Thus, management should establish a *timetable* that sets forth the sequence of activities to be followed in preparing the budgets and the *due dates* for each step of the budget preparation process. This timetable must also provide sufficient time for everything to be done. This varies for each organization but usually requires the process to start 4 to 6 months before the date the budgets are to be submitted to the Board of Trustees for its approval.

It should be stressed that the preparation of next year's budgets begins at the submission of this year's budgets. To prepare for the budgeting process for the next fiscal period management should review carefully the mission state-ment, the goals and objectives set for the organization, and the strategic plans and programs that have been established to achieve these goals and objectives. Preparation also includes a careful review of the changes that have occurred, are occurring, or will occur in the internal environment and the external environ-ment. Finally, data on how current operations compare with the budgets set for the current fiscal period should be gathered and analyzed. With this background preparation the management of the organization is now ready to begin the pro-cess of preparing the budgets for the next fiscal period.

Before beginning the actual task of developing the budgets management should decide on the basic approach for the budget process. What type and amount of participation will persons at each level of the organization have? Will they be expected to approach the budget preparation task as making *incremental* adjustments to the current year's budget, or to prepare a *zero-based budget* as if each activity was new to the organization?

There is no preferred basic approach, but significant participation by per-sons at all levels of the organization utilizes the expertise they have and in-creases their commitment to the final budget. One must recognize that the cur-rent year's budget and how well actual performance is matching that budget will be considered by everyone. It is, therefore, desirable to establish the expectation that all budget items will be examined with the attitude espoused in the zero-based budget approach—Is this item needed and if yes, at what level of expenditure?

Based on the results of the reviews of the environments and current operations described previously management prepares operating guidelines that will be used by all persons involved in preparing the budgets for the next fiscal year. These guidelines include statements in three areas:

1. *Operating decisions* made such as salary increases; projected change in total employment; adjustments in rates charged; addition, deletion, or modification of services or products offered.
2. *Assumptions about the external environment* stated in terms of their anticipated financial impact from the effect of the projected level of reimbursement by third-party payors including Medicare and contractual allowances to be given to preferred providers; impact of changes in activities by competitors such as establishing more outpatient clinics, urgent care centers, or adding new services to their hospital with the anticipated modification of the CON laws on gross revenues.
3. *Assumptions about operations* such as average length of stay for patients, number of total patient visits, expected changes in level of demand for particular services or products.

Once management has developed the initial statement of these guidelines, they should be discussed with all key persons in the budget preparation process. When there is some consensus on the guidelines these should be presented to the Board of Trustees (or Directors), or an appropriate group from the Board, for their review and acceptance. It is desirable to have this review and acceptance as the guidelines are important parameters within which the final budgets will be prepared and the Board must approve the budgets before they can be implemented.

When the task of preparing the guidelines is completed the actual work of preparing the detailed budgets within these guidelines begins. How this process is done can range from the financial people preparing budgets that are given to the various operating units for their review and comment, to having each operating unit submit a proposed budget. To gain the benefits of participation as described it is suggested that each operating unit be asked to submit a proposed budget. This starts an iterative process of submission, review, and adjustments between the operating unit and management until the final budgets are established. At this point the budgets are presented to the Board for their approval and to any outside agencies that have the right to review the budget because of state or local laws, or lease or loan agreements. Once these approval and review activities are completed the organization has its budgets for the next fiscal period.

Budgets as Standards

During the fiscal period the budgets serve two functions. They direct most of the decisions to be made and provide several standards by which to judge the performance of each operating unit and the organization as a whole. Even though management tries to anticipate fully the decisions and activities that have budget impact, it must provide some contingency funds in the operating budget for those unexpected situations that will arise. One can judge the quality of the budget preparation process by the number of these unexpected situations that arise and answering the question of how reasonable it is to expect management to have anticipated each of these unexpected situations in the budgeting process.

Perhaps the major function of the budget is to set performance standards by which to evaluate each operating unit and the total organization for the fiscal period to date. This evaluation is done by computing the *variance* for each budget item, that is, actual value minus budget value. In one sense all variances are unfavorable as actual performance does not equal budget. On the other hand, if actual revenues exceed budgeted revenues, or budgeted expenses exceed actual expenses, management would consider these to be favorable occurrences. Usually further analysis is made of these variances to determine if they occur as the result of changes in volume expected, average revenues received per patient visit, or the efficiency of personnel used. Once these detailed variances are known management must decide which variances represent conditions over which the responsible nurse administrator has some control and thus are ones for which he or she can be held responsible. Table 9–9 demonstrates the computation and evaluation of budget variances.

The above discussion has assumed *static budgets (fixed budgets)* that were not changed whenever any significant changes occurred in the environments described by the guidelines used as parameters for preparing these budgets. Given the rapid changes occurring in the health care field more organizations are now using flexible budgets in which adjustments are made to the budgets whenever these significant changes occur. The use of *flexible budgets* also requires that the relationships of a change in a particular guideline value to each budget item be known. With computers it is now easier to make the adjustments required for flexible budgeting. Because the budget serves as an operating standard against which to measure actual performance, it is essential that management, when using flexible budgets, only make changes in the budgets whenever a truly significant change in operating conditions occurs over which the nurse executive responsible for those budgets had no control. This is critical because the budgets must still be accepted as setting the standards against which evaluation of actual performance occurs.

Whether using static or flexible budgets management must examine carefully the results of the variance analyses to see if certain corrective actions should be undertaken that would bring future actual performance closer to that budgeted. If flexible budgets are correctly used, the explanation that the variances occurred because of conditions beyond the control of nurse executives has been

TABLE 9-9. ANALYSIS OF BUDGET VARIANCES AT GOODHEALTH CLINIC

	Budget	Actual	Total	Variances Price	Volume
Revenue					
Patient visits	$278,280	$262,773	($15,507)	($12,222)	($3,285)
Expenses					
Employed physicians	$130,000	$130,000			
RN-salaries	60,000	65,000	$ 5,000	$ 5,000	
Telephone	564	591	27	27	
Rent	24,000	24,000			
Supplies	24,044	25,316	1,272	1,528	$ (256)
Laundry	18,552	18,700	148	367	(219)
Custodian services	7,800	7,800			
Depreciation	10,000	10,000			
Totals	$274,960	$281,407	$ 6,447	$ 6,922	$ (475)
Excess of revenues over expenses	$ 3,320	$(18,634)	($21,954)	($19,144)	($2,810)

These facts were used by management in completing the variance analysis for the patient visits to the Goodhealth Clinic for the past year.

1. In determining the budgeted revenues it was estimated there would be 6184 visits at an average charge of $45 per visit. Analysis of the records show that there were 6111 actual visits at an average charge of $43.
2. Each of the two RNs was given an annual salary increase of $2,500, on July 1.
3. As of April 1 this year the monthly charge for each telephone line increased from $23.50 to $25.00 per line. The clinic uses two lines.
4. The cost of supplies was budgeted at the rate of $200 per month plus $3.50 per patient visit to the clinic. Analysis of the records shows that the variable cost of supplies per patient visit last year was $3.75.
5. Laundry was budgeted at the rate of $3.00 per clinic patient visit. Analysis of the records for the past year shows that the average cost for laundry per patient visit was $3.06.

removed. The executives know they are responsible to undertake corrective action for the amount and type of each variance.

Nurses with this knowledge understand their responsibility in the budgeting process and why what they do is important to the financial viability of the organization. Responsibility for the continued financial viability of the organization must share importance equal to the quality of care nurses give to their patients. With the present competitive conditions in the health care field nurses can no longer minimize this responsibility.

BIOGRAPHICAL SKETCH

Dr Lloyd M. DeBoer is Special Assistant to the President for Community Relations and Emeritus Dean of the School of Business Administration at George Mason University. He served as the first Dean of the school for 9 years during which time enrollment in the school grew from slightly more than 1500 to over 3600. The school had both undergraduate and graduate programs. He has served as a trustee of the Fairfax Hospital System for 9 years and as Chairman of its Board since 1983. This not-for-profit system has four hospitals with over 1200 beds, and has expanded to include other not-for-profit ventures—two nursing homes, home care, and several for-profit enterprises including seven urgent care centers and a durable medical equipment company.

SUGGESTED READINGS

Nurse Executive: Agency-wide Financial Management

Berman, H.J., & Weeks, L.E. (1982). *The Financial Management of Hospitals.* Ann Arbor: University of Michigan Health Administration Press.

Cleverly, W.O. (1986). *Essentials of Health Care Finance,* 2nd ed. Rockville, MD: Aspen Systems Corp.

Gillman, T.A. (1985). Hospitals recognize need to install or improve cost accounting systems. *Hospital Financial Management, 39* (11), 86–89.

J.K. Lasser Institute. (1984). *How To Read A Financial Statement.* New York: Simon & Schuster, Inc.

Mark, B.A., & Smith, H.L. (1987). *Essentials of Finance in Nursing.* Rockville, MD: Aspen Publishers Inc.

Middle Manager: Unit Budgeting, Staffing, and Control

Cushman, M.J. (1984). Program budgeting in home care agencies. *Nursing Economics, 2* (6), 409–412.

Finkler, S.A. (1984). *Budgeting Concepts for Nurse Managers.* Orlando, FL: Grune & Stratton, Inc.

Finkler, S.A. (1984). Electronic spreadsheets and budgeting: A case study. *Nursing Economics, 2* (3), 166–174.

Hoffman, F.M. (1984). *Financial Management for Nurse Managers.* East Norwalk, CT: Appleton-Century-Crofts.

Hoffman, F.M. Monthly column on financial management, in *Journal of Nursing Administration.*

Porter-O'Grady, T. (1987). *Nursing Finance.* Rockville, MD: Aspen Systems Inc.

Cost

Curtin, L. (1983). Determining costs of nursing services per DRG. *Nursing Management, 14* (4), 16–20.

Kirk, R. (1987). *Identifying Costs and Pricing Nursing Services—Practical Management Tools.* Rockville, MD: Aspen Publishers, Inc.

Shaffer, F.A. (Ed.). (1985). *Costing Out Nursing: Pricing Our Product.* New York: National League for Nursing.

Sources of Revenues

Averill, R.F., Kalison, M.J., Sparrow, D.A., & Owens, T.R. (1984). How hospital managers should respond to PPS. *Healthcare Financial Management, 38* (3), 72–74, 76, 82, 84.

Azarnoff, M. (1985). State, local governments scramble to find ways to pay for indigent care. *Modern Healthcare, 15* (1), 65.

Eastaugh, S.R. (1987). *Financing health care: Economic efficiency and equity.* Dover, MA: Auburn House Publishing Co.

Glaser, W.A. (1987). *Paying the hospital.* San Francisco: Jossey Bass, Inc.

REFERENCES

Cleverley, W.O. (1986). *Hospital Industry Analysis Report 1981–85.* Oakbrook, IL: Healthcare Financial Management Association.

Neumann, B.R., Suver, J.O., & Zelman, W.M. (1984). *Financial management: Concepts and applications for health care providers.* Owings Mills, MD: National Health Publishing, Rynd Communications.

CASE 9-1

Nursing Assuming Financial Control in a Tertiary Hospital

Gertrude L. Rodgers
Joyce Richardson

In reviewing the changes in nursing administration at Fairfax Hospital since 1980, a critical path emerges that is, we believe, representative of the entire health care industry. In 1980, the hospital was a 656-bed, suburban community, teaching hospital with inpatient and ER services. Management was organized with a Corporate Board of Directors, Hospital Administrator, and two parallel, separate divisions, business and patient care. The critical mission was to provide health care to the community as a public service. The major focus was on clinical issues; the finance and business offices were seen as ancillary. The financial office prepared and monitored budgets, arranged financing, and collected monies; the financial health of the hospital was its responsibility. The nursing office recruited, selected, and scheduled nurses and monitored the quality of nursing care; the clinical practice of nursing was the primary focus. The single fiscal responsibility of the nursing office was efficient use of personnel and supplies within its alloted budget.

Today, Fairfax Hospital is the flagship teaching hospital for INOVA, a Vir-

Note: This article was prepared on the authors' personal time and was not part of Joyce Richardson's official responsibilities with nor should it be attributed to the U.S. Army.

ginia Corporation, INOVA is a vertically and horizonally integrated health system comprising services that range from heart transplants to durable medical devices. Fairfax Hospital today continues as a 656-bed facility and is recognized especially for its centers of excellence in maternal and child health and cardiovascular surgery. Sophistication in management has grown along with sophistication in medical and health care. Restructuring of administration has decentralized many responsibilities, integrated clinical and business accountability, and expanded nursing's management focus from purely operational to also include strategic and tactical administration. Competency in business practice is a sine qua non of all nursing managers throughout the hospital. Quality care is the final measure of success. Nursing administration has been catapulted to levels of managerial and financial competency that they would have never thought possible or desirable in 1980.

How has the nursing division acquired the business skills to assume financial accountability? It has been a gradual process, requiring development of new skills and reporting systems at every level within the hospital and the nursing division. Financial management simultaneously became decentralized with data processing. Major training programs had to be designed and implemented. There has been a repetitive cycle of determining needs, designing means, training users, reinforcing and implementing changes, and refining the systems based on evaluations and changing needs.

The active involvement of nursing in the financial management of Fairfax Hospital has been an iterative process. We began by realizing the importance of nurturing a close relationship between nursing and accounting, data processing, finance, and top management. One long-term goal was to become an active partner in shaping budget assumptions, this made vital sense as nursing practice and patient services are virtually interwined. Before this goal could be achieved we needed to increase financial management credibility of the nursing office by visibly contributing to improve the budget process. We chose as our first move a system to collect evidence to predict the staffing needs throughout the hospital.

Initially, there was no system to review or attract resources or determine manpower needs. In addition, there was no patient classification system to determine hours of patient care or substantiate patient acuity. A system was needed to predict staffing needs and to ensure a consistent workforce. Over the years, we have made three significant changes to achieve this goal: (1) redesign recruitment, (2) establish accurate manpower predictors, and (3) restructure responsibilities of line staff and operational positions. These areas of change were critical. It is worthwhile to examine each further.

Redesign Recruitment

The first area of concern was measuring and controlling the rate of nursing turnover. In 1980, monthly turnover rates ranged from 29 to 32 percent. This high rate, although not unusual for a hospital, was unacceptable to top nursing administration. Stabilization of a lower rate was needed. Initially, recruitment, selection, and termination were done by nursing personnel without specialized education. The nurse recruiter received applicants on a walk-in basis through the use of recruitment ads in local newspapers. It was hoped that a nurse with specialized education could design and implement a more effective process. The decision was made to change the nurse recruiter position, which led to discussions of what educational qualifications and experience were needed and what responsibilities should be expected.

There was consensus that it was important that the nurse recruiter have a positive image representing the hospital and be able to analyze problems and design systems to solve them. She had to be able to balance the needs of the job applicants and nursing units, which would necessitate excellent communication skills. She needed to follow up nurse applicants to sense the levels of job satisfaction in the actual work environment. The nurse recruiter would work more closely with the high turnover units and concentrate recruitment efforts in those areas.

Once hired, the first priority for the nurse recruiter would be to design a system to anticipate vacancies. At that time, there was a time lag between termination and notification by the nursing office. The other two major priorities identified were: (1) identification of units likely to have high turnover and (2) involvement of nurse coordinators in recruitment, selection, and retention. By 1988 these priorities were met, thereby reducing the turnover rate to about 17 percent annually. The units most likely to have high turnover were medical units and the ICUs. One strategy the recruiter worked out with the nurses was to develop a program of internal recruitment. For the ICUs this involved the identification of staff nurses who had an interest in critical care and then providing an educational program for critical care preparation. The system we designed to anticipate vacancies included a variety of management reports. These are done on accounting periods and provide us with the capability for tracking vacancies.

A fully staffed office of Nursing Recruitment is now in operation. It works closely with the nursing administrators. Further, the nurse resource committee has been established, consisting of management, staff RNs, and the recruitment personnel. The members jointly evaluate recruitment needs and improve retention rates. The nurse resource committee is interested in the sensitive areas of nurse concerns and the treatment of the nurses in practice. This open forum permits creative responses to improving the work environment. Nurse coordinators now interview each potential applicant for their units. The nurse coordinators must include recruitment and retention activities in their yearly goals.

To meet our future needs and to control turnover the nurse recruiter developed new marketing skills and implemented them to gain a competitive advantage. The first step was to recognize and describe the competition, that is, hospitals that provided comparable services and educational programs in the Capital area. The nurse recruiter conducts a semiannual survey of salary–benefits among competing institutions and actively participates in the Metropolitan Area Nurse Recruiters Association. An extensive ''exit interview'' format is followed to glean factual updates of the market place and to spot trends useful for recruitment. Recent findings included salary, benefits, flexible working hours, awards and recognition, educational opportunities, work environment, nurse–physician relationships, and organizational status. Changes have been instituted to make our hospital more attractive to potential nurse applicants. Various committees and programs have been established to address these important factors. One example of improvement was establishment of the five level Clinical Ladder program to recognize clinical professional excellence. Each of the levels has a discrete job title and job requirement. Nurse coordinators diligently and effectively work with staff to plan career paths and to promote consistent achievements.

Another improvement was establishment of the collaborative practice committee, whose members include medical staff and various levels of nursing personnel, to review patient care and practice issues common to nursing and medicine. The objective is to develop stronger communication among medical staff members and primary nurses so that the patient may be the recipient of the best care possible.

Other programs developed to increase nurse job satisfaction focused on enhancement of educational programs. Plans were put in place to ease the transition of nurses to academic settings to respond to their needs for advanced education. Ongoing internal educational programs were also developed to enhance nurses career orientation with all-day workshops and conferences that involved a variety of nationally known speakers.

Exit interviews identified flexibility of hours of work as another important factor in job satisfaction. In response, staggering of shifts and implementation of flexible work hours to include 10- and 12-hour shifts was developed. Nurse coordinators worked more closely with staff to clarify their transportation, child care, and personal needs as they effect scheduling of work time. It was found that greater flexibility not only met the employee's needs but also contributed to better work flow. Exit interviews continue to be an excellent source of ideas for innovation.

Establish Accurate Manpower Predictors

With a centralized recruitment process in place, our concentration shifted to daily staffing problems. Objective data were lacking to support and justify staffing levels. At about the same time the hospital had begun to automate billing and nursing administration had acquired its own personal computer work stations. Position control, recruitment, and retention statistics were one of the first systems nursing automated. Our next step was computerized scheduling and manpower need determination. We again went through a process of need determination, means design, training of users, reinforcement of change and refinement.

The Nurse Executive Team while studying available management software products realized our manual prototype patient classification system was woefully inadequate. Scheduling software for the new computer system were chosen and customized. The next step was to outline what features we wanted in a patient classification system. The features are incorporated in the following decision grid (Fig. 9–1). These were the criteria on which presenting vendors were evaluated.

A request for proposals (RFP) was designed and sent to potential systems software vendors. This included a listing of desired features. The *proposal rating form* was the instrument used to select the best fit among those responding to the RFP. The software selected was quickly "Beta" tested (validated for this hospital) and subsequently implemented by a pilot unit followed by the medical–surgical and obstetrics units. Implementation then expanded to CCU, NICU, pediatrics, and psychiatry. There is now fully adequate and timely acuity data from our patient classification used to predict nursing schedules and to substantiate request for changes in manpower.

The training necessary to support the implementation of this program is extensive and requires continuous surveillance and support by the nursing administrators. Classes were presented to nurse coordinators on scheduling and once they were knowledgeable of the scheduling system, all personnel were educated on the patient classification system. This is now a continuous program for all new personnel entering the nursing division. As a means of reinforcement, periodic reliability checks are done to evaluate the results achieved from the patient classification system and a budget analysis for scheduling is done to verify the relationship between acuity and staffing.

It took months of serious work by the Director of Nursing Management Systems to design spreadsheets and aggregate report forms to refine the system so that nursing coordinators would have timely, easy to read, updates on actual, recommended, and budgeted staffing. Today, the nursing coordinators wonder how they explained budget variances and justified requests to change manpower levels before they had these reports.

Restructure Responsibilities

Simultaneously, with actions to decrease turnover and implement an acuity patient classification system for predicting staffing needs, the nursing office along with the rest of the hospital, restructured to decentralize management. A key strategy by the nursing office was the creation of a new position: Director of Nursing Management Systems. The nursing division needed its own financial and computer expert, ideally a nurse knowledgeable in accounting, finance, data processing, and computer systems. A search was done and a well-qualified candidate hired. She is an important member of the executive nursing team.

Before nurse coordinators could be educated to be fiscally responsible for their units, a budget process and the means to defend changes and monitor variances needed to be in place. The structure of reports and means for timely processing and receiving of information was necessary. Only then would educational programs be developed to train nurse coordinators in using these processes to think fiscally.

Although 89 percent of the coordinators had a master's degree in 1987, few

System: _____

Rater: _____

Specification/Criteria	Poor 1	2	3	4	Excellent 5	Comments
Theory of operation and Mathematical basis						
Validity of system (proven statistically)						
Reliability of System: Objective criteria						
Easy to train raters						
Proven homogeneity within groups (if the system puts patients in groups)						
Capability of integrating quality assurance program/ process						
Capability of integrating in care planning and nursing process						
Long-term integrity of classification components						
Maintenance and updating requirements						
Source for procedural definitions/standard times						
Applications to productivity system						
Applications to budgeting system						
Applications to microcosting						
Ability to interface with ANSOS						
Degree of ease of use and automation						
Comparative database (valid and demonstrable)						
Proven track record at other comparable facilities						

Figure 9-1. Proposal Rating Form.

had formal preparation in financial management. They needed to learn how to develop a budget, how to analyze variances, how to develop action plans based on variances, and more importantly how to communicate financial plans to their staff. They also had to understand their particular unit's financial allocation relative to the overall organizational budget. Therefore, a financial curriculum was developed and is taught to all nurse managers. Currently this financial curriculum is presented to new managers annually, before budget preparation. The curriculum is outlined in Table 9–10.

The unit manager, and the unit secretary play vital roles as the information flows. The unit manager is responsible for procuring and reviewing the daily management of unit supplies and its supporting data collection. The unit secretary has two critical functions: (1) as spokesperson for the hospital to patients and their families and (2) to compile the record of all services rendered in the chart on patient discharge. Timeliness of appropriate completion of the medical record has a major financial implication for today's hospital.

With new financial management skills the success of nurse managers in managing resources is a part of their performance review. These resources include salary expenses, capital expenditures, and supply expenses managed in relation to demand and productivity as determined by the patient classification system. Finally, to ensure the availability of managers who have the knowledge and operational ability to comply with set standards, ongoing review and educational reinforcement continues to be a top priority.

After the nurse coordinators assumed control of budget preparation, justification of variances, and preparation of financial proposals for new services, the nursing division was ready to cost nursing services to affix a charge to patients

TABLE 9–10. THE FAIRFAX HOSPITAL NURSING SERVICES DIVISION SEMINAR ON MANAGING RESOURCES SCHEDULE AND TOPIC OUTLINE

Date	Topic	Required Preparation
3/3	Introduction Definition of Terms Common Computations 1987 Budget—Flexible Budgets	Read Introductory Articles Bring 1987 Budgets Bring 13th Period Amherst
3/17	Developing Schedules Staffing Patterns Shift Rotations Position Control	Read Articles Provided Bring Latest Unit Schedule Bring Last Plan Sheet Bring Controller Printout
3/31	Patient Classification Worksheets Staffing Office Reports Impact of Classification on Budget	Bring Medicus Reports Bring ANSOS Reports
4/14	Variance Reporting Variable Billing Division Resources	Bring 1st Period Amherst Complete Case Study Read Articles Provided
4/28	Trends in Reimbursement	Read Articles Provided

for nursing care rendered. Implementation of this program is now in operation so that appropriate charges can be assigned to the care provided to each patient.

Today, nursing management reports include data on productivity monitoring, acuity monitoring, position control, utilization of floats and PRN pool personnel, and rate of turnover. The financial database of the nursing division has some unique features not included in the hospital-wide database, such as a breakout of PRN personnel to determine utilization by specific unit.

THE NURSE MANAGER TODAY

Today's nurse manager needs to be creative, innovative, and flexible. A nurse manager must also demonstrate the ability to assimilate new knowledge, design and implement changes as the need arises, and focus within the context of the total organization at all times. Communicating all of this to those nurses providing patient care is even more vital. Overall, managers must accept responsibility and accountability for all resources including materials, monies, and manpower. Often this requires upgrading of skills such as computing and financial management.

Manpower was not the only area of financial management in which nursing has increased its sophistication. However, it is a prime example of beginning small and expanding over time. Once we instituted a system to track turnover we realized a need for automation and collaboration with the personnel department and the accounting department to support effectively the delivery of hospital-based care. In turn, these supporting departments have grown in appreciating the clinical impact of their financial assumptions and practices. This broader perspective sensitized the Nurse Executive Team to new priorities for (1) tracking nurse manpower full-time, part-time, PRN, and float pool by unit; (2) for collecting internal comparative data of nursing and nonnursing functions; (3) for generating external comparative data on nursing salaries, benefits, and costs for hospital services; (4) for purchasing a valid, reliable patient classification acuity system as a base to identify needs for manpower; (5) for calculating the costs of nursing care for each service the hospital provides; (6) for restructuring of the nursing division and job descriptions to support recognition of excellence, management of information, and decision making; (7) for providing career development in both clinical skills and business skills; (8) for developing educational programs for our clinical nurses and managers that focused on financial management, computing, and the measurement of quality of care; and (9) for developing of standards of care with quantification of the costs associated with quality.

Does this open up a Pandora's box? Each objective attained sets higher standards and clearer insights to unmet needs. Many times, valuable suggestions have been supplied by unit coordinators or staff nurses. For example, they pointed out when they were responsible for costs that they could not control. This has led to upper management working to connect control and responsibility to increase accountability.

Manpower is inextricably connected to quality of care, hospital financial health, education and training, patient acuity, personnel policies and practices, strategic planning, job design, and humanistic management. Incrementally we have been addressing each of these areas and sense there has been substantial progress. The ultimate goal is for nursing to have the autonomy and authority to make changes in practice so that the work performed and the person responsible for performing it is correlated to appropriate financial allocations within given reimbursement patterns for care.

The steps taken in our manpower tracking and forecasting system, automated scheduling, patient classification and monitoring system, annual budget preparation and monitoring process, and management development programs have given the nursing office credibility throughout the institution. It has also increased the nursing office's participation and authority in hospital-wide financial and clinical decision making. These measures lead us to realize that new refinements are required in related systems and new needs we have not yet identified. Gaining financial control is a challenge and a never ending process.

BIOGRAPHICAL SKETCHES

Gertrude L. Rodgers has a diploma in Nursing from Saint Clare's Mercy Hospital in Saint John's, Newfoundland, Canada, a BS in Nursing Education and Nursing Administration, from Ottawa University, Ontario, Canada, and a master's degree in Nursing Administration, from Boston University, Boston, Massachusetts. Her positions in nursing administration have included: Assistant Director of Nursing, Malden Hospital, Malden, Massachusetts and Director of Nursing at Lynn Hospital, Lynn, at New England Baptist Hospital, Boston, Massachusetts, and at Prince George General Hospital, Cheverly, Maryland. She is especially recognized for extraordinary organization and management skills in a large and diversified health care organization. She is currently the Associate Administrator, Director of Nursing Services, Fairfax Hospital System, Falls Church, Virginia. She also serves as a member of the Board of Directors of INOVA Health Systems, the parent corporation that owns four hospitals and multiple other health care facilities. She is also active in ANA and serves on the Board of the Virginia Organization of Nurse Executives.

Joyce Richardson holds a BSN from North Carolina Central University, Durham, North Carolina. Joyce was enrolled at George Mason University, Fairfax, Virginia in the master's program in Nursing Administration when she co-authored this case. She has also completed the Army Medical Department Officer Basic and Advances Courses, at Academy of Health Sciences, Fort Sam Houston, Texas.

Joyce has been a staff nurse, army nurse recruiter, assistant head nurse, and head nurse for organ transplant services, emergency room, and outpatient department services, and surgical specialty units. She is currently an assistant chief nurse at Fox Army Community Hospital.

10

Organizations as Information Systems

Stephen R. Ruth

INFORMATION SYSTEMS IN HEALTH CARE

As computers permeate our society, there continues to be rapid continued development of automated systems in health care. For nurse administrators these systems offer increased opportunity to redefine, simplify, and extend the influence of the practice of nursing.

By the end of this decade, health care information systems will grow from a 4.5 to a 7 billion dollar industry. Inpatient systems are being further developed and replaced and automation is expanding to alternative health care sites outside the hospital setting. Between 1.5 and 2.3 percent of the operating budget of today's hospitals is spent on information systems. Fifty percent of that is spent on patient accounting systems (Knittle, Ruth, & Gardner, 1987). This allocation reflects the early stage of development of health care management information systems.

Clinical care areas including nursing, medical records, pharmacy, radiology, and laboratories are now the focus of new software development because of the issues of quality control, federal, state, and local regulations, and integration to decrease costs and identify areas for increasing profits. Simultaneously, new business applications for all industries are moving from automating routine functions to aggregating data into meaningful information for decision making.

The purpose of this chapter is to discuss information systems in health care and how nurse administrators can facilitate their jobs through the use of computers. It entails information on assessment of automation needs, system selection and implementation, and current and future applications in nursing administration. Computers are pervasive in health care and refinement is necessary for the future. Appropriate management of this resource as a tool is integral to the quality and progress of nursing leadership.

MANAGEMENT INFORMATION SYSTEMS

Cost Effectiveness

Although computer-based management information systems (MIS) have been part of most organizations activities for more than 30 years, there are many fundamental issues of MIS that are still as important today as they were at the outset of the computer revolution. The essential concept of MIS has always been to harness technology for the reduction of unit costs and improvement of productivity. The verb *harness* is particularly appropriate as it brings to mind the problems encountered by a farmer in the preindustrial era to bring an earlier technology—horses and mules—to productive use. Early uses were primitive and limited to a few jobs. Effective use of horses and mules involved farmers having detailed knowledge of both the animal's capabilities and the commands and training processes to improve productivity.

The harnessing of MIS requires similar knowledge. It has always been associated with the productive use of computer hardware, software, and computing experts along with the careful nurturing of the users of the computer system.

The fundamental importance of the concept of unit cost per service in MIS is shown in Figure 10–1. The vertical scale shows unit costs of delivery of a service and the horizontal scale reflects the total volume of services delivered. The horizontal line labeled manual system shows that the unit cost of a completely hand-operated process changes little over different ranges of volume. For example, a patient reporting system at every nursing station that involved writing down each entry with pen and paper would have a unit cost that varies little. Each nurse would be responsible for logging in as needed and the unit costs would be about the same at small as well as very large hospitals. But if automated systems are introduced, like the two downward-sloping lines in the diagram, there is an opportunity to seize major cost advantages—as long as there is sufficient volume to overcome the investment cost and to take advantage of the computer's relative speed in performing the task. These are the fundamental questions in purchasing systems—Will it be capable of reducing unit costs and how many ways may it increase unit productivity? Without this framework of decision making, the computer resource may be left unharnessed and many potential benefits never realized. In fact, it may be a poor investment.

It can also be seen from Figure 10–1 that points A and B represent the mini-

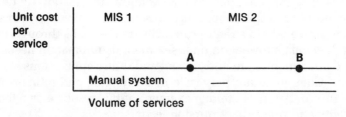

Figure 10-1. Effect of increased volume on unit cost per service.

mum volumes of services where automation will save money, using reduced unit cost of service delivery as the criterion. Notice also, automated system 1 and 2 are not the same. One is more expensive to operate than the other. The decision between purchasing system 1 and 2 would be based on cost and other criteria such as number of ways each may increase unit productivity. These criteria are discussed further later in the chapter.

Who Benefits from the MIS?

The original reason for the "M" in MIS was that the benefits were thought to accrue primarily to top management. In fact, it is now generally agreed that all levels of management benefit from a MIS. The first-line manager, often called the operational manager, is the individual responsible for day-to-day decisions. These decisions have a time horizon of days or weeks. In the nursing context this person would be the equivalent of a head nurse. The MIS would be used by that person for scheduling, budgeting, unit quality assurance, and patient classification.

The second level of management, tactical manager, has broader responsibilities and a longer time horizon for decision impact. The Associate Director of Nursing or even the Director of Nursing, whose job focuses on strategies for implementation of the strategic plan, are examples of tactical managers. These individuals have to make plans for months and even years ahead. They need aggregate data related to the performance of units, equipment, and facilities. They have input in major financial decisions affecting their functional area. They use MIS for reports on exceptions, projected budgets and variances, comparisons of costs and performance, and so forth.

The early MIS were directed toward meeting the needs of these two types of managers. They are capable of furnishing reports, inventory balances, shift data, patient comparisons quickly and accurately. In fact, nearly all the popular success stories of MIS were framed in the context of greater availability of timely summary data and the great improvements in productivity that have resulted.

But the most information-starved manager of all is at the third level. These managers called top management, executive management, or strategic managers had been little served by MIS. Nurse administrators have only recently entered this arena. They include many in Assistant Administrator, Executive Director, or corporate positions. Their decision time span is several years. They need information to support decision making about the organization's strategic plan. The executive has very different needs than those with primary responsibility for operations. Recently an entire class of MIS has been developed for them called either decision support systems (DSS) or executive information systems (EIS) (Albee, 1980; Ruth, 1987).

New Trends in MIS

The strategic manager with a planning spectrum measured in years needs information of a different character to guide the organization. This individual needs information about business and societal trends from outside the organization to speculate about alternative futures and their potential unit costs, where dollars are only one of several criteria, such as market position, potential growth, and societal values. A MIS is needed with the power to represent abstractions and vagaries of the organization within the context of its larger environment. New EIS seek to address these needs. They are distinguished by three characteristics: lack of internal transaction analysis, integration of complicated data concerning issues external to the organization, and utilization of widely varied symbolic and graphic input and output techniques.

The EIS offers the executive a lever to extend their information base in planning, organizing, selecting, and directing fundamental decisions in their organization's mission and philosophy to drive implementation strategies. In effect, the executive is attempting actively to shape the organization's future. This is not possible with information from a traditional MIS. The success of EIS is not yet clear. Many executives are reluctant to invest in EIS approaches, either because of an inherent skepticism of the appropriate role of any MIS in strategic decision making or a reluctance to master the associated technology (Martin, 1982).

A new technology for MIS that may have the most significant potential for the services sector is expert systems. These computer programs are intelligent, in that they capture the best decision behavior of an expert in some focused area of specialty. For example, if a person has developed over many years an ability to diagnose problems in scheduling, the decision behaviors of this individual can be extracted and institutionalized through incorporation in an expert system program. People without this expertise can then learn to solve the same problems using this program; experts can also use it to solve the same problems faster than without the assistance of the program. Expert systems are becoming a common element in many new MIS (Ruth, 1987).

The MIS Growth Cycle

Richard Nolan (1979), in his classic article, elaborated the six stages in the growth of MIS development. He also points out that different divisions in the same organization may be experiencing different stages of growth. This model has been widely applied to many disciplines, including nursing information systems (NIS) (Suding, 1984). Table 10-1 describes this cycle. It consists of six stages of data processing (DP) development, each characterized by behaviors in DP applications, DP planning and control, and user vs DP personnel involvement. Applications slowly expand from automation (stage I, II) to include management decision making (stages III–V) and then strategic planning (stage VI). Nolan argues that many organizations never even approach stage IV, where major benefits can be attained due to issues of user acceptance, control of information, and poor communication between programmers and users. Development of MIS growth needs to be periodically assessed by administrators for pervasiveness of functional applications and technological adequacy. Growth should be systematically planned using a DP steering committee in the early stages and placement of DP experts in executive management positions in the later stages.

TABLE 10-1. STAGES OF MANAGEMENT INFORMATION SYSTEM GROWTH

	I Initiation	II Contagion	III Control	IV Integration	V Data Administration	VI Maturity
DP applications	Financial automation	Widespread automation	Upgrade and restructure systems for data bases	Apply data base technology	Integration internal information	Integration internal and external information
DP plan and control	Financial application demonstrates savings	Facilitate and expand applications	Formalize planning and control over applications	Refine to match supply and demand	Network sharing data bases	Balance supply and demand
User vs DP personnel involvement	User: "hands off"; DP: accountable	Limited number of users receive data DP: controls and designs	User "more" active role but still DP dependent and few trained	User: defines needs DP: designs solutions	User: designs solutions DP: support	Joint user and DP accountability

DP, data processing.
Adapted from Nolan, 1979, pp. 115–126.

AUTOMATION OF ROUTINE WORK

The Automation Revolution

The computer age, beginning in the late 1940s has been described as a kind of new industrial revolution, freeing the office worker of drudgery in the same way that the industrial revolution in the 1800s reduced the drudgery of the craftsman and farmer. It is not clear whether office workers exchanged one kind of drudgery for another, but it is certain that the introduction of computer-based MIS in the 1950s changed their jobs forever. It also increased profits by reducing unit costs. Nowhere is this more evident than where tasks changed from monitoring each unit to monitoring exceptions—referred to as the *management by exception* principle. For example, pharmacy orders used to require the preparation of each order and invoice by hand for thousands of products each month with continuous review by the supervisor. With an automated system, orders and invoices are automatically produced by computer and checked against a specified standard such as previous orders. The supervisor receives a listing of all exceptions, that is, changes in quantity, drug concentrations, or vendors, for review. This change to computer-based, accurate, timely review of all orders with the supervisor reviewing only exceptions, has resulted in dramatic changes in the use of the supervisor's time and improvement in quality control. The identification of standards for quality review has become a key supervisory activity with a substantial reduction in routine tasks.

Automation of office work has also made a major contribution to the use of databases. Typically a database is a group of records, like patient records, that require frequent updating, sorting, merging, filing, copying, auditing, and many other actions by a population as varied as physicians, Medicare examiners, and tax analysts. Before automation, records were composed of many forms, each designed for a specific use, manually compiled and kept in envelopes, folders, and file cabinets using a logical labeling system and sorted in some sequence. Today's computer-automated hospital keeps databases, such as patient information, on disks or other storage devices instantly available through video display terminals (VDTs). Information is organized according to its own characteristics on one central database and then extracted using menus similar to paper forms for specific purposes. Such databases have resulted in many economies in unit cost for entry, handling, and storage. They have also allowed the economical creation of aggregate reports and analysis never before possible.

Perhaps the most notable of the economies produced by automation is due to the insistence that there be only one source record for every piece of information in computer databases. For instance, once the patient's name and Social Security number are entered in the system it should never be duplicated elsewhere in that database. This insistence on the integrity of databases has undoubtedly reduced error rates, improved integration of information, and saved entry time. However, it has also required more systematic planning and coordination in designing the databases so they will contain all the information that each user needs formerly found on their forms and reports.

The comprehensiveness of databases has also lead to recognition of the importance of data security and methods to control access to users on a need to know basis. In selecting MIS systems, administrators should pay close attention to how the vendor has designed security techniques and responses to security failures.

Microcomputers and MIS

One of the most significant opportunities that has emerged on the horizon of MIS automation has been the use of microcomputers. Although microcomputers (micros) have only been in regular use in MIS for less than 10 years, the possibilities they offer are dramatic. There are several reasons for this, all related to unit costs and benefits. The micro has become a multipurpose tool. It is capable of being used by the same client for the five major tasks occupying the majority of administrative office worker's time: data entry, spread sheet analysis, data communications, database management, and word processing. Recent advances in software applications, especially integrated packages that support all five tasks and require only moderate training, have made offices without micros anachronistic.

Previously many applications could only be done by mainframe computers by those with considerable computer expertise. One central processing unit (CPU) in a central location would occupy hundreds of square feet of space. This was connected electronically to multiple "dumb" video display terminals through which users entered programs, data, and read resultant output. Printed results were only available at central locations. A more recent development has been "smart" VDTs where users could still enter programs and data and read output from the mainframe CPU but could also, independently, do a local task using the smaller CPU within the terminal for preprogramed applications such as word processing.

Microcomputers each have their own CPU and can be used for a wide variety of tasks limited only by their memory and graphics capability. Recent advances in hardware engineering have greatly expanded their capabilities without increasing their size or cost. They do not have preprogrammed applications like smart terminals but use programs the user purchases separately. Thus, a complete micro system involves purchasing separate software program applications, data storage disks, and hardware components.

Perhaps the most important development for the use of micros in MIS has been hardware and software to link them to each other and a mainframe computer. By the use of modems and local area networks (LAN) hardware and software it has become possible to have the versatile micro used both as an individual work station and a terminal for the mainframe. A hospital example may be instructive. A few years ago a patient admitting office in the hospital would have used a "dumb" terminal linked to the admission software system of the mainframe computer elsewhere in the hospital. This VDT, while providing focused support of the patient entry function, was limited to only that one task. When a microcomputer linked by a LAN is installed for the same purpose, the result is a work station that can do patient entry, any other clerical tasks for which programs were purchased and directly communicate information to another micro in the LAN on a patient unit or elsewhere in the hospital. A smart terminal in the same location could do patient entry and any local task for which it was preprogrammed. See Table 10–2 for a comparison of dumb, smart, and micro VDTs.

Applications Software

The software packages that have given micros the potential for great contributions to MIS have primarily been the spreadsheet, word processing, and database management applications. Spreadsheet applications are dominated by LOTUS 123. These packages are far more than just means for rapidly doing accounting and mathematical procedures. They also offer powerful database management and graphics display of comparison data. Spreadsheets are used by nurse administrators primarily for budget preparation and comparison of "what if" changes for planning. For instance, a spreadsheet could be used to compare costs of one additional holiday to an increase in the shift differential to see which would be more expensive.

Like all good spreadsheet programs, LOTUS 123 requires extensive training for a user to become very familiar with all its potential applications. A recent study of over a thousand users of LOTUS 123 in a large county government agency, indicated that there were only about 20 persons capable of developing applications that used the full range of LOTUS 123's capabilities. Everyone else was more or less operating at a clerical level, able to enter and output data, and perhaps create a simple spreadsheet with simple mathematical formulas but lit-

TABLE 10-2. COMPARISON OF DUMB TERMINALS, SMART TERMINALS, AND MICROCOMPUTER TERMINALS

	Terminals		
Characteristics	Dumb	Smart	Microcomputer
1. Data entry and output from mainframe	X	X	X[a]
2. Own CPU		X	X
3. Preprogrammed application programs		X	
4. Uses purchased application programs			X
5. Drives a workstation printer	X	X	X
6. Download and upload information to and from mainframe		X	X
7. Download and upload information from other terminals			X[b]
8. Cost per unit	Lowest	Highest	Middle
9. Training required to use	Lowest	Middle	Highest
10. Cost to expand and add new applications	Unable	Highest	Lowest
11. Versatility	Lowest	Middle	Highest

[a]With a modem or terminal emulation program.
[b]With a local area network.

tle more. Such a result is not necessarily a serious problem if the organization uses those 20 persons as experts to consult with other managers and develop applications. Due to the specialization of different areas of today's knowledge organizations, such as health care agencies, however, all managers need to assume the responsibility for knowing their own information needs and how these may potentially be met by a spreadsheet or database management program.

With the lack of universal expertise, there is a danger that the diseconomies of the earlier MIS applications could result, where a central design agency did most of the programming and the users accepted the results with little understanding or input. MIS outputs were often not very useful and managers had to hunt through reams of data to create meaningful reports.

Spreadsheet programs can become major advantages for the organization of MIS if they can be used to the full potential of their capabilities (Bellinger & Laden, 1985) and integrated into the larger system. This requires a large investment, not only in micros and software, but also training of management and secretarial personnel. Otherwise spreadsheets and other applications programs will be used only casually and for their simplest features throughout the organization except for a small group of interested, self-trained employees. The investment for the software (often over $500 per program per work station) can be wasted and the unit costs of the limited, isolated successful applications will be excessive.

Word processing micro-based software, aside from being the most prevalent application, has been the most successful. There are literally scores of word processing packages. Packages vary in capabilities like editing features, text manipulation, spelling and thesaurus supports, transportability, user friendliness, file management, and cost. Many offices with automated work stations use them primarily for word processing. This development would seem to be of fundamental importance for MIS in organizations, making functional integration of information a realistic, cost effective goal.

Word processing packages used in micro work stations should be chosen to include the capability to communicate with other word processing packages, spreadsheets, and database management programs. This is a common feature in the more powerful packages, such as Word Perfect, Word Star, and Multi Mate. With such a package, it is completely feasible for a person who is using the micro for a spreadsheet application to shift directly to a word processing program and compose a letter to a client including data accumulated in the spreadsheet (Finkler, 1985). The potential for saving time and improving the quality of letters and reports is obvious.

Division of Labor

The automation of work stations for the manager and secretaries has led to changes in the division and flow of work. For instance, a manager used to have to compose letters manually or dictate them. Letters were then typed and proofread by the secretary, signed by the manager, and then sent by the secretary. The alternative was an impersonal form letter. With micros in a LAN each exchange can be done electronically—the manager outlines a letter or provides individualized information and sends it to the secretary who then inserts this information into one of many form letters stored in the microcomputer files. The letter is then sent back to the manager who edits as necessary and returns it for the secretary to print, have signed, and send.

Secretaries now enter data to updata spreadsheets that were designed by managers, sometimes with the assistance of an expert. Secretaries may also download data from the mainframe database and then enter it in spreadsheets that are used for various unit budgets. The manager can then use this data for analysis and reports already organized in a relevant format on spreadsheets.

Database management of information relevant to that manager's area of accountability is also a function that a secretary can update and maintain for use by the manager. Employee performance information, patient classification, quality assurance data, and risk management data, can all be available for analysis and reports at the manager's request. Design of the database, sources of information, and reporting menus are the responsibility of the manager, possibly with consultation from an expert.

Many managers make the mistaken assumption that a computer is only an improved typewriter and thus a secretary's tool. Nothing could be more incorrect. Data entry and printing are secretarial duties that parallel typewriter use. Computer applications go far beyond these functions. To harness the technology effectively, managerial personnel need training and their own work stations. As specialists they know what data will provide them with the information they need for their tasks. With automation, their positions have gone from information poor to being deluged with information. They must design the aggregation of these data to provide information for decision making for planning, controlling, and budgeting or experience data overload and information blackout.

SELECTION

Key Variables

The basic ground rules for the selection of an MIS have changed fundamentally during the past 10 years. The crucial issues up to that time had been hardware and software costs with a heavy emphasis on the former. Until recently, hardware capability and reliability were the critical limiting factors that received the wise buyer's utmost consideration.

In designing an optimal MIS, managers need to consider both people and computer variables. These may be summarized (Emery, 1987):

People variables

- Availability of relevant inputs
- Timeliness of the database including response time between an event and its recording in the database

- Accuracy, agreement between stored and actual data
- Backup redundancy, frequency that copies are made to provide protection against loss
- Adequacy of training programs

Hardware variables

- Variety of transactions that can be handled
- Flexibility, relative ease with which the system can be modified
- Reliability, probability that the system will operate satisfactorily without breakdowns
- Availability of support and maintenance personnel, often supplied by contract from the vendor.
- Space and special environmental requirements such as air conditioning and electricity demands
- Peripherals available, input and output devices
- Cost to purchase and to maintain

Software variables

- Robustness, the extent that the system safeguards against user errors
- User friendliness, degree of familiarity with computer programming that the user needs in learning the system
- Security, protection against unauthorized access or loss of system resources
- Generality, range of functions provided
- Degree of "intelligence" or complexity of logical steps the programs can perform
- Availability of packaged programs versus programmer-created programs
- Transportability of programs between computers and information between programs
- Lack of errors in the source code (program itself)
- Maintainability or ease of updating and correction

In recent years, MIS selection has been affected by the major change in the cost characteristics of hardware and software development and maintenance. In 1955 over 80 percent of the cost of a MIS system was hardware; by 1985 this had reversed with indications that software services would command 90 percent of costs in the near future (Boehm, 1982). As a result, hardware selection is now less critical in the sense that its unit cost and unit quality are less variable and its total share of the data processing budget has decreased substantially. Currently, the crucial variables for consideration by a potential buyer are software related.

Software Selection Considerations

Although difficult to measure explicitly, software quality has been generally considered to be a measure of the ratio of the total number of completely correct lines of source code compared with the total number of lines of source code in the program. Japan has been especially successful in generating high quality source code. MIS implementations are frequently delayed for long periods due to errors in the programs as different parts of systems are brought on line, due to the low quality of source code by the original programmer (Knittle, Ruth, & Gardner, 1987). Most of the errors are in the logic of the program rather than in the syntax. The errors in programming language usage and organization, called syntax errors, are relatively easy to identify and most programming languages have automatic error checking features that alert programmers to these errors for easy correction. Logic errors refer to commands to direct the computer to do the wrong function. Unless the programmer has documented each step of their logic in writing a program, these errors may be very difficult and time consuming to discover and correct. For example, a hospital MIS may have a module that is supposed to calculate the average number of days of a hospital stay that will be covered by diagnostic related group (DRG) payments for Medicare patients. Detecting the source of faulty results requires a programmer tediously tracing the logic in writing the program, a DRG specialist checking all the standards used in programming, and possibly an analyst checking the databases used for retrieving the information. This could have been avoided if scrupulous attention was given to technical documentation through coordination of efforts of the programmer, experts, and analysts during analysis, design, and implementation. This quality issue underlines the importance of a potential buyer asking the vendor if the programs they will use are installed and running elsewhere with the same computer system. If so, they should request references and arrange to make site visits before signing a contract. If not, some major delays can be anticipated and concessions should be made by the vendor for this expense.

Maintainability of MIS software refers to the ability of the system to be easily changed or repaired. The typical MIS development center dedicates about 80 percent or more of its efforts to maintaining previously developed programs and the rest to developing new programs. Good documentation facilitates finding logical errors and training of new users. Good documentation includes: (1) extensive use of a high level programming language, (2) detailed operator and user instructions written in jargon-free language, and (3) logical indexes for quick reference (Nolan, 1979; Emery, 1987).

Finally, the MIS programs should be transportable, meaning that it must be relatively easy to adapt the programs to a new hardware and data communications environment. Early MIS were written in computer languages that were specific to only one computer. As long as the vendor provided support for that particular computer the MIS was satisfactory. As advances were made in hardware engineering, however, vendors changed computers to incorporate new features and frequently abandoned support of outdated computers. The hardware modifications were relatively inexpensive but each change necessitated totally rewriting the MIS. This was very expensive.

Later, more advanced computer languages were designed to be transportable between machines. They are procedure-oriented, that is, each was designed for a specific class of procedures such as business or scientific applications. The source code is written using English-like words that would be understandable to even casual users. This makes searching for logic errors dramatically easier. A truly transportable MIS may not only be easily adapted for use with later models of computers made by the same vendor, but also for computers made by different vendors. Advanced computer languages are often used to create multipurpose integrated programs that include all five of the functions most used in office automation: word processing, database management, spreadsheet, data communications, and data entry.

Some hospitals are now facing decisions to lose their entire investment in an outdated system or to stay with a vendor and computer system that may not have hardware or software with all the features they prefer. The majority of the MIS for sale today are written in advanced computer languages, but the wise purchaser will inquire as to transportability of the MIS.

FUTURE DIRECTIONS

Future Organizational Management Information System Objectives

In the preceding sections key issues that have led to the success of MIS have been described. The recommended view that has been stressed throughout has been the importance of harnessing MIS to take advantage of the recent advances and reduction in unit cost of computer hardware through extensive use of micros and a LAN and to be aware of the key criteria for selecting software with recognition of its current domination of system costs. The visionary administrator will make decisions with these futuristic objectives in mind (Emery, 1987).

Organizational Integration. The MIS must permeate the organization to provide help at operational, tactical, and strategic levels. Thus, the executive team must include the MIS director. Also, several levels of nursing should be on the MIS team.

Modular Design. Rather than massive central MIS systems, it will become crucial for rapid adaptation to break MIS into linked, free-standing elements using micro-based software and advanced computer languages. Modular information centers may replace central mainframes. Work stations are replacing dumb terminals.

Availability of Personal Work Stations. For MIS to flourish and meet its potential in an organization, it must be available to all levels of management, clinicians, and clerical support services. This means multifunction work stations capable of offering the full range of developmental and operational software in numbers so that people are not waiting in line for access.

Computer Literature Personnel. Computing is not the responsibility of data processing experts and secretaries alone. Micros represent a low cost way to make terminals available to all members of the organization. An integrated MIS requires interaction of managers and clinicians as fully functioning participants in the organization's use of advanced computer-based automation. This requires a high investment in training as many adults are not computer literate. Training efforts are being reinforced by the tens of millions of microcomputers families are purchasing for home use. Many large corporations are providing home computers to executives as an inducement to become computer literate.

Satisfaction of All Users' Information Needs. Many managers have never had timely data to use in decision making. As MIS makes information available they will come to recognize new information needs and ask for more system capabilities to meet these needs. In time MIS will be capable of providing information across all organizational levels and boundaries, both vertically and horizontally. The MIS will expand rapidly in the next few years, changing both the structure and the managerial functions of personnel.

Incorporation of MIS in Strategic Planning. Executive information systems will continue to develop and increasingly link interorganizational information. Organizations will routinely compare themselves to competitors and use EIS for marketing to tailor goods and services to meet consumer needs and desires. Information on the economy, social values, demographic characteristics, and other societal trends will be accessible for use in strategic planning. Currently, most organizations regard the MIS as a cost center used by tactical and operational managers. This will change over time to centers that serve all levels of management.

More Rigorous and Rapid Managerial Decision Making. Expanded use of exception reporting and data aggregate systems in MIS will support program evaluations, clinical and operational decision making, and selection procedures. New artificial intelligence (AI) and expert system (ES) applications will become routine parts of future MIS development. Managers will be guided by decision rules developed by experts to weigh alternatives. Expert systems will lead them to seek comprehensive, relevant information for decisions, and to sharpen their logic.

Management Information System in Nursing: Management Skills are Crucial

With respect to MIS that are used in the nursing profession, it would appear that the prospects are particularly bright, as the hardware and software advances described are not yet used to a great degree. There are indications that the nursing profession has a large number of, as yet unrealized, MIS opportunities

(Farlee, 1978; Zielstroff, 1985). To harness MIS within nursing, administrators need to become familiar with potential MIS applications for patient classification, statistical analysis, scheduling staff, preparing and monitoring budgets, and quality assurance. They also need to design new nursing roles that incorporate use of the MIS and design training programs to prepare nurses to assume these roles.

Increasingly, health care organizations are expanding their MIS to include integrated patient information for financial and clinical purposes. The key to successful implementation of these systems is nurse manager involvement. There are a number of case examples published where MIS for nursing and patient care have had the support of state of the art hardware and software but have been failures due to lack of involvement of nurse managers in analyzing, designing, and implementing MIS. Full-time nurse managers, in control of the entire process from feasibility analysis to selection, design, and implementation appears to be the distinguishing feature of successful outcomes. At the time of initiation nurse managers may not be an expert in MIS, but through self-study and interaction with the team they will make a valuable contribution. They are the pivotal persons to communicate nursing and other clinical needs and anticipate problems in both system and work station design. Many avenues for learning about MIS are available through publications, workshops, courses, and networking.

Nurse administrators need to actively seek automation of their work stations and training to be able to harness the power of the health care agency's MIS to improve both tactical and operational management within nursing. They also need to recruit or internally train a member of their management team to be an expert in MIS to have someone who knows its full potential to spearhead the design, implementation, and monitoring of the nursing information system. The first step is awareness of MIS potential to support data-based decision making within nursing administration.

As nurse administrators become increasingly involved in strategic management for the total organization, they also need to strongly support MIS development and training throughout the agency. The challenge of MIS will always be one of integrating people systems and computer systems to increase productivity and quality while decreasing unit cost. Only through keeping this challenge as a top organizational priority will the MIS of the future become a reality.

BIOGRAPHICAL SKETCH

Dr Stephen Ruth is Professor of Decision Sciences at George Mason University. He is a graduate of the U.S. Naval Academy (BS) in 1955, of the Navy Post Graduate School (MS with distinction) in 1964, and the University of Pennsylvania (PhD) in 1971. His areas of specialization are Business Applications of Artificial Intelligence and Expert Systems, Decision Support Systems and Human Factors in EDP-related settings. Dr Ruth is the author of over 100 journal articles, books, and monographs and he has planned and/or delivered over a

100 automation-related seminars and lectures aimed at managers from government and industry on four continents. In 1984, Dr Ruth served as a Visiting Professor of Business at Georgetown University. He consults extensively with companies and government agencies involved in developing training programs for all levels of management. In 1985 and 1987, he was named senior Fulbright lecturer to Argentina, and, in 1986, Distinguished Professor at George Mason University. In 1987, he was one of thirteen professors named Outstanding Professor in the State of Virginia.

SUGGESTED READING

Basic Information on Computers

Hopper, G.M. & Mandell, S. (1984). *Understanding Computers.* New York: West Publishing Company.

McWilliams, P.A. (1983). *The Personal Computer Book.* Los Angeles: Prelude Press.

Sweeney, M.A. (1985). *The Nurse's Guide to Computers.* New York: Macmillan.

Productivity

Bush, R., Knutson, L., & Eric, K. (1978). Integration of corporate and MIS planning: The impact on productivity. *Data Base, 9* (3), 4–8.

Drucker, P. (1988). The coming of the new organization. *Harvard Business Review, 66* (1), 45–51.

Rushinek, A., & Rushinek, S.F. (1986). End user satisfaction of data base management systems: An empirical assessment of mainframe, mini, and micro computer-based systems using an interactive model. *Data Base, 17* (2), 17–27.

Skinner, W. (1986). The productivity paradox. *Harvard Business Review, 64* (7), 55.

Expert Systems

Carroll, J.M., & McKendree, J. (1987). Interface design issues for advice-giving expert systems. *Communications of the ACM, 30* (1), 14.

Laborde, J.M. (1984). Expert systems for nursing? *Computers in Nursing, 2* (8), 130–135.

MIS Components and Design

Austin, C.J. (1983). *Information Systems for Hospital Administration.* Ann Arbor: Health Administration Press.

Canter, S.J. (1983). Database: The application implementation decision. *Data Base, 15* (1), 4–10.

Gilhooley, I.A. (1986). A methodology for productive systems development. *Journal of Information Systems Management, 3* (1), 36–41.

Heath, F.R. (1976). Guidelines for identifying high payoff applications. *Data Base, 7* (3), 7–17.

Turn, R. (1975). Cost implications of privacy protection in databank systems. *Data Base, 6* (4), 3–9.

Microcomputers and MIS

Egyhazy, C.J. (1984) Microcomputers and relational database management systems: A new strategy for decentralizing databases. *Data Base, 16* (1), 15–20.

Finkler, S.A. (1985). Microcomputers in nursing administration: A software overview. *Journal of Nursing Administration, 15* (4), 18–23.

Keen, P.G.W., & Woodman, L.A. (1984). What to do with all those micros. *Harvard Business Review, 62* (5), 142–150.

Health Care Applications

Alfirevic, J., Kroman, B., & Ruflin, P. (1987). Informational needs for a product line management system. *Health Care Financial Management, 34* (3) 6–8, 42–43.

Cox, H.C., Harsanyi, B., & Dean, L.C. (1987). *Computers and Nursing,* Norwalk, CT: Appleton & Lange.

Computers in Nursing. Philadelphia: Lippincott.

Christensen, W.W., & Stearns, E.I. (1984). *Microcomputers in Health Care Management.* Rockville, MD: Aspen Systems Corp.

REFERENCES

Albee, S.L. (1980). *Decision Support Systems: Current Practice and Continuing Challenges.* Reading, MA: Addison Wesley.

Bellinger, K., & Laden, J. (1985). Nurse use of general purpose microcomputer software. *Nursing Outlook, 33* (1), 22–25.

Boehm, B. (1982). Software engineering. In Cougar, J.D., Colter, M.A., & Knapp, R. (eds.): *Advanced System Development Feasibility Techniques.* New York: John Wiley and Sons, p. 97.

Emery, J.C. (1987). *Management Information Systems: The Critical Strategic Force.* Oxford, England: Oxford University Press.

Farlee, C. (1978). The computer as a focus of organizational change in the hospital. *Journal of Nursing Administration, 8* (2), 20–26.

Finkler, S. (1985). Microcomputers in nursing administration. *Journal of Nursing Administration, 15* (4), 18–23.

Knittle, D., Ruth, S., & Gardner, E. (1987). Establishing user-centered criteria for information systems: A software ergonomics perspective. *Information and Management, 10* (6), 163–72.

Martin, J. (1982). *Applications Development Without Programmers.* Englewood Cliffs, NJ: Prentice Hall.

Nolan, R. (1979). Managing the crises in data processing. *Harvard Business Review, 57* (2), 115–126.

Ruth S. (1987). Expert systems in universities: A shell game. *Interfaces, 9* (4), 42–48.

Suding, M.J. (1984). Decision making: Controlling the computer input. *Nursing Management, 15* (7), 44–52.

Thomas, A.N. (1986). Management information systems: Determining nursing requirements. *Nursing Management, 17* (7), 23–26.

Walters, Shirley (1986). Computerized care plans help nurses achieve quality patient care. *Journal of Nursing Administration, 16* (11), 33–39.

Zielstroff, Rita. (1985). Cost effectiveness of computerization in nursing practice and administration. *Journal of Nursing Administration, 15* (2), 22–26.

CASE 10–1
Automating a Patient Classification System
Nurse–Vendor Collaboration

Raymond D. Hylton
Joyce E. Johnson
Mary Jo Moran

Automation in hospital nursing departments can exert a profound impact on patient care, on the ability of nursing administration to cost-out and control services, and on the development of nursing's professional body of knowledge (Donaho & Hess, 1984; Happ, 1983; Kiley, et al, 1983). Automation systems must not only meet nursing's current information requirements but also provide flexibility to accommodate future needs. Creation of a successful system requires nursing input at each stage of activity, beginning with vendor selection and continuing through system development and training.

The nursing team at the Washington Hospital Center (WHC), an 821-bed, nonprofit, tertiary care facility in Washington, D.C., played a pivotal role in the hospital's selection of a computer vendor in 1982. Through a complex process of requesting proposals, developing an evaluation instrument, conducting site visits, and sorting through reams of documentation and interview material to develop a final evaluation report, nursing was able to make its voice heard in the hospital's choice of a vendor. The system selected not only had a "user friendly" order entry system and the capability to generate useful financial and personnel reports, but also the ability to develop "new applications, such as staffing and scheduling systems, nursing care plans and Kardexes, and even automated charting." High on nursing's priority list was expansion and automation of the patient classification system (Weaver & Johnson, 1984). The choice of a vendor who was actively developing nursing systems provided an opportunity for nursing to play a significant role in the development process.

By early 1984, the computer vendor had installed financial, personnel, and order entry applications. The next task facing nursing was to collaborate with the vendor in developing a totally automated patient classification system. The groundwork for this project was already solid as the hospital had a manual patient classification system in place. The automation of this system meant a transfer from a lead pencil manual system of classification to a light pen automated system. It was imperative that the new system not take nurses away from the bedside and that it improve patient care.

From Raymond D. Hylton, Joyce E. Johnson, and Mary Jo Moran, Automating a patient classification system: Nurse-vendor collaboration. *Computers in Nursing, 4* (1), 27–31. Reprinted by permission of J.B. Lippincott Company, Philadelphia, PA.

Nursing also wanted to integrate patient classification into a comprehensive nursing management information system (NMIS). Such a system had to interface efficiently with future automated scheduling, care planning, and charting capabilities. It needed the potential to provide a rich source of patient care data and to provide the capability to analyze patient acuity data as they related to diagnosis related groups (DRGs) established under Medicare's prospective payment system. Nursing wanted to be able to carry out other complex analyses of finance, budget, and position control as they related to patient acuity. In summary, nursing visualized a flexible, expandable system that could meet both planned and unanticipated needs during the next decade.

ASSOCIATE ADMINISTRATOR'S ROLE

The Associate Administrator for Nursing participated in the initial vendor selection process and contract negotiations. As a result, nursing ensured that patient classification "would be developed according to definite time frames and would meet WHC's individual specifications" (Weaver & Johnson, 1984, p. 34). In January 1984, the computer vendor selected WHC as its alpha site for primary development of its patient classification system. In renewed negotiations with the vendor, the Associate Administrator for Nursing secured assurances that WHC would be eligible to benefit from subsequent refinements of the system. The Associate Administrator also assessed the economic impact and risks involved in developing the system; she again secured guarantees from the vendor that the system would be flexible enough to conform to WHC specifications and that serving as the alpha site would offer substantial financial benefit to the hospital. As an alpha site, the hospital participated in the designing, testing, and the evaluation process for the new nursing application. The vendor provided all software programming and their expertise in system design.

ROLE OF THE TASK FORCE

The Associate Administrator for Nursing selected an Automated Patient Classification Task Force, headed by the Associate Director of Nursing Systems. A former head nurse at WHC, the Associate Director analyzed the impact that the automated patient classification system would have on patient care delivery. The Associate Director also served as a linking-pin, securing input from the Associate Administrator for Nursing, the four directors of decentralized nursing divisions, and head nurses and staff nurses. Also on the team were a graduate student intern in nursing administration and two experienced management-engineering consultants. Liaison representatives from the hospital's information systems department were responsible for supporting nursing's automation systems.

Self-education was ongoing throughout the development process. Task force members invited other vendors to give demonstrations, participated in computer workshops, took courses at local universities, read product brochures and specifications, conducted literature searches, and talked with the management and engineering consultants on the team and with colleagues involved in automation. This process enabled task force members to assess what the vendor had to offer, to communicate with vendor representatives in their own language, and to determine what standards of system capability were reasonable and wise to demand. In this way, the task force was able to use a common sense, business approach in negotiating with the vendor.

Task force members met before each encounter with the vendor to set strategy. They frequently met again after conferring with the vendor as well. These sessions helped team members to validate what had transpired in these long and complex meetings and to clarify issues. Several task force members kept meticulous notes, which proved invaluable in helping task force members to recall details of discussions. This documentation served as source material for a list of unresolved issues that task force members pursued to resolution. In addition, the notes were useful in maintaining accountability to the task force's nursing constituency.

The task force formed an alliance with nurses at another hospital who also were developing a similar automated patient classification system with the same vendor. This collaboration provided even more opportunities to keep abreast of the tasks at hand, to validate information, and to pool resources. Maintaining this relationship among colleagues also gave nursing at each hospital more leverage in vendor negotiations.

All these activities served the task force and nursing well. Task force members kept themselves fully abreast of the development process and always validated information provided by the vendor with other sources. In this way, they were able to set priorities, to allocate their resources effectively, to negotiate knowledgeably, to collaborate effectively, and to compromise appropriately.

FEATURES OF THE AUTOMATED PATIENT CLASSIFICATION SYSTEM

The vendor proposed a two-tiered system that was developed by the two separate vendor teams. The first tier involved the actual classification process by the nurse on the unit terminal. The second tier involved a download of the classification data to a microcomputer in the nursing office from which staffing and management reports were generated. A separate audit function allowed nurse auditors to compare their classification of a selected patient with that of the caregiver, thereby ensuring that patients were classified accurately. Three mainframe reports were developed. (1) The "latest patient classifications" report listed the most recent patient classification by date, time, and person classifying. This report would allow managers to make sure that classifications were being listed as total care hours for each patient each day during a hospital stay so that staffing could be updated promptly. (2) The "cumulative patient classifications for stay" report listed changes in required care hours tracked over time. (3) The "cumulative audited classifications" report listed all classification audits and provided point variances between the original classification and that of the auditor. The system retained detailed classification data on each patient for the total patient hospitalization. Another component of the system, the master patient file, retained the care hours required for each day but did not retain detailed classification data.

To calculate staffing needs, summary information to each unit was downloaded into a microcomputer (IBM-XT) that produced daily and summary staffing reports, acuity summary reports, and productivity reports. This personal computer application came on-line after the automated patient classification application was in place.

DEVELOPING THE SYSTEM: A PROCESS OF COLLABORATION AND COMPROMISE

The vendor representatives made a presentation of their proposed plan and then the real work began. First, a conference group consisting of the nursing task force and vendor representatives who were developing the patient classification application outlined all the work to be done. Group members devised a Gantt chart outlining all the major target dates. The nursing task force agreed to deliver algorithms and descriptions of aspects of care and nursing care factors, and to train nurses by certain deadlines. The vendor agreed on dates for completion of the computer programming, and delivery of the patient classification screens to the hospital.

The next phase of activity was programming and system development. The nursing task force began the monumental task of listing and coding 32 aspects of care and over 600 nursing care factors. Each aspect of care was coded so that the vendor could program the computer to allow unlimited choices from certain aspect-of-care categories and limited choices from others. Other aspects of care were coded and required the classifier to make at least one choice before moving to the next screen. If the nurse selected more or less than one of these care factors, an error message appeared at the bottom of the screen stating that exactly one item must be chosen within that category. Furthermore, behind every classification screen, a "help" screen told the nurse the selection parameters for each aspect of care on that screen. To access the help screen, the nurse pressed one education key on the keyboard. This feature of the system eliminated selection errors that had occurred with the manual system and kept all system documentation on-line (see Appendix for details).

The task force also wanted to be able to retain and track detailed data for use in research. For example, not only did nursing want to analyze the mean number of care hours associated with a particular nursing diagnoses or DRG, it also wanted to determine if particular nursing care factors were significantly associated with these variables. Toward this end, each nursing care factor was assigned a unique code so that it could be tracked through the system.

Storage was another problem. Because new data were constantly being entered, the mainframe computer only retained detailed information for the patient's length of stay in the hospital. Although interested in possible nursing research applications, after considering the cost versus the benefits of several storage methods, nursing chose to forego the taping of the details of each classification. The sequential retrieval of this data from tape would be difficult as the classification is but one small part of the patients' total database. The entire database would have to be stored to keep the details of classification. Disk storage proved to be too expensive. As a result, only the daily required care hours for each patient were taped in the historical file.

Another difficult decision involved computer printouts of the classification tool. The manual classification tool was a part of the nursing care planning Kardex and served as a communication tool for nurses. Nurses frequently made detailed written notations on it. The automated patient classification tool would allow entry of only 30 characters of free text from the terminal because the vendor had not yet begun to develop the nursing care planning or charting applications. Knowing that it would be an unnecessary duplication of work for nurses to recopy their handwritten notations daily onto a computer printout, the task force decided to retain the handwritten Kardex as a communication tool. This manual tool could also function as a backup if the automated system malfunctioned.

Although the traditional handwritten Kardex remained, the task force wanted to explore other uses for the computer printout, and it, therefore, piloted the use of computer printouts of the classification tool on one unit. This option allowed for experimentation with hard copies of the tool and provided data on their use in planning future automated charting applications.

Report formats were also an important issue. Nursing lobbied for uncluttered staffing reports that contained the relevant, required information. Because the vendor planned to market this system, however, its representatives were reluctant to delete items from report formats that other hospitals might require. Finally, the task force and vendor reached a compromise. Some standard staffing reports were revised, other reports would be revised if they were unacceptable after a reasonable trial period. An "ad hoc report writer," a software program written in Data Base III, was selected for the microcomputer so that nursing could tailor reports to changing needs.

The "give and take" process between the vendor and nursing was ongoing during the development of the system. Task force members convinced the vendor to provide a variety of classification–tool screen layouts that nurses could evaluate for readability and usability. The nursing task force was also able to secure special audit reporting capabilities. When the patient classification tools were audited, a special portion of the system would display and print out a grid indicating discrepancies between the auditor's classification and that of the caregiver's. Once certain patterns of classification errors were identified, nursing could introduce measures to resolve the problem.

Unique patient care situations occurred from time to time at WHC; for example, gynecological patients were occasionally transferred to surgical or medical units. It was necessary that the system accommodate such cases. The task force asked the vendor to design the system so that all seven patient classification tools could be called up if needed. The vendor was able to accommodate this adaptation.

Nursing made some concessions along the way. For example, we were not successful in securing unit-specific calculations of budgeted hours in the initial phase of the automated system. The system can only incorporate hospital-wide averages into calculations, and this limits the precision of certain report data. The task force was unable to secure a staffing reporting system with both centralized and decentralized functions in the alpha process. Nursing wanted five automated printers that could produce hospital-wide staffing reports in the central nursing office and division-specific staffing reports in the four decentralized divisions. The vendor offered nursing an either/or option: either nursing could have a centralized reporting function or a decentralized function, but not both. The task force chose the centralized reporting function. Nonetheless, it also began to explore the possibilities of purchasing a local area network to provide automated decentralized staffing reports as well as an NMIS. This turn of events demonstrated to task force members the validity of a classic dictum of business strategy: if the vendor cannot provide all that is needed in a reasonable time frame, compatible services should be investigated elsewhere. Nursing successfully negotiated some objectives. Not only was a strong auditing mechanism developed at their request, another important step was accomplished. The task force wanted the option to view certain staffing reports on the microcomputer without necessarily receiving a printout of the report. After first stating that this option was not feasible in the time-frame, the vendor later accommodated this request.

When important decision-making points were reached, such as when the vendor made claims that it could not provide certain design features, task force members educated themselves to the services that other vendors could provide. This negotiating strategy gave the task force great leverage in gaining a number of concessions. (Because the vendor made concessions on the major issues and was willing to compromise on other issues, the task force opted to continue project development with this vendor rather than seek a new contract with another.)

PLANNING FOR IMPLEMENTATION

Another key assignment of the task force was to plan for orderly implementation of the system. The patient classification system would require that nurses spend time at computer terminals on each nursing station; however, time spent away from patients had to be minimal. To accommodate a large number of new users efficiently, additional terminals and computer cables had to be approved and installed by the information systems department.

The biggest challenge was planning to train almost 1000 nurses to use the system. Each nurse was issued a user number and a password that gave access only to the nursing applications of the computer system. Most of the nurses had little or no experience with computers. The vendor took responsibility for train-ing 12 in-house personnel to educate nurses in the uses of the system. Each staff nurse required an average of 1½ hours of training, and the entire project took 12 part-time trainers a period of 3 months to complete.

The task force planned a staggered implementation program. After the ini-tial three pilot units were on-line, units in the rest of the hospital were "brought up live" in three groups over 1½ months at 2- to -3-week intervals. In this man-ner, task force members could troubleshoot problems on each unit as nurses became familiar with the classification system. An educational nursing forum was held early in the implementation period to share information and experi-ences with the new system and to plant the seeds for creative uses of the system by nurse managers and staff.

Finally, the task force began to evaluate the impact of the system on patient care. One purpose of the automated system was to save time. Could the time saved, however, be devoted to patient care? Would classifying patients on the computer, while keeping similar information on a manual Kardex for communi-cation purposes, take more or less time? Would some nurses resist the system? Would they begin to "nurse the computer instead of nursing the patients" (M. Flaherty, personal communication, July 19, 1984)? Would increased automation create unanticipated ethical problems or dehumanize care (Happ, 1983)?

Many of these questions remained unanswered until the system was fully operational for a length of time. In anticipation of problems in this area, how-ever, the task force, at the suggestion of a colleague (M. Flaherty, personal com-munication, July 19, 1984), looked for a way to address the effects of computeri-zation on the humanizing aspects of patient care. During the automation process, the hospital held a seminar on "humanizing patient care." The nursing staff was encouraged to participate.

In fact, the automated system was accepted extremely well by nursing staff because it saved them time and effort. No longer did they have to total points for their patients. They made selections from the screen, and the computer did the work.

The task force used a firm and canny business approach in negotiations. They always validated claims made by the vendor and strived to become as knowledgeable as the vendor to obtain maximum benefit from the capital outlay expended.

SUMMARY AND RECOMMENDATIONS

In planning for developing and installing a prototype of an automated patient classification system, the Associate Administrator for Nursing at WHC negoti-ated firm guarantees from the vendor that the system would meet WHC specifi-cations and selected a competent task force engaged in a continuous process of self-education, collaboration, compromise, and problem solving with the vendor.

Putting the system into operation involved planning for a staggered program of training, implementation, and troubleshooting. The 12-month process involved a lot of hard work; at the same time, it was exciting and challenging to be at the vanguard of efforts to cost-out nursing services, to facilitate nursing research, and, most important, to exert a positive impact on patient care.

The Nursing Automation Task force at the WHC came to believe firmly that nurses should take the lead in defining their automation needs and participate in the decisions involved in every effort of developing such systems. Ours is but one approach that may be used in collaborating with a vendor in developing an automated nursing system. This approach was profitable for nursing and may serve as a guide to others.

BIOGRAPHICAL SKETCHES

Mr Hylton is acting Associate Chief Nurse, Acute Psychiatric Hospital, St. Elizabeth's Campus, D.C. Commission on Mental Health Services in Washington, D.C. He received his BA degree from the College of Wooster in 1971 and subsequently earned a BSN at St. Louis University in 1977 and an MSN at the Catholic University of America in 1984. He participated in this project as practicum experience while earning his MSN.

Dr Joyce E. Johnson is Vice President, Division of Nursing at the Washington Hospital Center. Dr Johnson obtained her master's and doctoral degrees from the Catholic University of America and has held administrative positions in Nursing since 1971. In 1984, she attended the Johnson & Johnson Wharton Fellows Program. She has participated in a variety of educational programs at Catholic University, Marymount University and George Washington University. She is the editor of a book on creating business plans for nurse executives.

Ms Moran is Assistant Administrator, Nursing Systems Department at the Washington Hospital Center. She participated as a member of the task force to design and implement both the manual and automated patient classification systems at the hospital. She is well known as a speaker on nursing information systems and business planning. She has a masters degree in General Administration with a Health Administration specialty from the University of Maryland where she also earned her BSN.

REFERENCES

Donaho, B., & Hass, J. (1984). On the scene: Sisters of Mercy Health Corporation–The development and implementation of a corporate patient classification system. *Nursing Administration Quarterly*, (2), 12–15.

Happ, B. (1983). Should computers be used in the nursing care of patients? *Nursing Management, 14*(7), 31–35.

Washington Hospital Center

Nursing Kardex A (Med/Surg)

Patient Profile (History) _____

Referrals: _____

Discharge Planning: _____

Diet:

NPO			2
Feeds self/family feeds			2
Feeds self with help		Special/Q2H	5
Total feeding by staff			14
Cont tube/gastrostomy			
Feeding with checks	Q6H		5
	Q4H		8
	Q3H		11
	Q2H		16
Inter tube/gastrostomy			
Feeding with checks	Q6H		10
	Q4H		15
	Q3H		20
	Q2H		30

Vital signs:

TPR & BP	TID	3
	QID	4
	Q4H	7
	Q2H	13
Close observation		
Neuro/vascular eval	Q8H	1
	Q4H	3
	Q2H	6
	Q1H	12
CVP reading	Q_H	2
Telemetry maintenance		1

Treatments

Dressings/decubitus care		
Simple		
Medium		
Complex		
T E D stockings		
ACE bandages		
Psoriasis treatment		
Hot/cold packs		

Activity

Out of bed		
Dangle _____		
Pre op scrub		
Enema		0
Until clear		2

Treatments

Pre op check list			2
Peritoneal dialysis			
Manual	TID	2	80
Cycler	QID	9	34
Isolation	Q4H	15	
[ ] Strict [ ] Protective		20	18
		30	
[ ] Wound & skin precautions		1	9
[ ] Radiation [ ] Enteric [ ] Respiratory		3	3
Formal teaching/	BID	10	
Emotional support	TID	15	5
		7	

Sensory Aids

	2
	4
Dentures [ ] Upper	9

Toilet/output / Activity / Treatment — Manual Patient Classification Tool

Fluids (PO) D E N
Force ___ ___ ___
Restrict ___ ___ ___

Toilet/output   I&O [ ]
Item		Points
Toilets without help		1
Toilets with help		5
Constant supervision		8
Commode/urine/bedpan		6
Foley catheter care with output	QS	5
	Q1H	14
Intermittent catheter Q_H		13
Incontinent care		7
Urine f s ___		4

Hygiene
Item	Points
Bathes self	3
Bathes self with help	5
Bathed by staff	7
Roto bed/bath	30
Shave/shampoo	2

Classification points ___
Date ___
1 PM ___

Item		Points
Chair with help		3
Walk with help		5
Complete bed rest		0
Turns self		
Turn & preventive skin care	Q4H	10
	Q2H	20
Circo electric/stryker		40
Preventive skin care		7

Medications/IVs
Item		Points
Routine light (4a or less)		2
Heavy (5a or more)		6
PRN/special meds		5
IV meds	QD/B1D	2
	T1D/Q1D	4
	Q4H	5
	Q2H	11
Heparin lock		6
Blood/dextran		5
Cont IV/hyperal		5

Item		Points
Ostomy bag change		3
Colostomy irrigation		5
Sitz bath in room		
Sitz bath & const attend		0
Weigh ___	Scale	1
Thach cane	TID	7
	Q1H	10
Tach suction	Q1D	7
	Q4H	9
	Q3H	11
	Q2H	15
	Q1H	27
Oral suction		4
N G suction		5
Cough/deep breathe	Q1D	3
	Q2H	10
Sterile irrigations	Q_H	4
Ortho leg exercises		5
Specimen collection		1

[ ] Lower
[ ] Glasses [ ] Contacts   2
[ ] Hearing aid   7
Prosthesis ___   5
___   12

Sensory deficits
Speech ___   1
Hearing ___   7
Vision ___   10
Mental status ___   7
Restraints ___   9
___   11
___   4

Side rails ___

Mode of transport
[ ] Walks [ ] Wheelchair
[ ] Stretcher [ ] With IV

Special considerations

Code status ___

Figure 10–2. Manual patient classification tool for Med/Surg nursing units.

Kiley, M., Hollaran, E. Wester, J., Ozbolt, J., Werley, H., Gordon, M., Giova-netti, P., Thompson, J., Simpson, R., Zielstroff, R., Fitzpatrick., J., Davis, H., Cook, M., & Grier, M. (1983). Computerized Nursing Information Systems (NIS), *Nursing Management 14*(7), 26–30.

Weaver, C., & Johnson, J. (1984), Nursing participation in computer vendor se-lection. *Computers in Nursing 2*(2), 31–34.

APPENDIX

Details of the Patient Classification System

A manual patient classification system was developed in 1982 using a methodol-ogy that defined appropriate care factors for each nursing area.

At that time, individual classification tools were developed for medicine and surgery, shock trauma, obstetrics and gynecology, psychiatry, medical ICU, the neonatal nursery, and the intensive care nursery (Figure 10–2).

In addition, formulas (or algorithms) were developed for each unit which reflected its physical layout, unique workload, and amount of indirect care pro-

```
CLASSIFY PATIENT ON 1D BED 1D01-A              MED/SURG (KARDEX A) 08/06/85 1314
              SVC INT DR                          DX PULMON EMBOLISM/INFA
- - - - - - - - - - - - - - - - - - - - - - - - - - - - - - - - - - - - - - - - - - - - - -
PROBE UNASSIGNED FACTORS TO ADD THEM. PROBE ASSIGNED FACTORS TO DELETE THEM.
       DIET                    "   TOILET/OUTPUT         "    HYGIENE
       ? NPO                   "                         "    ? BATHES SELF
  *    ? FD. SELF/FAM. FD      "   ? TOILET W/O HELP      "
       ? FD. SELF W/HELP       "   ? TOILETS W/HELP      " *  ? BTH SELF W/HELP
  +    ? TOT. FD. BY STAFF     "   ? CNST SUPERVISN      "
       CONT. TUBE/GASTROSTOMY  " * ? COMMODE/UR/BEDP     "    ? BATHED BY STAFF
       ? W/CHECKS Q6H          "                         "
       ? W/CHECKS Q4H          "   - -FOLEY CATHETER CARE- -  "    ? ROTO/BED BATH
       ? W/CHECKS Q3H          "   ? W/OUTPUT QS         "
       ? W/CHECKS Q2H          "   ? W/OUTPUT Q1H        "    ? SHAVE/SHAMPOO
       INTER. TUBE/GASTROSTOMY "                         "
       ? W/CHECKS Q6H          "   ? INTERMITTENT        "
       ? W/CHECKS Q4H          "      CATHETER           "
       ? W/CHECKS Q3H          "   ? INCONTINENT CRE     "
       ? W/CHECKS Q2H          "   ? URINE FX            "

       ? FORCE FLUIDS          "                         "
- - - - - - - - - - - - - - - - - - - - - - - - - - - - - - - - - - - - - -
  ! EXIT          PRESS PF24 FOR HELP          ! EDUCATION          ! CONTINUE
E4357: PLEASE SELECT 01 OR FEWER FACTORS WITHIN DIET/FEEDING: MEAL/FEEDING/TUBE
```

Figure 10–3. Automated patient classification screen with error message.

vided, such as charting and coordinating care. These formulas and patient classification tools were adapted to a fully automated system. Each day nurses select care factors for their patients on the cathode ray tube (CRT). By touching a light pen to the screen, the nurses make relevant selections pertaining to each patient. Major classification categories such as Diet, Hygiene, Medications, and Treatments contain nursing care factors. For example, three nursing care factors appearing under Diet are "Feeds self," "Feeds self with help," and "Total feeding by staff." The nurse can select only one care factor in this category. Because each item is limited by coding to certain parameters, the nurses must select only one item. If the nurse selects more than one, an error message appears and the screen will not change until the error is corrected (Figure 10–3). This process assures correct usage of the system.

The CRT displays the classification choices made by the caregiver until the patient is reclassified. Quick review screens enable the nurse to classify patients in less than 1 minute.

07/29/1985 12:17   DAILY STAFFING REPORT
                      Last Download: 07/29/1985 12:59

5F/MED - AVG PCH: 7.56   07/29 EVENING   15:00   Shift AVG PCH: 2.49

Projections (07/29/85 12:59)   ADM: 3 D/C: 5 T/I: 0 T/O:0 OTH: 0

Census ACT (UND)	REC PCH	Other Hours	SKL	[----Staff----] SCH	REC	VAR	ACT Staff	Comments
13 (0)	32.42	−5.20	RN	2.0	2.3	−0.3		
			SLN	2.0	1.1	0.9		
			TOT	4.0	3.4	0.6		(Utilization = 85.1%

07/29 NIGHT   23:00   Shift AVG PCH: 1.89

Census ACT (UND)	REC PCH	Other Hours	SKL	[----Staff----] SCH	REC	VAR	ACT Staff	Comments
13 (0)	24.56	0.00	RN	2.0	2.1	−0.1		
			SLN	1.0	1.0	0.0		
			TOT	3.0	3.1	−0.1		(Utilization = 102.3%)

07/30 DAY   07:00   Shift AVG PCH: 3.17

Census ACT (UND)	REC PCH	Other Hours	SKL	[----Staff----] SCH	REC	VAR	ACT Staff	Comments
			RN	4.0	3.5	0.5		
13 (0)	41.27	0.00	SLN	1.0	1.7	−0.7		
			TOT	5.0	5.2	−0.2		(Utilization = 103.2%

Figure 10–4. Daily staffing report showing care hours needed for the nursing unit and the utilization rate of the staff.

```
┌─────────────────────────────────────────────────────────────────────────┐
│                                                                           │
│ AUDIT CLASSIFICATION: REVIEW                        MED-SURG 08/06/85 1317 │
│                  SVC INT DR                         DX PULMON EMBOLISM/INFA│
│ ------------------------------------------------------------------------- │
│ ASPECT          DESCRIPTION              ASPECT        DESCRIPTION          │
│ --------    -----------------------     --------   --------------------    │
│ AM 1        BED REST/TURNS SELF                                            │
│ AM 2        PREVENTIVE SKIN CARE                                          │
│ DT 1        FEEDS SELF/FAMILY FEEDS                                        │
│ HC 1        BATHED BY STAFF                                                │
│ MD 2        PRN/SPECIAL MEDS                                               │
│ MD 4        ROUTINE LIGHT: 4X OR LESS                                      │
│ TO 1        BEDPAN/URINAL/COMMODE                                          │
│ TX 2        DRESSINGS/DECUBITUS CARE: SIMPLE                               │
│ TX 2        FORMAL TEACHING/EMOT SUPPORT                                   │
│ VS 1        TPR BP TID/Q8H                                                 │
│ VS 2        CLOSE OBSERVATION                                              │
│                                                                           │
│     !  NEXT PAGE          DISCREP: 1 2 3 4 5 6 7 8           COMMENT        │
│ ORIGINAL CARE POINTS:    36.00        ×             AUDIT                   │
│ AUDITOR CARE POINTS:     38.00    TYPE: A    LVL:    ! ENTER COMMENT        │
│ ! DIET/TOIL/HYGIENE      ! VS/ACTV/MEDS   ! TREATMENTS                      │
│ PCCLSFAR                                             PRESS ENTER TO ACCEPT  │
│                                                                           │
└─────────────────────────────────────────────────────────────────────────┘
```

Figure 10-5. Audit review screen.

The staffing application runs on a microcomputer in the nursing office. Reports can be generated on a printer (Figure 10–4) or viewed on the screen.

Nursing units can be analyzed individually, in groups, or in relation to the entire hospital to determine staffing needs. At first, the vendor said it would not be possible to have a screen view option in the first phase, but later they accommodated this request.

A special audit function tracks errors and variances in order to ensure proper use of the system. A review screen at the end of each audit reflects the difference in points between the auditors classification and the caregivers classification. A grid demonstrates the aspect of care in which the error occurred (Figure 10–5).

11

Organizations as Work Flow Systems

Theodore Gessner

One characteristic that contributes to the effectiveness of an organization is the division of labor. Complex tasks are often carried out more easily if they are subdivided into parts. There are several ways to subdivide a job so that it can be carried out more efficiently; managers often adapt to this dilemma by accepting traditional ways of defining job characteristics. "This division of labor has worked in the past, so it is appropriate here" (e.g., a physician's primary task is to diagnose and order a medical regimen; a nurse's primary task is to carry out the physician's orders). This reliance on traditional approaches is often economical in simple static organizations but it can present serious problems for complex dynamic organizations.

The traditional job description is an important starting point for job design, but there are numerous factors that must be weighed in the deliberate designing of the division of work. Work in complex organizations does not occur in isolation. Each person's work is interdependent with the work of others and is subject to evaluation by others. When designing a job, therefore, it becomes important to consider both the characteristics of the task and how the task is embedded in the sociotechnical fabric of the organization.

JOB ANALYSIS

When performing a job analysis, there are three major dimensions to be considered: the job content, the job functions, and the interpersonal component. *Job content* refers to the general nature of the task and includes job variety, complexity, difficulty, the autonomy and task identity or completeness of the task. *Job functions* refer to the requirements and methods involved in each task. Job functions include job responsibility, authority, work methods, information flow, and coordination requirements. The *interpersonal component* of the job includes the amount of interaction required, the teamwork requirements, and the acquaintance potential.

In addition to these three major job design dimensions there are job issues concerned with the value placed on the work. These include job evaluation at the organizational level, the employee's evaluation of task accomplishment, and the direct and indirect feedback about task accomplishment.

Efforts directed at job design should closely evaluate the importance of each of these dimensions. These are the more concrete aspects of the task of job design. One must also be cognizant of the integration of the entire system within which a job is embedded and the assumptions made about work by administrators and workers within that system. The history of job design represents a lesson in the importance of the systems view and highlights the types of changes that have been made in job design over time.

HISTORY OF SYSTEMATIC JOB DESIGN

The history of systematic job design can be divided into three major periods. The first period was between the early 1900s and the beginning of the 1950s. Most of the job design effort in this period was directed toward job simplification. This was the heyday of the assembly line, and the task of job design was to break the job into its simplest parts. The second period lasted until the early 1960s and was an era of job enlargement. This change was a reaction to the morale problems that had resulted from job simplification. The third period, which extends from the 1960s until the present, involves the redesigning of jobs to allow for personal and professional growth of the workers.

Job Simplification

The concept of *scientific management* has been attributed to Taylor (1910). This approach focused on the simplification of jobs through standardization of work to increase efficiency. The major method is to observe the efficient worker and analyze the component parts of each task in a job. The concepts supporting this approach are very simple. The workers are more efficient if their work is standardized and broken into simple discrete components. The smaller, standardized units of work may then be easily learned, supervised, and rewarded. Using this approach, work can be more precisely planned by managers. The parts of the job can be prescribed and the timing of the task can be calculated, controlled, and coordinated. This is an approach from which efficient production lines were made.

Scientific management represents an important movement in modern organizational thought and in terms of job design was the preeminent model for over 50 years. The primary value of this approach was that it provided managers with tools for controlling the quantity and speed of production. Deviations from expectations could be identified and corrected with direct action. The planning and scheduling of work becomes a rational enterprise. The negative effects of this approach were recognized as associated with workers' perceptions that they were being treated as cogs in a machine. Jobs were designed to be simple and routine (mechanical), low in skill requirements, and involving little interaction. Workers often felt that their jobs were boring, unchallenging, and meaningless. They had little control over their work. Many people reacted with a lack of pride or care as to the quality of their work.

Job Enlargement

After World War II there was increased recognition that many jobs had become so routine and boring that they were causing serious worker morale problems. Low productivity and high turnover became serious management problems. New job design techniques were developed to deal with these problems by introducing variety in unskilled jobs.

In job rotation the tasks performed by the workers were considered to be simple and interchangeable. Unskilled workers could be rotated from one simple task to another without extensive retraining or a detrimental slowing of production. There was no major change in job functions but the worker gained a variety of skills. It was expected that job rotation would reduce both fatigue and boredom and increase job meaning and involvement as workers participated in an entire task through rotation.

Usually the process of job rotation resulted in only short-term gains. The jobs in the rotation were usually very similar and very routine. It took a little longer for the worker to become fatigued and bored. The most important impact of this method was that it considered the worker's morale in job design.

The next step in the evolution of job design was the work on job enlargement. Proponents of job enlargement recognized that the small simplified parts of a job could be connected into larger more complex jobs to be carried out by a simple worker. The worker's job then increased in task variety and complexity. This approach was designed to increase job satisfaction, but like job rotation it proved to be only a short-term solution. It did little to increase the meaning of work or the personal involvement of workers. The enlargement and job rotation approaches enjoyed relative success, and they opened the way for more complex and theoretically based approaches to job design.

Job Enrichment

The phase of job design referred to as job enrichment involved three major theoretical contributions. They were: Herzberg's theory (Herzberg, Mausner, & Snyderman, 1959) of job motivation, and expansion of this theory by Hackman and Oldham (1975), and the sociotechnical design approach (Trist, 1981) to job design.

The concept of job enrichment is grounded on the theoretical framework developed by Herzberg (1966). The theory identified two sets of motivational factors: hygiene factors and motivators. Hygiene factors are the external characteristics of the job (e.g., pay, job content, security, benefits). The job rotation and enlargement approaches dealt with hygiene factors. These factors are important because they reduce job dissatisfaction, but according to Herzberg's theory they do not result in an increase in satisfaction. Job dissatisfaction and satisfaction are viewed as two separate dimensions related to the two motivational factors. It is the motivators (e.g., job challenge, autonomy, responsibility) that are the basis for the feelings of job satisfaction. The motivators are important for all jobs, but they take on greater importance in professional jobs where job challenge, autonomy, and responsibility are expectations of both the employee and the employer.

Job enrichment approaches are concerned with changing the motivators. In job enrichment an increased sense of achievement and involvement is the goal. Worker accountability and responsibility is increased and feedback is provided. The job is not just increased in terms of complexity but there is the opportunity for the worker to shape the job and experience personal growth. The thrust of this approach is that enlarging the job vertically as well as horizontally will increase job satisfaction and there will be a concomitant increase in quality of production.

The cost of this approach from the managerial viewpoint is that there is greater investment in each employee and less control as each employee participates in decision making. More skill is required to carry out the enriched job, and there is greater investment of time, training, and pay in each worker. The success of a job enrichment program is measured by reduction in absenteeism and turnover. Savings result from reducing the costs of recruiting and training of replacements.

The idea of job enrichment is to deal with both the hygiene factors and motivators to reduce sources of dissatisfaction and increase sources of satisfaction. Basically it considers the skills and needs of the employee in the design of the job.

The approach of Herzberg was modified by Hackman and Oldham (1975), and is based on the idea of altering core job dimensions to fit the specific needs of the employee (Fig. 11–1). In this approach the core job dimensions are linked to specific psychological states. The psychological states are linked to specific production and work behavior outcomes. The total linkage between job dimensions and productivity are moderated by the employee's needs.

The five core job dimensions are skill variety, task identity, task significance, autonomy, and feedback. Skill variety refers to the degree that the job requires different skills and talents. Task identity is the extent to which the job requires the completion of a visible, identifiable product. Task significance is the extent to which the product impacts on others or is valued within and outside the organization. Autonomy is the extent to which the employee can exercise discretion in how and when the job will be done. Feedback is the extent to which the job and the organization provide clear information about the employee's performance.

When the core job dimensions of skill variety, task identity, and task significance are maximized the employee experiences the critical psychological state of meaningful work. When autonomy is maximized the individual experiences a

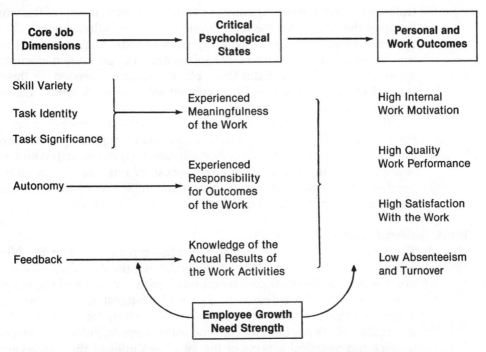

Figure 11-1. Relationships among core job dimensions, critical psychological states, and on-the-job outcomes. Copyright © by the Regents of the University of California. *(Reprinted/ condensed from the* California Management Review, *Vol. 17, No. 4. By permission of The Regents.)*

sense of responsibility for the work outcome. When feedback is increased the person has knowledge of work activities. The theory predicts that the combination of these three critical psychological states results in high productivity and job satisfaction.

The caveat in this theory is the assumption of a clear linkage between core job dimensions, personal and work outcomes, and the needs of the employee. If the employee is concerned primarily with work meeting lower order needs (*hygiene factors*) the attempts at job design are likely to be resisted. If the employee places a high value on meeting higher order needs (Herzberg's motivators) through their work, then the attempts at job design are more likely to increase job satisfaction and reduce absenteeism and turnover. There is some evidence that over time employees can be trained to change their expectations of their work to include meeting higher needs.

Work Group Design

The sociotechnical approach (Trist, 1981) focuses on the work group as the appropriate place for job redesign. The task of the group is defined, but the methods used to accomplish the task are determined by the members of the work group. With this type of approach the work group becomes the unit that controls the planning and assignment of work. The performance of the work group becomes the criteria for the distribution of pay and other rewards. Within this approach there is change in both the work of individuals and the structure of the organization. One of the most successful and best known examples of this approach is the design of the Volvo plant in Kalmar, Sweden. In this situation the replacement of assembly lines with autonomous work groups increased morale and reduced turnover.

The major lesson that can be garnered from the theories of job design is that there is not a single best approach or clear set of guidelines. The literature on the effectiveness of job design is basically case history research with no rigorous studies comparing the relative effectiveness of one job design strategy over another. These case studies have been done in different industries, and few of the studies have been concerned with service organizations.

Work Roles of Nurses

The foundation of modern nursing practice can be found in the Nightingale School of Nursing (Kelly, 1981). This model identified two types of nurses: the nurse educator/administrator/community health clinician and the hospital ward nurse. The hospital ward nurse is of particular interest because it is on this foundation that the traditional job description of the hospital nurse is built. The job description of the Nightingale hospital ward nurse included personality characteristics and technical aspects of the job. The duties of the probationer are included in Table 11-1. The role of the nurse was to keep the ward hygienic and to provide for the technical care of the patient while remaining virtuous.

This job description did not change much for the next 80 years. Although during this time there were definite changes in nursing in the United States. The major change came in terms of trying to provide adequate training for nurses. The major mechanisms for training were the hospital-affiliated nursing schools and the incorporation of nursing into the curriculum of colleges and universities. Despite educational upgrading, nursing was perceived as an occupation without much status.

During World War II, the job of the nurse increased in value. There was a shortage of trained nurses that was felt on both the battlefield and the homefront. Nursing was beginning to be recognized as a legitimate occupation for women. Licensure laws were passed and attempts were made to standardize the training of nurses. After the war, medical technology made some spectacular advances in the treatment and cure of disease and the role of the nurse experienced a concomitant expansion. There was expansion of the role of nursing both within the traditional hospital setting and within the community. With the role expansion came improvement in education. More people began to talk about nursing as a profession.

At the present time there are problems facing nursing because of the increased emphasis on professionalism. Nurses are trained to be professionals, but the organizations where nurses are employed treat them as semiprofessionals (Gross & Etzioni, 1985). Nurses get little respect in many health care organi-

TABLE 11-1. DUTIES OF PROBATIONER UNDER THE "NIGHTINGALE FUND."
ST. THOMAS'S HOSPITAL, 1860

Your are required to be

Sober	Punctual
Honest	Quiet and Orderly
Truthful	Cleanly and Neat
Trustworthy	Patient—Cheerful, and Kindly

You are expected to become skillful

1. In the dressing of blisters, burns, sores, wounds and in applying fomentations, poultices, and minor dressings.
2. In the application of leeches, externally and internally.
3. In the administration of enemas for men and women.
4. In the management of trusses, and appliances in uterine complaints.
5. In the best method of friction to the body and extremities.
6. In the management of helpless patients, i.e., moving, changing, personal cleanliness of, feeding, keeping warm, (or cool), preventing and dressing bed sores, managing position of.
7. In bandaging, making bandages, and rollers, lining of splints, etc.
8. In making the beds of the patients, and removal of sheets whilst patient is in bed.
9. You are required to attend at operations.
10. To be competent to cook gruel, arrowroot, egg flip, puddings, drinks, for the sick.
11. To understand ventilation, or keeping the ward fresh by night as well as by day; you are to be careful that great cleanliness is observed in all the utensils; those used for secretions as well as those required for cooking.
12. To make strict observation of the sick in the following particulars: The state of secretions, expectoration, pulse, skin, appetite; intelligence, as delirium or stupor; breathing, sleep, state of wounds, eruptions, formation of matter, effect of diet, or of stimulants, and of medicines.
13. And to learn the management of convalescents.

zations, and they are often disillusioned. This condition has been called reality shock (Kramer, 1974). As a result of reality shock, research has shown that the professionally oriented nurses are more likely to leave the profession.

McClure and colleagues (1983) studied well-managed hospitals to try to determine what these "magnet hospitals" do to retain staff nurses. The staff nurses in these hospitals value the fact that they are treated as professionals. The management in these hospitals is perceived as participatory in style, there is a recognition of professional standards of performance, and the nurses have a sense of autonomy. These hospitals are seen as supporting the professional development of their nursing staffs. This study suggests the type of changes that the nursing administrator should consider in the design or redesign of the role of nurses within a complex organization. Nurses want to be treated as professionals and it is the responsibility of the administrator to work for these goals even though within many health care organizations there are serious impediments to this kind of change.

JOB DESIGN IN NURSING

The history of scientific job design helps to elucidate the major strategies of job design, but it does not directly address the specific problems that are faced by the nurse administrator. Nursing is at a critical point in its history. It can continue in a semiprofessional status or it can adopt models of nursing practice that increase the recognition of the professional status of nurses. This second alternative will be readily accepted by most nurses. It is, however, an alternative that requires an active process of job design and it is an alternative that will have impact on the structure of health care organizations.

Historically nursing had been under the administrative control of physicians and, more recently, the professional hospital administrator. The nurse has been a key care provider but there has not been acceptance of the nurse as a professional member of the staff by many hospital administrators. The nurse carries out the orders of the physicians as well as other tasks; the services of the nurses are paid for out of daily operating budgets. The responsibility of the staff nurse is seen by many administrators as using skills only within the constraints of the prescribed medical regimen. The nurse provides the routine medical care that is too time consuming for the physician to perform. The nurse is viewed as a physician extender with little recognition of the nurse's independent functions. The physician's job has been simplified through delegation of certain tasks to nurses. In these hospitals administration views the physician as having the professional part of the job (e.g., diagnosis, treatment planning, prescription) and the nurse as having the semiprofessional part (e.g., monitoring the patient, delivering medications). Decisions about the patient's care are seen as the primary responsibility of the physicians. This job distinction has been clearly codified in the structure of many health care organizations and in some licensing laws.

The question that faces the nurse administrator is how can the professional status of the nurse be either established or enhanced within a complex organization? Within the nursing profession there are a number of models of nursing practice that provide the basis for executing a program of job design within an organization. Some of the models that can be considered are nurse extenders, service-line managers, primary care nursing or case management, clinical ladders, shared governance, and nurse administered units. Each of these models provides the structure upon which a comprehensive program of job design can be built. Each of these models have strengths and weaknesses that should be considered before they are applied and other professionals in the organization may well place practical restraints on the choice of the model.

The *nurse extender* model is one of the easiest models to implement. This model may best be employed to deal with situations where there is a shortage of nurses or where the organization has to economize to survive. Nurse extender programs can be implemented relatively quickly and efficiently. The strategy is one of job simplification. The job of the nurse on a unit is analyzed into its component parts and the more routine aspects of the jobs are assigned to Liscensed Practical Nurses, nursing aides, or medical technicians. For example, on an ICU unit instead of assigning a single nurse to monitor each patient, the monitoring of equipment might be assigned to medical technicians and a nurse may supervise a number of medical technicians and provide direct nursing care.

The job design task becomes a matter of deciding what tasks can be most easily and legally carried out by the paraprofessional and what kinds of training the paraprofessionals need to do these jobs and nurses need to monitor them. These kinds of programs do have an immediate impact on the professional status of the nurse because they free the nurse to perform the more challenging parts of the job and they increase the responsibility of nurses to include more direct supervision and training of the paraprofessionals. These kinds of changes are usually not met by much resistance within the organization as they are a response to immediate crisis and they do little to alter the structure of the organization other than to increase the supervisory responsibility of the staff nurse.

The major problem with this type of job design is that it has very little impact on the structure of the organization and does very little to change the autonomy and responsibility of the nurse in the process of determining the care of the patient. It may in some cases remove the nurse from direct involvement in patient care resulting in both a reduction in stress and a reduction in job satisfaction. It may also increase stress if the nurse does not receive legitimate authority commensurate with the responsibility of supervising the paraprofessionals.

The *service-line manager* model (Bruhn & Howes, 1986) is a job design strategy that offers potential for increasing the responsibility of the nurse within the organization. In this model of patient care delivery, the nurse acts as a manager of services to patients who are admitted for a particular type of problem such as opthalmic surgery. The nurse becomes a boundary spanner who is not tied to one service but is responsible for coordinating the total range of services required by that class of clients. This strategy increases the job variety and responsibility of the nurse and the duties of coordinating service may represent an increase in autonomy within some systems.

This type of change does involve a change in some areas of the institution's chain of command and from a status perspective can be seen as enhancing the professional status of nurses. One drawback of this kind of approach, however, is that if the services provided for a particular type of patient are fairly routine or if any change in routine requires the permission of a physician, then there may be no reason for this type of function to be carried out by a nurse. If no clinical judgment is needed, there is no reason that the job needs to be done by a nurse.

Another model of job design is *primary care nursing* or *case management* (Grau, 1984; Zander, 1985). Within this model, as in the service-line manager model, there is a central concern with the movement of the client through the health care system. The two approaches seem to differ on the level of responsibility of the nurse. The primary care nursing model is tied more closely with the traditional setting of nursing care. This model of nursing care is an extension of the traditional nursing role. The primary care nurse becomes an administrator who has the autonomy and the responsibility to provide patient care without losing the rewards that come from being directly involved in the providing of care. The job is enriched in terms of task, responsibility, and autonomy. The staff nurse has to exercise professional judgment and is accountable for that judgment. This model of nursing care increases the meaningfulness of the work because the primary care nurse must oversee and evaluate the total treatment process and follow-up.

Case management is sometimes referred to as second-generation primary nursing. Here, the nurse is assigned a patient upon admission and becomes a case manager for the entire course of treatment for that admission. The responsibilities of the case manager are to oversee the process of providing treatment within the health care setting and to provide for continued treatment outside of the setting. The nurse plays an active role in the planning, the providing of treatment, cost monitoring the evaluation of treatment effectiveness, and the provision of aftercare.

The implementation of either primary nursing or case management involves organizational change. The nurse administrator is further removed from direct involvement in the provision of patient services, and new responsibilities for evaluation and advocacy will have to be learned. In addition to change in the nursing roles, these models affect the roles of other professionals (e.g., social workers, other nurses, physicians) and paraprofessionals (e.g., medical technicians, rehabilitation therapists), and these changes may present an impediment to the implementation of this program of job design.

Another model of nursing care that can provide the foundation for increasing the professional status of nurses is the *clinical ladder* (American Nurses Association Cabinet on Nursing Service, 1984). Two problems noted in the nursing turnover literature are that the nurse quickly reaches the salary ceiling and that advancement within many organizations involves becoming an administrator. The clinical ladder in its prototypic form differentiates the lines of advancement into a clinical track and an administrative track. To implement this type of system, criteria for advancement including both skill and education must be developed, and within the organization the pay scale of the nurse must be modified to accommodate the differentiation of skills within the nurses' work.

This model affects the organization in that it modifies the pay ceiling primarily for the clinical nurse. It also does contribute to the professional status of nursing because it codifies the responsibilities and duties that are performed by the nurse. The problem of the model is that there is a great deal of work and soul searching involved in developing the criteria and except for the pay schedule changes and some organizational recognition of the status of nurses, there is little concomitant change in the organizational structure.

The *shared governance* for nursing (Peterson & Allen, 1986a,b) is the most radical and idealistic of the job design models and its focus is on the modification of the organization. The job of the nurse is defined in terms similar to the terms used in primary care nursing. Within this model, however, the changes that must be accomplished are in the very structure of the health care organization.

Most health care organizations are hierarchical bureaucracies where decisions are made through a rigid chain of command. The alternative health care organization that is proposed within this model is the professional practice organization that is organized as a matrix organization. In this kind of organization there is a flattening of structure. Decisions are made in a more democratic and collaborative fashion. The skills of each profession and the interdependence between professions are recognized. Lateral communication is fostered and the joint decision making is the rule rather than the exception.

As a job design strategy the shared governance approach differs from the others in its organizational focus. Its primary methods involve changing the decision-making and communication channels within the organization. A primary mechanism for organizational change are joint practice committees that carry out the job of defining the work of the organization and open the process of professional communications so that a more equalitarian structure can evolve. A major impediment to the implementation of the shared governance model is the nurses' power within the organization. This approach involves not just self-change but extensive organizational change. This kind of job design involves a substantial and long-term effort in organizational development.

The final model that is considered is the *nurse administered unit* (Dear, Weisman, & O'Keefe, 1985). In this model there is increased self-governance for the nurses. In this particular example of the model a group of nurses who are hospital employees develop an informal contract with the hospital for the total management of the unit. The contract involves a budget, agreements about amounts of hospital support, and specification of criteria for quality of care. In effect in this model a team of nurses negotiates a contract with the organization, and within that contract the team of nurses is free to develop a system for providing a program of health care. The nursing team experiences increased responsibility, autonomy, control, and accountability. The redesigning of the nurses' job is not as sweeping a change as envisioned in the shared governance approach, and it can be implemented more quickly because it is localized within the contracting unit. Its success is dependent on both the acceptance of accountability by the nurses and cooperative working relationships with physicians and other professionals working on the unit.

IMPLEMENTING JOB DESIGN

Job design can be as simple as changing the duties of a single nurse or as complex as redesigning the role of nurses within an organization. There is no correct way to design the nurses' job. Under ideal conditions the decision about job design can be incorporated within the long-term planning processes of the organization. Ideal conditions, however, rarely exist in complex organizations, and the nurse administrator has to make decisions that are at best only partial solutions to complex problems. This should not stop the process of job design. Many of the activities that have been included under the title of job design are not exotic activities for an administrator. They are frequently routine responses to problems that arise within the day-to-day commerce of an organization. It is obvious that if health care activities continue to grow in complexity and the supply of trained professional nurses continues to decline that job design activities will have to be more radical in nature than these day-to-day adjustments. Job design will become a necessity to attract new nurses, to retain trained nurses, and to respond to changes in organizational structure.

Job design should not be looked at as a single discrete event but as an ongoing process. Understanding this process involves awareness of what is happening within the organization, the profession, and the health care industry. At the organizational level there is a need to know how the organization is structured and what plans are being made for continued and innovated services. At the professional level there is the need to know the major trends in the provision of nursing care. There are a number of models of nursing practice that can provide the skeleton upon which nursing and nursing-related jobs can be shaped. At the level of the health care industry it is necessary to identify the new technologies and services that are being developed.

The process of job design that involves changing the model of nursing services can be conceived as an organizational developmental process. To carry out a program of *organizational change* it is necessary for the nurse administrator to engage in a systematic program that can be conceptualized as involving three stages of planning, implementation, and evaluation. Each of these stages involves a great deal of effort and the success of any program of organizational change requires attention to detail at every stage.

Planning Stage

The planning stage can be seen as having four steps. The first step is to perceive a need for change. The second step is to identify the existing problems within the organization. The third step is to select and modify a specific model for change. The final step in the planning stage is to systematically plan for the implementation of the change. The careful execution of the steps in this first stage can reduce, although not eliminate, problems in the implementation and evaluation stages.

The first step in planning for job redesign is to be aware that the redesigning of the nursing job is possible. *Perceiving the need for change* is not as simple as it appears. Within organizations the daily demands on an administrator of a large service are frequently both exhilarating and exacerbating. The demands on time and resources can limit one's ability to look at an organization objectively. There are constant problems to be dealt with and often there is neither the time nor resources available to plan for the long term. Without consideration of long-term objectives the process of job redesign turns out to be a crisis intervention and not a thoughtful enhancement of the jobs of the people within the organization. Many administrators hire consultants to assist in diagnosing problems and planning job redesign. The ability to perceive the need for change involves an acute awareness of both the organization and the total environment within which that organization is embedded.

The second step in the planning stage is the identification of problems. *Diagnosis of problems* within a nursing staff requires knowledge of the nurses' professional concerns and their views of their job duties and responsibilities. This information is sometimes available through the normal interaction between the nurse administrator and the staff nurses, but as an organization gets larger informal methods of obtaining information are often inadequate. Other methods are needed to obtain information. Structured group techniques can be used to clarify the concerns of staff nurses. These might include routine procedures, such as staff meetings, or more directed interactions, such as quality circles or focus groups. These techniques provide a way to learn about staff concerns and they encourage staff participation in the planning, which can prove invaluable for garnering support for institutional change. In addition to group interaction approaches there is often the need to collect more precise empirical data about the staff and their views of nursing and the work that nurses do.

At the level of measuring attitudes toward the work there are measures already developed to look at the attitudes of nurses (Kramer, 1974; Prestholdt Lane, & Mathews, 1987). In addition to the attitudinal measures, there are structured measures of the staff member self-reports of their work such as the job diagnostic survey (Hackman & Oldham, 1975) or the multimethod job design questionnaire (Campion & Thayer, 1985). These questionnaires provide a relatively cheap and effective method to assess the nurses' evaluations of their work. Another source of information is the behavioral assessment of nursing staff productivity (Rantz & Hauer, 1987). This method involves taking a time sample of the nursing staff at work, and it gives a complete picture of how nurses actually spend their working time.

The diagnoses that are made by the nurse administrator are only as good as the information on which they are based, and the nurse administrator has to make conscious choices about the amount and quality of the information that is necessary to identify problems of the nursing staff. In most cases it is prudent to collect information using more than one method, and if job design is an ongoing process, routine collection of this type of data should be considered.

The next step after problems have been identified, is to develop *methods to remedy* or *reduce the problems* identified. The information collected about the nursing staff and the organization become important data for the planning of change. The choice of an alternative design of nursing duties and responsibilities should be based on a realistic assessment of the attitudes and needs of the nursing staff and with full awareness of organizational constraints. The models of job design developed within the nursing profession can provide both structure and justification for organizational change, but any model of the nursing job must be molded to fit the needs of that particular nursing staff and organization. At this step in the planning it is important to involve professional staff in the decision-making process.

The final step in the planning stage is to plan for the *implementation* of the job redesign. At this point the plan begins to move from an abstraction to a concrete reality, and it becomes necessary to deal with resistance to change. This resistance comes not only from management but also from the nursing staff. Change represents a threat to established patterns of relationships, and when there is animosity between management and staff the threat posed by change is magnified by the lack of trust and communication. One strategy that can be helpful in overcoming this resistance is to include organizational staff in this choice process. The treating of professional staff in a professional manner by involving them in the choice process can increase both their involvement and investment in the change process. The short-term costs of this approach is that it often broadens the scope of the changes, but in the long term it reduces some of the resistance. It keeps the new program from being perceived as being imposed by the administrators, and the people included in this planning stage become in many cases the core group of the implementation phase.

Implementation Stage

The implementation stage is the major action component in organizational change. In most cases the success of this stage is dependent on the thoroughness of the planning and the involvement of middle management. It also depends on the ability of the administrators and staff to translate plans into action. Often insufficient resources are allocated to this stage resulting in fragmented implementation. For example, deadlines have to be established, staff members must be trained, responsibilities of staff and management must be defined, mechanisms must be established to deal with the problems that inevitably arise, and methods for obtaining feedback from the staff and communicating information to the staff must be established. The implementation is not a one-time occurrence, but an ongoing process.

Evaluation Stage

The final stage is evaluation of the effectiveness of the job redesign. This involves measuring the impact of the changes on staff, clients, and the organization. The measures should be chosen to reflect the stated goals of the job redesign effort. These measures should include measures of clients (e.g., quality of care, client satisfaction), staff (e.g., absenteeism, turnover, job satisfaction), and organizational effectiveness (e.g., cost–benefit analysis). The job redesign program has been designed and implemented to improve the organization and it has involved a great deal of effort. Thought and effort alone, however, do not insure that the job redesign will work. The evaluation component of organizational change is designed to provide objective standards for justifying continued implementation and for identifying components of the effort that require modification. The administrator must realize that the job redesign usually will not fulfill all of the stated goals, and there will be the need for modification over time.

As health care organizations are becoming market driven their structures are changing both to accommodate increasing complexity and to employ more sophisticated business practices such as strategic planning. Simultaneously pressures for cost containment and a scarcity of nurses to meet demand are reshaping service delivery. Nurse administrators must act to take advantage of this time of change to redesign nursing systems and to enhance the professional practice of nursing.

BIOGRAPHICAL SKETCH

Dr Theodore Gessner is an Associate Professor of Psychology at George Mason University. Dr Gessner received his PhD in Social Psychology from the University of Maryland. Before joining the faculty at George Mason University, he was employed as a research psychologist in both public and private mental hospitals. His research interests include adaptation to organizations, sex roles, impression management by psychiatric patients, and evaluation research. Dr Gessner teaches undergraduate social psychology courses and industrial/organizational and human factors engineering courses in the doctoral program in psychology. He also does management and program evaluation consulting with psychiatric facilities.

SUGGESTED READINGS

Hackman, J.R., & Suttle, J.L. (Eds.). (1977). *Improving Life at Work: Behavioral Science Approaches to Organizational Change.* Santa Monica: Goodyear.

Joiner, C., & van Servellen, G.M. (1984). *Job Enrichment in Nursing: A Guide To Improving Morale, Productivity, and Retention.* Rockville: Aspen.

Porter-O'Grady, T., & Finnigan, S. (1984). *Shared Governance For Nursing: A Creative Approach to Professional Accountability.* Rockville: Aspen.

REFERENCES

American Nurses' Association Cabinet on Nursing Service. (1984). *Career Ladders: An Approach to Professional Productivity and Job Satisfaction.* Kansas City: American Nurses Association.

Bruhn, P.S., & Howes, D.H. (1986). Service line management: New opportunities for nursing executives. *Journal of Nursing Administration, 16*(6), 13–18.

Campion, M.A., & Thayer, P.W. (1985). Development and field evaluation of an interdisciplinary measure of job design. *Journal of Applied Psychology, 70*(1), 29–43.

Dear, M.R., Weisman, C.S., & O'Keefe, S. (1985). Evaluation of a contract model for professional nursing practice. *Health Care Management Review, 10*(2), 65–77.

Grau, L. (1984). Case management and the nurse. *Geriatric Nursing, 5*(8), 372–375.

Gross, E., & Etzioni, A. (1985). *Organizations in Society*. Englewood Cliffs: Prentice-Hall.

Hackman, J.R., & Oldham, G.R. (1975). Development of the job diagnostic survey. *Journal of Applied Psychology, 60*(1), 159–170.

Herzberg, F. (1966). *Work and the Nature of Man*. New York: World Publishing Company.

Herzberg, F., Mausner, B., & Snyderman, B. (1959). *The Motivation to Work*. New York: Wiley.

Kelly, L.Y. (1981). *Dimensions of Professional Nursing*, 4th ed. New York: Macmillan.

Kramer, M. (1974). *Reality Shock: Why Nurses Leave Nursing*. St. Louis: Mosby.

McClure, M.L., Pulin, M.A., Sovie, M.D., & Wandelt, M.A. (1983). *Magnet Hospitals: Attraction and Retention of Professional Nurses*. Kansas City: American Nurses' Association.

Peterson, M.E., & Allen, D.G. (1986a). Shared governance: A strategy for transforming organizations, Part 1. *Journal of Nursing Administration, 16*(1), 9–12.

Peterson, M.E., & Allen, D.G. (1986b). Shared governance: A strategy for transforming organizations, Part 2. *Journal of Nursing Administration, 16* (2), 11–16.

Prestholdt, P.H., Lane, I.M., & Mathews, R.C. (1987). Nurse turnover as reasoned action: Development of a process model. *Journal of Applied Psychology, 72*(2), 121–127.

Rantz, M., & Hauer, J.D. (1987). Analyzing acute care nursing staff productivity. *Nursing Management, 18*(4), 33–44.

Taylor, F.W. (1910). *The Principles of Scientific Management*. New York: Harper & Row.

Trist, E. (1981). The evaluation of sociotechnical systems as a conceptual framework and as an action research program in A.H. Vandiven & W.F. Joyce (eds.) *Perspectives in Organizational Design and Behavior* New York: Wiley. Wiley Interscience 19–75.

Zander, K. (1985). Second generation primary nursing: A new agenda. *Journal of Nursing Administration, 15*(3), 18–21.

APPLICATION 11-1

Decentralizing a Nursing System

Phillipa Ferguson Johnston

This scenario illustrates how job redesign might be accomplished in a community hospital. Valley Hospital is a 350-bed hospital in a large urban area. Changes in reimbursement have resulted in shorter lengths of stay and decreased occupancy. In addition, a new hospital 15 minutes away has resulted in the loss of 15 physicians who were previously high admitters to Valley. The

hospital faces extensive competition for beds, physicians, nurses, and other resources. The Board of Directors is concerned about survival of the hospital. One
year ago they hired a new Chief Executive Officer (CEO), who was given a mandate to assure that the hospital was competitive in the market place.

Although the institution is generally well run, there are sufficient problems
within the ranks of nursing to warrant concern. Turnover is approaching 40
percent. Physicians complain that there are not enough nurses and that their
patients are not properly cared for. Physicians say that they do not understand
what went wrong, but in the last 2 years nursing care at Valley Hospital has
diminished in quality. This decline in care is a factor in their change to the new
hospital. If things could be improved they would consider returning to Valley.
The CEO wants the hospital to be perceived as a quality institution for patients
and physicians and a good place to work for employees. He is concerned that
nursing has so many problems, because nursing is critical to the success of the
institution.

The CEO attempts to work with and support the incumbent Vice President
for Nursing of 15 years, but finds that she is unable to design strategies to improve the nursing department. He replaces her with another experienced nurse
administrator coming from an institution that once had similar problems. She
accepts the mandate for change and sees the hospital as having great potential.
She spends the first 3 months completing an assessment of the organization by
talking to nursing staff, physicians, patients, other administrators and her peers
in other cities with similar problems.

The nursing organization is presently decentralized into three divisions
headed by three assistant vice presidents who report to the vice president for
nursing. Three to four head nurses report to each of the division directors. The
head nurses have 24-hour accountability and responsibility for patient care on
paper, but in practice have not actualized these responsibilities. Each head nurse
has one to three assistant head nurses. The staff reports through the assistant
head nurses to the head nurse and consists of registered nurses, nursing assistants, and unit clerks. Supervisors cover the nursing division on evenings,
nights, and weekends.

Regarding staffing, budgeted FTEs are adequate. The ratio of registered
nurses to ancillary staff is 80 to 20. Staffing is based on patient classification, but
because of vacancies actual FTEs are frequently less than indicated as required.
Each head nurse schedules nurses differently and there is little control of agency
nurse utilization. Recruitment of nurses is haphazard and turnover is high.

There is confusion and conflict concerning accountability among head
nurses, assistant vice presidents, and supervisors. There is role conflict and confusion among registered nurses and nursing assistants as well. Poor relationships exist with medical chiefs and attending physicians. Nursing practice is
task oriented.

Interviews with nursing staff identify concerns related to the following
issues:

- Job importance and recognition: Nurses are not respected especially by physicians.
- Pay is low: Nurses should be paid more for working weekends; other financial incentives are needed.
- Advancement opportunities: The only way to improve pay is to become a manager.
- Occupational tedium: Nursing seems to be routine and not very much fun.
- Morale is poor: Contributes to high turnover.
- Head nurses treat certain staff preferentially.
- Support systems do not work properly, especially pharmacy and housekeeping.
- Nursing assistants do not do their jobs.

Based on this assessment, the vice president for nursing identified four broad objectives:

1. Improve the clinical practice of nursing.
2. Create participative management.
3. Improve physician–nurse relationships.
4. Improve employee morale.

The first step in meeting these objectives is to ask the question, "what is the best structure to accomplish these objectives?" The vice president for nursing systematically considered first nursing work, and second, how to structure work to meet her four objectives. When necessary, jobs were redesigned, with consideration given to degree of control over work, accountability and improved communication. In all instances new standards of performance were created.

Assistant Vice President Role

The assistant vice president layer of management was eliminated. The assistant vice president role was preventing the head nurses from having access to the vice president of nursing and immediate access to the information necessary to make crucial decisions. In addition, decision making was delayed because of the requirement to go through the assistant vice president. This hospital is not so large that the span of control for the nurse executive will be unwieldy.

Head Nurse Role

The head nurse position was elevated to department head status. A salary survey and comparison with other department heads within the organization revealed the head nurse salary substantially lower than other department heads. A salary adjustment modified this inequity and the job was redesigned to include the following functions:

- Management of patient care and supervision of patient care providers.
- Selection, performance evaluation, and discipline of nursing and clerical staff.
- Budgeting, development, and monitoring of staffing levels, unit inventory, and capital improvements.
- Planning and unit policy formulation to support the strategic plan.
- Quality assurance.
- Development of working relationships with medical chiefs.
- Participation on hospital and medical staff committees and task forces.
- Participation in the tactical decision making body, the nursing executive council.
- Input for marketing plans for services on their units.
- Educational preparation by a management development series was necessary to actualize the new job. In addition, the vice president for nursing coached and counseled the incumbents to assure success in the new roles. New head nurses would be expected to have or be enrolled in master's degree programs in administration. Current head nurses without master's degrees must include a plan for achievement in their yearly goals.

This job redesign resulted in:

- Twenty-four-hour accountability for patient care.
- Greater flexibility in working hours.
- Authority and power to manage employees and patients.
- Recognition as a department head.
- Clear definition of role and responsibilities.
- More money and hopefully greater job satisfaction.

Assistant Head Nurse Role

The assistant head nurse role was previously considered a "desk job." The assistant head nurses (AHNs) functioned as charge nurse on days and "acting head nurse" on off shifts. As charge nurse, assistant head nurses basically completed orders and coordinated discharges and transfers. The AHNs were not expected to actually monitor or direct patient care or as a resource by the staff for clinical problems. The AHNs complained that these positions had a title but no authority. Caught between the head nurse and the staff, they sometimes were confused as to their role and responsibilities. The assistant head nurse role was redesigned to a clinical manager role. Order completion and discharge coordination responsibilities were delegated to unit clerks. Critical elements added to the role were:

- Clinical expertise to manage patient care and staff activities.
- Case management and multidisciplinary discharge planning.
- Plan and carry out all orientation of new staff and unit in-services.

- Specific managerial functions such as payroll, scheduling, input to quality assurance, input to performance evaluation, carry out performance evaluations on off shifts.
- Resolution of operational day-to-day problems and conflict between nurses and physicians.
- Participation on hospital and medical staff committees.

Again, education and training were necessary to complete the transition from charge nurse to assistant head nurse. New AHNs would be expected to have or be enrolled in a baccalaureate nursing program. Current AHNs without a bachelor's degree must include a plan for achievement in their yearly goals.

Staff Nurse Role

Staff nurses previously functioned as team leaders and members with inconsistent patient assignments. There were frequent complaints of being overworked and evidence that clinical and organizational skills were often lacking. An overall feeling that physicians did not respect nurses was fueled by the lack of communication with physicians. Registered nurses are not enjoying much success. In addition, pay was inadequate.

The staff nurse role was redesigned with a focus on clinical excellence and problem solving. The importance of the staff nurse role was communicated to all members of the nursing division. New expectations were communicated in the new performance standards:

- Specific continuing education requirements.
- Participation in quality assurance activities.
- Participation in division, unit, and/or hospital committees.
- Participation in the planning and decision making regarding nursing practice.
- Initiate communication with physicians concerning patient care.
- Accountability for delivery, documentation and care planning for assigned patients.

This change in expectations meant an opportunity to participate in determining one's own practice, professional growth and recognition, and a chance to move away from the bedside for brief periods of time. With new expectations the vice president for nursing negotiated and obtained increased differentials for less desirable shifts and a higher ceiling on staff nurse pay to recognize excellence and experiences.

Other areas of concern were addressed as well. Specific functions and expectations were defined for team leader and charge nurse to clarify actual activities during the shift. Head nurses reviewed the documentation system to be certain that it was efficient and properly utilized by the staff. A committee began working to develop a clinical ladder to recognize expertise. A collaborative practice committee brought nurses and physicians together to discuss expectations and resolve concerns. New performance standards were presented at medical staff meetings.

The problems with support systems were reported to the vice president of this area. He agreed to have the support department heads work with nursing to identify and resolve problems.

Nursing Resource Coordinator Role

The vice president for nursing created this department head position to manage recruiting, staffing, scheduling, budgeting, and secretarial staff for the nursing department. Her first priorities were (1) to begin using an automated scheduling and position control system purchased 2 years ago, (2) establish a nurse retention committee of staff nurses to identify specific financial and job design incentives to improve retention, and (3) competitor analyses of salary structure and benefits. The nursing resource coordinator serves as a liaison to the nurse recruiter who reports to personnel.

This position also supervises PRN nurses, supplemental agency nurses, student affiliations, and nursing supervisors. The coordinator also works closely with the Director of Hospital Education who manages both clinical and hospital education.

Nursing Assistant Role

The nursing assistant role required no changes. Head nurses now give more attention to clarifying job expectations with each nursing assistant to eliminate conflict between registered nurses and nursing assistants. Each nursing unit has an objective of improving the working relationship between these two groups and are instructed to involve nursing assistants in developing the plan to meet these objectives.

Nursing Supervisor Role

Previously reporting to the vice president for nursing, all supervisors have greater than 15 years experience with the institution. They have seen their position move from the acting administrator on off shifts to where the supervisor calls to consult with the head nurse. This loss of power to the head nurse has resulted in conflict between the two roles. The reporting mechanism for supervisors was changed from the vice president to the coordinator of nursing resources as one of their major functions is assigning supplemental staffing of evenings, nights, and weekends.

In addition to clarity regarding reporting and role and responsibilities, these functions were added to the job:

- Counseling, coaching, and discipline after consultation with the head nurse.
- Input into performance evaluations.
- Monitoring of patient care and participation in quality assurance activities.
- Specific yearly education requirements.

- To improve communication and participation in decision making, supervisors were expected to attend the nursing executive council meetings.

    The vice president first met with the executive team and discussed her plans, their costs and the impact of these changes on each department, physicians and other professional roles, and patients. With full support of the executive team she then planned the training necessary to implement the plan and asked for input from the entire nursing management team on how to best implement the change, deadlines for changes, and probable barriers and resistance. She sought support from the physicians through their committee structure: the change over took 1 year, the evaluation report reflects an improvement in turnover, absenteeism, and reduced conflict among nursing staff and between nurses and physicians.

BIOGRAPHICAL SKETCH

Phillippa Johnston is currently Nurse Executive at Capitol Hill Hospital in Washington, D.C. Having worked as Nurse Executive in two other hospital systems she has extensive experience in the management of health-care services. Born in Fort Worth, Texas, Mrs. Johnston received her BS in nursing from Hampton Institute in 1969 and her MS in nursing from the University of Maryland in 1978. She has completed postgraduate work at the Washington Public Affairs Center of the University of Southern California and is currently a doctoral student in nursing at George Mason University. She has appeared on several Washington television talk-shows to discuss health care issues and has written a number of articles addressing patient care for such publications as *The Hospital Medical Staff, Nursing Forum, Journal of Nursing Administration,* and *Nursing Administration Quarterly.* She is currently president of the capital area chapter of the American Association of Nurse Executives.

PART IV

Nursing Administration

12

The Organization of Nursing Care Delivery

Roberta M. Conti, Jennifer Burks

PLACEMENT OF NURSING IN THE OVERALL STRUCTURE

> One of the most critical concerns of modern society is how to create and maintain organizations which are rational and adaptive (so as to minimize unpredictability of behavior and uncertainty of outcomes while taking full advantage of the benefits of an advanced technology), economically efficient, and satisfying to their members, clients, and communities.—Basil S. Georgopoulas

Although millions of hours of nursing service are delivered daily, there continues to be an abundance of questions as to its efficiency and effectiveness by both those internal and external to the profession of nursing. Health administrators, nurses, physicians, the Joint Commission on Accreditation of Health Care Organizations, government regulatory agencies, and the public are all shareholders with a vested interest in how nursing service is to be structured and practiced.

At the same time, administrators within the health care delivery system are struggling to deal strategically with the changes that are occurring in the newly competitive environment with shifting sources and methods of payment and to choose successful survival strategies. Nurse administrators take a part in this struggle along with the nursing profession as a whole. Nursing services are perceived as a necessity by all, but the boundaries between physicians, professional nurses, technical nurses, and support services is unclear. Also, historically, the majority of nursing services have been provided within hospitals, which were professional bureaucracies whose executives until very recently have not included nurses.

Pearce and Robinson (1982) identify three levels of decision making within corporations. The first level consists of the governing board, the chief executive officer, and the administrative directors. It is at this executive or corporate level that the major thrust of strategic decision making is taking place. Other authors refer to this level as strategic managers. Today, the nursing executive is a significant member of this corporate team, whose responsibility it is to determine the business in which the hospital should be involved. In turn, that includes responsibility for a profitable financial performance in a very complex, competing environment.

The second level of decision making identified by Pearce and Robinson is the business level. This level consists of managers whose responsibilities are to interpret the strategic corporate plans into functional objectives for their divisions. Other authors refer to this group as tactical managers. It is at this level that nursing administrators have functioned for years and developed expertise in implementing the corporate mission statement for the delivery of quality patient care, education for providers, and in some instances medical research. Today, this business level is the second level within the structure of nursing organizations, requiring individuals who can devise business strategies to deliver clinical services. It is significant to note, however, that many nursing executives find themselves straddling both the executive and the business level as in many structures their role has not yet fully moved to the executive level.

The third level of decision making is the functional level (Pearce & Robinson, 1982). This level personnel manages the direct service or product. Other authors refer to this as the operational managers. It is here that strategies are implemented. At this level quality assurance is crucial as well as fiscal efficiency and effectiveness. Today, head nurses are the managers at this level and act as the visible corporate representatives to the consumer along with nurse clinicians and other service providers.

Hospitals have been described as professional bureaucracies by Mintzberg (1979). These bureaucracies have an inherent clash of cultures, which has historically been contained by separate administrator and clinical decision-making structures. Raelin (1986) identifies the conflict as between the corporate culture and the professional culture.

The corporate culture is localized in that organization and reflected in its mission statement. Its strongest adherents are the organizational administrators; their first loyalty is to the organization. Each health professional was socialized into their discipline to value their purpose and technologies. Their first loyalty is to the professional services they provide to the patient.

The nurse administrator is forced to face the uncompromising dilemma of being intimately a part of both the corporate culture and the professional culture. Professional job responsibilities, as elaborated in accreditation and professional standards, focus on practice issues. Administrative job responsibilities as elaborated in the mission statement, strategic plan, and policies and procedures focus on organizational issues.

The nursing staff, as professional employees, also experience the conflict between the two cultures. Corwin (1961) in a study of professional nurses identified the fundamental areas of conflict to be: (1) the degree of standardization of procedures, (2) the degree of authority, and (3) the relationship of the individual to the goals and means of the organization. These conflicts continue to be the major concern of nurse administrators as they try to create a balance between these two cultures. Currently, two trends are evident in the restructuring of hospitals. The integration of business and clinical decision making and the reduction in levels of management moving responsibility downward. Thus, administrators and clinicians are experiencing increased cultural conflict.

The nursing literature is replete with what is wrong with nursing's structure within organizations and within itself (Fine, 1982). Much is basic to this clash of cultures. Throughout our history, some nurse administrators have taken great professional and organizational risks in attempts to restructure their departments to improve working conditions, autonomy of work, and the status of staff nurses. Progress has been uneven because top nurse administrators have traditionally been at the business level of the organization. Major decisions on organizational structure have been controlled at the executive level. Thus, nursing was dependent on administrators who did not share their professional culture to design structures to facilitate professional practice. The first step in proactive placement of nursing in the overall structure is placement of the top nursing administrator at the executive level.

Strategy

Strategy is the match between an organization's resources and skills; the environmental opportunities and risks it faces; and the purposes it wishes to accomplish (Hofer & Schendel, 1978).

Increasing rates of environmental change have accelerated the rate of internal change in health care organizations. The concept of strategy is one of top management's major tools for coping with both external and internal changes. Today's nursing service administrators need a futuristic orientation supported by formal analytical processes to periodically formulate explicit strategic plans consistent with organizational plans.

A strategic plan provides the needed integration for subunits to contribute to total organization objectives. A strategic plan acts as a motivational tool as most groups and individuals perform better if they know what is expected of them and how they contribute to the overall plan of the organization.

Strategy is the major link between the goals and the objectives the organization wants to achieve, and the infrastructure.

Peter Drucker (1954) was among the first to describe strategy as a business issue. To him, an organization's strategy was the answer to the dual questions: "What is our business?" and "What should it be?" The next major development was Alfred Chandler's landmark study (1962) delineating choice of structure as a function of strategy. Chandler found a common strategy–structure sequence consisting of: (1) the choice of a new strategy; (2) the emergence of administrative problems, a decline in performance; (3) a shift to an organizational structure more in line with the identified strategy; and (4) the improved execution and profitability.

Two observations from Chandler's research are: first, all forms of organizational structure are not equally effective in implementing different strategies, and second, existing structures limit administrator vision and ability to perceive potential benefits of change (Pearce & Robinson, 1982). For hospitals and nursing services, the question is how to restructure the organization to execute effectively its strategy for survival in the competitive market place. Nursing services are a scarce commodity that administrators must learn to use more effectively. Vision of macrostrategies that include dramatic structural changes will be needed to provide effective quality care cost.

Corporate strategy is a tool for integrating the hospital organization's diverse functions into coherent patterns designed to create competitive advantages in the market place. Strategy formulation has displaced policy formulation as the principle component of managerial work. This is a significant new idea for hospital organizations and nurse administrators. "What set of businesses should we compete in?" is a new perspective for health care administrators. They are also learning to ask "How should we complete?" Finally, they are realizing that professionals are an integral part of all service products. How can the organization increase their productivity? These three questions will be the focus for future structural decisions. A major priority in choosing strategies will be a planned organizational structure that is sensitive to supporting professional practice while monitoring their use of resources and quality of service.

Alternative Structures

Structure should not be an end in itself; it is a means to an end. The research by Lorsch and Allen (1973) supported Chandler's findings that the choice of structure makes a difference in the achievement of strategy. Choice of structure should involve assessment of the size and complexity of the organization; what influence that configuration has on career paths; the impact of the structure on the management information system and locus of strategic, business, and functional decision making; creation of competitive or cooperative stances between departments and the interdependence of those departments; and the impact on strategic planning, implementation, and accountability.

The five most common structures illustrated in Figure 12–1 were discussed by Pearce and Robinson (1982) in relation to their implication for strategic man-

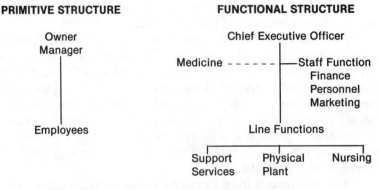

Figure 12–1. Alternative organizational structures.

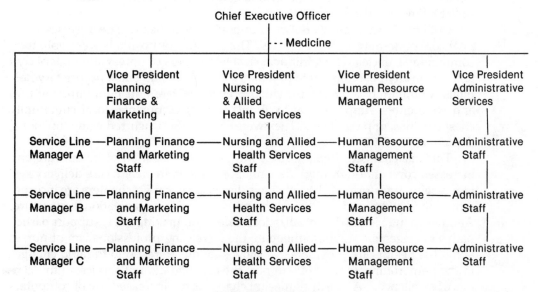

DIVISIONAL STRUCTURE

Chief Executive Officer

Vice President —————— Vice President
Administrative Services   Support Services

Medicine – – – – – – —————Vice President
                                            Nursing

General Manager General Manager General Manager
    Division A   Division B   Division C

–Personnel   –Personnel   –Personnel

–Accounting   –Accounting   –Accounting

–Planning   –Planning   –Planning

–Marketing   –Marketing   –Marketing

–Nursing   –Nursing   –Nursing

–Operations   –Operations   –Operations

STRATEGIC BUSINESS UNIT STRUCTURE

The same as the divisional structure with the insertion of another administrative level. Strategic business units (SBU) are groups of divisions. Each SBU is headed by a Vice President who reports to the Chief Executive Officer.

MATRIX ORGANIZATIONAL STRUCTURE

Chief Executive Officer

- - Medicine

	Vice President Planning Finance & Marketing	Vice President Nursing & Allied Health Services	Vice President Human Resource Management	Vice President Administrative Services
Service Line Manager A	Planning Finance and Marketing Staff	Nursing and Allied Health Services Staff	Human Resource Management Staff	Administrative Staff
Service Line Manager B	Planning Finance and Marketing Staff	Nursing and Allied Health Services Staff	Human Resource Management Staff	Administrative Staff
Service Line Manager C	Planning Finance and Marketing Staff	Nursing and Allied Health Services Staff	Human Resource Management Staff	Administrative Staff

Figure 12-1. *(continued)*

agement. Strategic managers use the long-range plans of the organization as a framework to guide business and functional decision making. The three structures that best support strategic management are the divisional structure, the strategic business unit structure, and the matrix organizational structure.

Primitive organizational structures are used by small "family-like" organizations such as free-standing urgent care centers, pharmacies, and small nursing homes. Functional structure has been the most common in hospitals since their inception with line authority by professional occupation rather than service groupings. It is also common in health departments and larger nursing homes.

Divisional structure, also called product line or service-line management, facilitates coordination and decision making by service grouping within large, diverse organizations. Major authority is delegated to the divisional managers for the strategic management of a business or service entity. It is their responsibility to respond to the competitive environment and manage the accurate assessment of profit and loss.

The strategic business unit structure is a variation on the divisionalized form. It adds another layer of management to handle groups of divisions. The strategic business unit is partitioned according to broad related market segments, such as maternal–child health or geographic areas.

The matrix organizational structure involves dual lines of authority, service delivery, and evaluation. The vice presidents represent functional areas and the service-line managers represent service areas.

Adaptations of these five structures are also possible. The significant issue is which one of these structures would be the most efficient and effective for the entire organization to achieve its strategy. Structure concepts may also be applied to an entire multiple organization corporation, which introduces other issues and increased complexity.

Until the 1980s there were two common types of health care agencies—hospitals or community health agencies. The majority of hospitals were voluntary community agencies with additional sizable numbers of university medical centers, urban city hospitals, state psychiatric hospitals, and small proprietary hospitals. Community agencies provided preventive care and home nursing care and were either supported by local and state governments, local community chest charities, or patient fees. They were commonly structured using functional departments.

This has changed dramatically with the corporatization of health care and increased competition through deregulation. The entire health care delivery system is being transformed. Two changes discussed in earlier chapters are incorporating marketing and strategic planning into the organizational structure. Another change is the decentralization of decision making to (1) support participative management, (2) accommodate the increasing professionalism of nurses and other health care providers, (3) allow subunits to respond to rapid changes in their environments, and (4) support the consolidation of services into "centers of excellence." A fourth significant change is the increased use of computers for management information systems and automation providing administrators with more timely information for decision making. Finally, nursing is increasingly recognized as a scarce resource that can no longer be used as an amorphous service doing both nursing and multiple other patient related services. As the wages of nurses rise, their jobs will be redesigned to use their time more effectively to deliver nursing care.

The structures that are emerging in the health care industry in response to these changes are the division structure and the matrix structure. These structures enable hospitals and community agencies to develop a system of operations and management that focuses activity on the delivery of defined groups of services. Nursing is being restructured to delineate professional and paraprofessional activities, as well as more sharply define nursing and nonnursing services.

The traditional functional hospital structure, with parallel lines of power for physicians and administrators, is declining due to the following limitations: (1) diminished ability to competitively position services in the market place, (2) administration of related services by different units making marketing awkward, (3) a lack of program integration and accountability, (4) process management making coordination across functions ineffective, and (5) poor utilization of nurses. Community health agencies with lines of authority by discipline were encountering the same limitations leading to restructuring.

ORGANIZING NURSING CARE DELIVERY AT THE UNIT LEVEL

The six most common modes of nursing care delivery are case load, function or task, modular or geographic catchment area nursing, team nursing, primary nursing, and case management. Other systems are usually modifications or combinations of the basic six. Dividing work by *case load*, each nurse is responsible for giving care to a patient or to a group of patients for one tour of duty. Using the *functional or task method*, each nurse is assigned to a function such as taking vital signs or doing treatments, for one tour of duty. The *modular or geographic catchment area system* assigns work to nurses by the patient's location for a tour of duty. The systems that are used most frequently today, however, are team nursing, primary nursing, and case management.

Team Nursing

In team nursing, several nursing personnel, usually representing several levels of preparation, are assigned to care for a group of patients for one tour of duty. The team leader is a registered nurse who is ideally the best prepared through both education and experience. The role of the team leader is to: (1) plan and update nursing care plans with other team members, (2) delegate specific tasks or patients, or both, to others on the team, (3) provide some professional nursing care, and (4) supervise, coordinate, and evaluate care provided by the team members (Shukla, 1981). Most team leaders consider themselves caregivers, but actually the amount of time spent giving care is usually less than the amount of time spent supervising others and doing paper work. This mode also does not provide for continuity of care planning for the entire length of stay.

Primary Nursing

The primary nursing system of care was first developed at the University of Minnesota Hospitals. In this system a single nurse is accountable for maintaining the nursing care plan for a patient from admission to discharge. The primary nurse provides nursing care when he or she is on duty. Other nurses provide care when the primary nurse is off duty using his or her care plan. The change-of-shift report, care conferences, and other means of communication are also used. Primary nursing increases the time the registered nurse is at the bedside giving direct care. Other levels of nursing personnel may be assigned to work with a primary nurse or they may be assigned to nonnursing tasks.

Research Findings Concerning Team and Primary Nursing

A comprehensive review of the literature (Young et al., 1981) has revealed more than 150 articles and reports on primary nursing. Almost 80 percent of these articles are descriptive or nonresearch based and are overwhelmingly in support of primary nursing. The remaining articles, which are research based, are also generally supportive of primary nursing. No rigorous studies, however, comparing the six modes of nursing care delivery have been done. Inconsistencies have been found in how different agencies structure each mode and even different providers on the same unit perceive themselves to be organized in different modes (Alexander & Bauerschmidt, 1987).

Initial studies concerning primary nursing found positive perceptions of nurses and positive associations with job satisfaction (Marram, Schlegel, & Bevis, 1974; Mills, 1979). Recent studies also found job satisfaction positively associated with primary nursing (Blair et al., 1982; Sellick, Russell, & Beckman, 1983). In recent years, however, there have also been reports indicating that there is no statistical significance between the job satisfaction for team nurses and primary nurses (Giovannetti, 1980, 1981; Joiner, Johnson, Corkrean, 1981; Alexander, Weisman, Chase, 1981; Betz, 1981). Other studies findings were inconclusive (Collins, 1975; Hymovich, 1977; Young, Giovannetti, Lewison, 1981).

Findings of studies that measured patient satisfaction were also not consistent. Most of the studies done on quality of care concluded that primary nursing improves the quality of care provided to patients (Felton, 1975; Collins, 1975; Jones, 1975; Kent, 1977; Hegedus, 1979; Eichhorn & Frevert, 1979; Steckel, Barnfather, & Owens, 1980). Hamera and O'Connell (1981), however, found that the number of contracts patients had with nursing staff and the amount of time patients spent with members of the nursing staff did not increase with the introduction of primary nursing. Also, Haussman, Hegyvary, and Newman (1976) found that the units with the highest quality scores were smaller, better coordinated, and had a high proportion of registered nurse hours per patient day. These units also tended to be primary nursing units, but the researchers pointed out that the greater proportion of variance of quality scores was explained by other variables.

On the issue of cost effectiveness, again the research findings are not in agreement. Marram and colleagues (1976) found that primary nursing was more cost effective than team nursing. The cost differences, however, could be explained by staff seniority rather than by unit organization. Jones (1975) concluded that primary nursing was more cost effective because primary nurses can be instrumental in reducing the cost of the stay to the patient by contributing to early recovery and discharge. Considering cost per patient day and the acuity of patients, Betz, Dickerson, and Wyatt (1980) found that primary nursing is less costly.

On the other hand, Collins (1975) found the cost differences between primary and team nursing were negligible. Shukla (1982a, 1982b, 1983) compared nurses on modular units, team units, and primary units. Results indicate that the primary nurses were the least productive and the cost per patient day on the primary nursing units was about 2 dollars per day more than on the team units.

Alexander, Weisman, and Chase (1981) found a significantly lower turnover and absenteeism rate for primary nurses in one of the hospitals they studied. Betz (1981) found turnover rates to be higher on primary nursing units, but orientation costs were lower on these units. Joiner, Johnson, and Corkrean (1981) found absenteeism and turnover rates were highest in primary nursing units.

The inconsistency in research findings may be explained by the fact that there is no agreement as to the operational definition of any nursing mode making comparisons between studies of dubious value. Primary nursing in one facility may be very different from primary nursing in another.

The other major flaw in these studies is the lack of comparability of the settings. Many factors influence quality of care, job satisfaction, patient satisfaction, and cost effectiveness besides structure of nursing care delivery. Shukla (1982b) has identified two contingencies that may explain some inconsistencies in research findings—the efficiency of nursing support systems and the patients' dependence. Primary nursing is most effective when the efficiency of support systems is high and when patients' dependence on nurses is high. Thus, there may not be one best mode of nursing care delivery. Different modes may be ideal for different staffing mix of registered nurses, licensed practical nurses, and nursing aides, different adequacy of support systems, and different levels of patient dependence or other characteristics.

Case Management

As health care delivery restructures, the role of the clinical nurse is frequently evolving to include case management in both hospital and community settings. The term *case management* has been used for years, but it was only recently identified as a nursing role. Case management is a set of logical steps and a process of interaction within a service network that assures that a client receives needed services in a supportive, effective, efficient, and cost effective manner (Weil & Karls, 1985). Application of this concept enlarges the scope of nursing service provision by emphasizing the nurse's responsibility to connect patients to a variety of essential services and to coordinate the sequencing of those services. A case manager assumes a variety of essential services and coordinates the sequencing of those services. A case manager assumes a variety of roles including problem solver, advocate, broker, diagnostician or assessor, planner, community or service organizer, employee and system boundary spanner, service monitor and system modifer, record keeper, evaluator, consultant, colleague and collaborator, service coordinator, counselor or therapist, and expeditor (Weil & Karls, 1985). Many of these roles have been a part of the traditional clinical nurse's roles. For example, nurses have always been problem solvers, advocates for patients, assessors, planners, record keepers, evaluators, and so on. A case manager, however, takes on additional roles to include community resources and to be aware of the cost of services recommended. For example, as a system modifier, a nurse might identify that patients had to remain hospitalized for an additional day or perhaps longer because the radiology department was not available for certain tests on Saturday afternoons and all day on Sunday. Knowing that increasing the patient length of stay increases hospital costs the nurse would share that information with the administrator. This might lead to a task force on weekend services that he or she would be asked to serve on. The task force would study the situation and take the necessary action to keep costs down. This has not been a traditional role for staff level clinical nurses. Usually the only concern of clinical nurses for costs of patient care were the amount and type of supplies used. Also the role was seen as patient focused on immediate care. This will change as organizations decentralize and reorganize.

As a broker, a clinical nurse case manager arranges for and sets conditions for service delivery. For instance, when scheduling diagnostic tests for a patient with severe respiratory disease, she may select a mid-morning time rather than an early morning time, to allow the patient time to wake up and clear collected secretions from the lungs before the procedure.

As a service organizer, the clinical nurse case manager would negotiate with ancillary departments so that needed services could be scheduled in a particular sequence that would facilitate early discharge from the hospital.

Colleague and collaborator is another role that has traditionally not been implemented well in our nursing care delivery systems. A nurse who needs to collaborate with someone regarding a patient care problem now usually seeks either a doctor or a nursing administrative person. Increasingly, clinical nurse case managers would consult with other expert peers to resolve nursing care problems.

As hospitals reorganize along specialized service lines, patients with acute exacerbations of chronic problems will most likely be admitted each time to the same unit and remain on that unit throughout their hospitalization. We are developing systems that allow nurses to be assigned as case managers for multiple admissions.

ROLES IN NURSING ADMINISTRATION

Nurse executives in the new structures must augment their nursing skills with broader business skills in financial management, marketing, and strategic management. They must prepare themselves to participate fully in executive decision making. They will often be the only woman and only clinician on the executive team. Their business skills will be crucial for acceptance of their competence and creation of opportunities to use their depth of knowledge concerning the clinical implications of financial decisions.

As organizations restructure, new staff administrative roles for nurses will emerge, such as quality assurance/risk management coordinator, nursing information systems coordinator, financial systems coordinator, and special systems design/research. The nurse executive will create these positions as a result of strategic planning and be responsible for their effectiveness.

It is also probable that service lines may be administered by nurses. These positions will also require formal management preparation in marketing and fiscal management. Nurses will have to compete with other health administrators for these positions.

Nurse managers at the operations level now frequently have responsibility for fiscal management, marketing, human resource management, and quality control.

Administrative Support Structures

One vital aspect of administration is creating an environment to support productive professional practice. Efficient support systems for professionals are an important aspect in planning a care delivery system. The responsibility of administration is to maintain and improve the work environment of professional providers (Zander, 1985).

Organizations can facilitate professional provider productivity by implementing new technology. Computers are being used to order supplies and document care, microprocessors are used to monitor the drip of intravenous lines, and equipment used for treatments is steadily being improved. Accompanying adoption of new technology is the need for training to use it effectively and changing roles to support that use.

Administrators can also facilitate productivity by standardization of routine work. This can be done through the use of appropriate technology such as written standards, policies, procedures, guidelines, chart forms, standard care plans for routine situations, and job descriptions. Examples include a one-time entry documentation system; clear, concise, convenient, written procedures available for review; and precisely written policies.

COSTING NURSING RESOURCES

As nursing is integrated into the emerging strategic structures of organizations, financial reporting and accounting will also be restructured at the macroorganizational level. As health care organizations are restructured into service grouped (product-line) units, financial reporting will be decentralized by service rather than function. At the unit level, the cost of functions by service will be critical data. For example, individual patients receiving the same services require varying amounts of nursing resources. The ability to measure this variability is increasingly critical to determine nursing costs per patient per diagnostic related group (DRG) (Mowry & Korpman, 1986). Likewise pharmacy, dietary, laboratory, and diagnostic imaging costs will be calculated not as cost centers but as costs by patient grouped by DRG for each service/product-line cost center. The entire service/product-line will be evaluated on profitability, which would include the cost of all human and material resources necessary to provide the service and the resulting financial gain over costs.

Future financial questions for nursing will focus on the value of nursing care expended in providing services. Profitability of service/product-lines will be of primary consideration as well as how service/product-lines relate to others (provide internal referrals) and relate to the centers of excellence of the organization.

Nursing Cost Methods

Nursing costs are now being determined. Historically, nursing costs were assumed to be between 30 and 40 percent of room rate reimbursement, but this was never investigated. Hospital administrators, rate regulators, and others, over the years have used this information in decision making without costing out nursing services.

Hospitals have now developed nurse-costing methodologies. Simultaneously, many are also pricing nursing services using a patient acuity classification system. This had lead to changes in figures used for nursing costs in hospital budgets. For instance, in November, 1986, the Medicus Systems Corporation announced the results of "The National DRG Nurse Costing Study." The major finding was that direct, variable nursing costs represent an average of 17.8 percent of the Medicare reimbursement for each of the 40 top DRGs (McCormick, 1986).

The literature describes a variety of methods used to examine the costs of nursing (Walker, 1982; Heggerson & Van Slyck, 1982; Staley & Luciano, 1983; Mason & Daugherty, 1984; Sovie et al., 1985). Commonalities among the methods are: (1) time-based units, (2) identified lists of inputs in providing care, (3) validity and reliability as certification processes, and (4) discrete levels of classification comparable across services (DiVestea, 1985).

The issues of stability and accuracy of patient classification systems are extremely important. As with any measuring device, some estimate of assurance of both reliability and validity must be established before they can be used with any confidence (Giovannetti, 1978).

Validity involves the extent to which a tool measures what it is intended to measure. No patient classification tool in existence can measure a patient's actual needs with complete validity. The purpose of a patient classification system is not to determine actual needs, but to group patients in terms of nursing care needed according to a predetermined standard (Giovannetti, 1979). Validity is established in tool development. In purchasing a tool the results of validity studies and criteria for whether this tool is valid for this agency should be provided by the vendor. Frequently, establishment of local validity requires on site time and motion studies, and small group interviews with nurse clinicians.

The reliability factor most important in patient classification tools is equivalence, between raters and with the same rater over time. Ongoing monitoring of reliability is vital to an effective patient classification system.

The central problem in costing nursing care has been the development of a valid and reliable method with standardized measures for comparison between agencies. Patient classification systems were developed as predictors of staffing based on patient intensity, as a result of being a requirement in the standards for nursing service of the Joint Commission on Accreditation of Health Care Organizations (Rutkowski, 1987). Because the major purpose of patient classification systems has been to assist individual hospitals with the complex task of staffing unique nursing units, there has been little or no incentive for developing standards for comparability. Thus, the definitions of nursing hours in the patient classification system is unique to each agency, even those using the same vendor's system. Therefore, studies that claim to determine the costs of nursing by merely gathering data on numbers of patients classified at each level by DRG are using uncomparable data and result in spurious conclusions. Universal definitions of each time unit of nursing care are needed.

Another related issue is whether time and motion methods and time units are appropriate methods for valuing nursing services. Dijkers and Pardise (1986) point out that these methods do not address expertise in clinical decision making or the multiple parallel tasks that nurses simultaneously perform.

Another method for comparing nursing costs between hospitals is lengths of stay of patients per DRG assuming nursing is a fixed percentage of daily costs. These data on every patient are available in the Medicare cost reports annually submitted to the Health Care Financing Agency (HCFA) that administers Medicare. Research by Atwood, Hinshaw, and Chance (1986), however, identified that (1) DRGs predict the average patient's nursing care requirements reasonably well for ICUs but they do not predict well for patients on general units, (2) DRGs with high variability in complexity of nursing care requirements cluster into groups of similar diagnoses, (3) charging a flat rate for nursing services by DRG would be equally as insensitive as charging a portion of the room rate. Sovie and colleagues (1985) found similar results and that DRGs coupled with patient classification data allowed a budget prediction that reflected 87 percent of the actual adjusted expenditures.

In summary, the cost of nursing care has been found to vary by DRG depending on the mix of staff, the physician's prescribed treatment pattern, the acuity level, and the way calculations were made (Rutkowski, 1987). Thus, comparisons between hospitals by DRGs without methods weighting differences in nursing costs are invalid. Development of these weights by participation in local, regional, and national studies should be a high priority for hospitals recognizing the importance of comparison data for market research and strategic planning.

The internal and external forces at work in today's fast changing health care delivery systems require the nurse executive to think differently about the organization of nursing services. As form should follow function, restructuring should follow changes in nurse's bedside roles. These changes, however, in function must meet corporate, consumer, and professional needs.

The structure for nursing care delivery chosen by nurse administrators must fit the current three major health care business strategies of (1) orientation to the market; (2) decentralization of decision making; and (3) the use of information/accounting systems to provide productivity/effectiveness data. Chosen structures must also use effectively nursing resources in the face of shorter periods of service for cost containment and fewer nursing professionals available due to the shortage.

The placement of nursing leadership within the organization will determine to a great extent the degree of inclusion of nursing in the corporate and business decision making within health care. Nursing leadership at all levels must recognize and seek accommodation of the conflict between business and professional value systems in health care delivery. The greatest challenge to health care in the next 10 years will be to achieve that accommodation. Nursing administration must play a key role in evolving a health care climate that is acceptable to both.

BIOGRAPHICAL SKETCHES

Roberta M. Conti RN, MSN, FAAN, is an accomplished nursing service administrator, having held executive level positions in two 400-bed hospitals and a large comprehensive rehabilitation center in Maryland over a period of 13 years. Her career includes numerous professional activities including the Maryland Governors Commission on Nursing Issues, the Maryland Board of Examiners of Nurses, President of the Maryland Organization of Nursing Executives, Chairperson of the ANA Council of Nursing Administration, Board Member of the Commission on Graduates of Foreign Nursing Schools, and the only nurse serving on the Northern Virginia Health Planning Council. The balance of her career includes health care consulting, medical case management, and academic teaching. She is an assistant professor and doctoral student at George Mason University, School of Nursing.

Jennifer Burks RN, MSN, is a graduate of the Medical College of Virginia baccalaureate program and the Catholic University of America graduate program. She has worked in intensive care and medical/surgical environments in large government hospitals and in a community hospital. As a middle manager she was responsible for a 100-bed service at the National Institutes of Health Clinical Center during the implementation of their medical information system. She also implemented a computerized patient classification and quality assurance program at a community hospital. Her experience as a middle manager and as an educator has prepared her for her current position as a health care and management consultant.

SUGGESTED READINGS

Levels of Organizational Decision Making

Pearce, J.A., & Robinson, R.B. (1982). *Strategic Management*. Horeward, IL: Richard D. Irwin, Inc.

Corporate Strategy

Drucker, P. (1954). *The Practice of Management*. New York: Harper & Row.

Nursing Care Delivery in Inpatient Units

Zander, K. (1985). Second generation primary nursing: A new agenda. *The Journal of Nursing Administration, 15*(2), 18–24.

Weil, M., & Karls, J.M. (1985). *Case Management in Human Service Practice*. San Francisco: Jossey-Bass Publishers.

Nursing Executive Role

Stull, M.K., & Pinhuton, S.E. (1988). *Current Strategies for Nursing Administrators*. Rockville, MD: Aspen Publishers, Inc.

Nursing Costs

Mowry, M.M., & Korpman, R.A. (1986). *Managing Health Care Costs, Quality, and Technology*. Rockville, MD: Aspen Publishers, Inc., pp. 35–55.

Patient Classification Systems

Schmult, N. (1982). Patient classification systems. In Marriner, A. (ed.): *Contemporary Nursing Management*. St. Louis: C.V. Mosby Co., pp. 150–159.

REFERENCES

Alexander, J., & Bauerschmidt, A. (1987). Implications for nursing administration of the relationship of technology and structure to quality of care. *Nursing Administration Quarterly, 11*(4), 1–10.

Alexander, C.S., Weisman, C.S., & Chase, G.A. (1981). Evaluating primary nursing in hospitals: Examination of effects on nursing staff. *Medical Care, 19*, 80–89.

Atwood, J.R., Hinshaw, A.S., & Chance, H.C. (1986). Relationships among nursing care requirements, nursing resources, and change. In Shaffer, F.A. (ed.): *Patients and Purse Strings: Patient Classification and Cost Management*. New York: National League for Nursing, pp. 99–119.

Betz, M. (1981). Some hidden costs of primary nursing. *Nursing and Health Care, 2*, 150–154.

Betz, M., Dickerson, T., & Wyatt, D. (1980). Cost and quality: primary and team nursing compared. *Nursing and Health Care, 1*, 150–157.

Blair, F., Sparger, G., Walts, I., & Thompson, J. (1982). Primary nursing in the emergency department: Nurse and patient satisfaction. *Journal of Emergency Nursing, 8*, 181–186.

Chandler, A. (1962). *Strategy and Structure*. Cambridge, MA: MIT Press.

Collins, V.B. (1975). The primary nursing role as model for evaluating quality of patient care, patient satisfaction, job satisfaction, and cost effectiveness in acute care settings. Dissertation Abstracts International, 36, 1655B. (University Microfilms No. 75-22, 117)

Corwin, R.C. (1961). The professional employee: A study of conflict in nursing roles. American Journal of Sociology, 66, 604-615.

Dijlers, M., & Pardise, T. (1986). PCS: One system for both staffing and costing. Nursing Management, 17(1), 25-34.

DiVostea, N. (1985). The changing health care system: An overview. In Shaffer, F.A. (ed.): Costing Out Nursing: Pricing Our Product. New York: National League for Nursing, pp. 29-36.

Drucker, P. (1954). The Practice of Management. New York: Harper & Row.

Eichhorn, M.L., & Frevert, E.I. (1979). Evaluation of a primary nursing system using the quality of patient care scale. Journal of Nursing Administration, 9(10), 11-15.

Felton, G. (1975). Increasing the quality of nursing care by introducing the concept of primary nursing: A model project. Nursing Research, 24, 27-32.

Fine, R.B. (1982). Creating a work place for the professional nurse, Chapter 11. In Marriner, A. (ed.): Contemporary nursing management. St. Louis: Mosby, pp. 96-109.

Georgopoulos, B. SD. (1972). Organizations Research on Health Institutions. Ann Arbor, MI: Institute for Social Research.

Giovannetti, P. (1980). A comparison of team and primary nursing care systems. Nursing Dimensions, 7(4), 96-100.

Giovannetti, P. (1981). A Comparative Study of Team and Primary Nursing Care. Unpublished doctoral dissertation. John Hopkins University, Baltimore, MD.

Giovannetti, P. (1978). Patient Classification Systems in Nursing: A Description and Analysis. Pub. No. (Hra) 78-22. Washington, D.C.: Department of Health, Education and Welfare.

Giovannetti, P. (1979). Understanding patient classification systems. Journal of Nursing Administration, 9(2).

Hamera, E., & O'Connell, K. (1981). Patient-centered variables in primary and team nursing. Research in Nursing and Health, 4, 183-192.

Haussman, R.K.D., Hegyvary, S.T., & Newman, J.F. (1976). Monitoring Quality of Nursing Care. Part II: Assessment and study of correlates (HRA Report No. 76-7.) Bethesda, MD: Department of Health, Education and Welfare.

Hegedus, K.S. (1979). A patient outcome criterion measure. Supervisor Nurse, 10(1), 40-45.

Heggerson, N.J., & Van Slyck, A. (1982). Variable billing for services: New fiscal direction for nursing. Journal of Nursing Administration, 12(6), 20-27.

Hofer, C.W., & Schendel, D. (1978). Strategy Formulation: Analytical Concepts. St. Paul, MN: West Publishing Company.

Hymovich, D.P. (1977). The effects of primary nursing care on children's, parents' and nurses' perceptions of the pediatric nursing role. Nursing Research Report, 12(2), 6-7, 11.

Jones, K. (1975). Study documents effects of primary nursing on renal transplant patients. Hospitals, 49(24), 85-89.

Joiner, C., Johnson, V., & Corkrean, M. (1981). Is primary nursing the answer? *Nursing Administration Quarterly, 5*(3), 69–76.

Kent, L.A. (1977). *Outcomes of a Comparative Study of Primary, Team, and Case Methods of Nursing Care Delivery in Terms of Quality of Patient Care and Staff Satisfaction in Six Western Region Hospitals.* Boulder, CO: Western Interstate Commission for Higher Education.

Lorsch, T.W., & Allen, S. (1973). *Managing Diversity and Interdependence: An Organizational Study of Multidivisional Firms.* Boston, MA: Graduate School of Business Administration, Harvard University.

Marram, G.D., Flynn, K.T., Abaravich, W.J., & Carey S. (1976). *Cost-Effectiveness of Primary Nursing and Team Nursing.* Wakefield, MA: Contemporary Publishing.

Marram, G.D., Schlegel, M.W., & Bevis, E.O. (1974). *Primary Nursing: A Model for Individualized Care.* St. Louis: Mosby.

Mason, E. J., & Daughterty, J.K. (1984). Nursing standards should determine nursing's price. *Nursing Management, 15*(9), 34–38.

McCormick, B. (1986). What's the cost of nursing care? *Hospitals, 60*(21), 48–52.

Mills, M.E.C. (1979). A Comparison of Primary and Team Nursing Care Systems as an Influence on Patient and Staff Perceptions of Care. Unpublished doctoral dissertation. John Hopkins University, Baltimore, MD.

Mintzberg, H. (1979). *The Structuring of Organizations.* New York: Prentice Hall.

Mowry, M.M., & Korpman, R.A. (1986). *Managing Health Care Costs, Quality, and Technology: Product Line Strategies for Nursing.* Rockville, MD: Aspen Publishers, Inc.

Pearce, J.A. II, & Robinson, R.B. Jr. (1982). *Strategic Management.* Harewood, IL: Richard D. Irwin, Inc.

Raelin, J.A. (1986). *The Clash of Cultures, Managers and Professions.* Boston, MA: Harvard Business School Press.

Rutkowski, B. (1987). *Managing for Productivity in Nursing.* Rockville, MD: Aspen Publishers.

Sellick, K.J., Russell, S., & Beckman, B. (1983). Primary nursing: An evaluation of its effects on patient perception of care and staff satisfaction. *International Journal of Nursing Studies, 20,* 265–273.

Shukla, R.K. (1981). Structure vs. people in primary nursing: An inquiry. *Nursing Research, 30*(4), 236–241.

Shukla, R.K. (1982a). Nursing care structures and productivity. *Hospital and Health Services Administration, 27*(16), 45–58.

Shukla, R.K. (1982b). Primary or team nursing? Two conditions determine the choice. *The Journal of Nursing Administration, 12*(11), 12–15.

Shukla, R.K. (1983). All-RN model of nursing care delivery: A cost-benefit evaluation. *Inquiry, 20,* 173–184.

Sovie, M.D., Tarcinale, M., Vanputta, A.W., & Stunden, A.E. (1985). Amalgam of nursing acuity, DRGs and costs. *Nursing Management, 16*(3), 22–42.

Staley, M., & Luciano, K. (1983). Eight steps to costing nursing services. *Nursing Management, 14*(10), 35–38.

Steckel, S.B., Barnfather, J., & Owens, M. (1980). Implementing primary nursing within a research design. *Nursing Dimensions, 7*(4), 78–81.

Walker, D.D. (1982). *The Cost of Nursing Care in Hospitals.* In Aiken, L. (ed): *Nursing in the 1980s: Crises, Opportunities, Challenges.* Philadelphia: Lippincott, pp. 131–143.

Weil, M. & Karls, J.M. (1985). *Case Management in Human Service Practice.* San Francisco: Jossey-Bass Publishers.

Young, J.P., Giovannetti, P., & Lewison, D. (1981). A Comparative Study of Team and Primary Nursing Care on Two Surgical Inpatient Units. (HRA Report no. 232–78–0150). Baltimore, MD: Johns Hopkins University. (NTIS No. HRP–0900642/0)

Young, J.P., Giovannetti, P., Lewison, D., & Thomas, M.L. (1981). *Factors Affecting Nurse Staffing in Acute Care Hospitals: A Review and Critique of the Literature* (DHEW Publication No. HRP 0501801). Hyattsville, MD: Department of Health Education and Welfare.

Zander K. (1985). Second generation primary nursing: A new agenda. *Journal of Nursing Administration, 15*(2), 18–24.

CASE 12–1

Nursing Administration in a Product Line Environment
Patricia J. Graham

Product line management is a concept and term that originates from business management techniques. Its application to the health care environment is a recent event thought to be initiated and driven in response to health care's changing conditions: prospective payment systems and their regulations, escalating competition among hospitals, ongoing struggles of profit versus quality, and increasing need for a customer orientation. *Product line,* sometimes called service line, is a term used to describe a specifically defined hospital service, or group of services that are related to each other, and that focuses on meeting the needs of particular markets (i.e., consumer groups such as the elderly, children, cancer patients, outpatient clients). In a product line organization one batch of services, which are logically related, are combined into a business division referred to as a product line. Services within that line are planned, managed, marketed, and evaluated as a defined group, rather than as individual activities or departments.

This type of organizational commitment requires organizational restructuring. One model discontinues functional divisions, such as nursing and finance, and creates product line divisions such as gerontology or oncology. An alternative structure retains functional divisions and creates product line staff responsibilities in a matrix structure. Other models mix divisions, some functional and some product-oriented.

Dependent on the specific organization, product line responsibilities are being designated to a variety of job categories: to unit managers, to newly developed staff positions, to nurse clinical specialists, or to administrators as additional duties. The responsibilities of a product line manager are broad and generally entail ongoing analysis of financial return; clinical quality reviews of the service; trend forecasting related to the specific product line(s), including user's demographics (patient profiles) and production resources required; and knowledge of the scope of the services that are offered and potentially can be added. The product managers should also have a clinical understanding of the services to which they are assigned. In general, the product manager plans for future product line development, serves as a primary source of information and reference point on each service in the line, and is the main coordinator of resources for all the integral components of the product line. Obviously the assumption of a product line structure and allocation of responsibilities can have a dramatic impact on the delivery and administration of nursing services in any organization where it is adopted.

IMPLEMENTATION OF PRODUCT LINE MANAGEMENT

Product line management at Mount Vernon Hospital (MVH) was conceived in 1986 as a response to increased competition in the local hospital industry and to answer the needs for better development and coordination of services. Although a member of the Fairfax Hospital System, a multihospital health care system, it is the only one that is presently organized around product lines.

As a first step in its implementation plan the management team at MVH selected its product lines. These selections have been based on demographic needs identified in the market analyses of our primary and secondary service areas and the abilities of current services (products) to meet these needs. In conjunction, the relative strength of the competitive providers in our service area in each of these identified areas was analyzed. The next action involved the development of a new table of organization that incorporated the management of these product lines and enhanced the flow of daily operations (Fig. 12–2). Three divisions were delineated: surgical services, medical services, and specialty services. Each division has several product lines.

Some product lines were already managed as one program (i.e., rehabilitation), whereas others required reorganization (i.e., women's services). Next, departmental responsibilities were reallocated depending on their placement in a specific product line. As shown in Figure 12–2, our product lines are clustered as:

Surgical Division	**Medical Division**	**Specialty Division**
Surgical orthopedics	Cardiology	Rehabilitation
Vascular surgery	Oncology	Psychiatry
Ambulatory services	Women's services	Emergency services

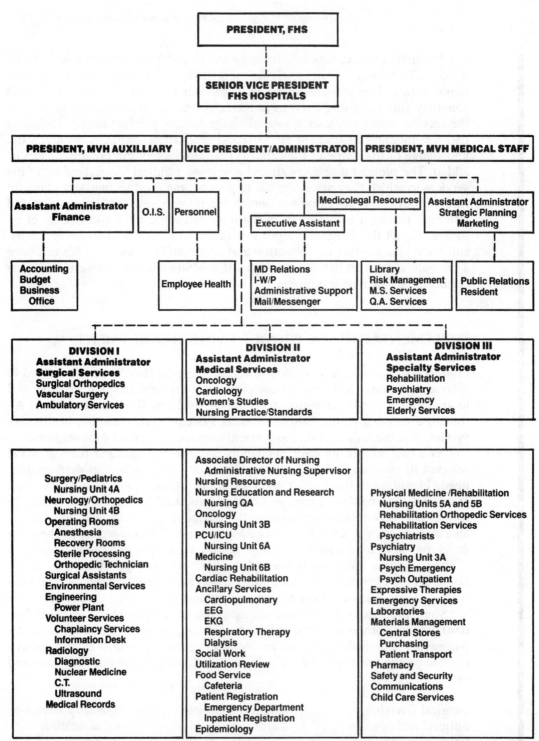

Figure 12–2. Fairfax Hospital System Table of Organization, Mount Vernon Hospital. C.T.: computed tomography, Emp. Health, FHS: Fairfax Hospital System, I-W/P, M.S. Svcs., MVH: Mount Vernon Hospital, O.I.S., PCU/ICU, P.R.: Public relations, Q.A. Svcs. *(Reprinted by permission of Mount Vernon Hospital, Fairfax Hospital System, Fairfax, Virginia.)*

INTEGRATION OF NURSING SERVICES WITHIN THE PRODUCT LINE STRUCTURE

Perhaps the greatest challenge was to determine how to pursue the organization/integration of nursing services into the new structure. Traditionally, at MVH, nursing units were centrally responsible to the executive nursing manager. To better facilitate the communication and coordination within product lines, this traditional organization was changed. The nursing units were placed within the division that best represented their clinical population, as shown in Figure 12–2. Realizing that nursing expertise and responsibility for the centralized nursing functions of education, quality assurance, staffing, and practice/standards was necessary, it was determined that one of the assistant administrators would also serve as the Director of Nursing. This required that at least one of the three assistant administrators have nursing administrative education and experience. Maintaining an identifiable director of nursing was deemed necessary for regulatory agency liaison, accreditation, and maintenance of professional nursing practices.

The responsibilities of each assistant administrator/division director may be broken down into (1) direct line management of the functional hospital departments assigned to his or her division and (2) product line management of the specific services of his or her designated product lines. In addition, the assistant administrator/director of nursing assumes the responsibility for the previously noted centralized nursing functions and represents nursing at the corporate level of the hospital system or at external events requiring nursing expertise. The responsibilities of the two remaining functional assistant administrators for finance and strategic planning/marketing are being maintained as before the changes but with the added emphasis of having information monitored and presented based on product lines in addition to departmental operations.

Presentation of the proposed system change was discussed with each department director through formalized forums and informal individual sessions. The concerns of the Director in the early stages of implementation revolved around (1) narrowing the emphasis the administrators place on the product line to only their designated programs versus all programs, (2) division of the nursing departments across the assistant administrators, and (3) the lack of general understanding of product line management and its concepts.

Presentation to the medical staff was done essentially through departmental channels and the routine meeting structure. In December, 1986, product line management was initiated through implementation of the new table of organization and resultant reassignment of reporting mechanisms. In addition, product line teams were established to plan and initiate development of services.

ASSESSMENT OF THE IMPACT OF PRODUCT LINE ORGANIZATION

After 12 months of using the new system, daily operations at the unit level are essentially unchanged. Divisional meetings of assistant administrators with their department directors are being held monthly. Nursing unit directors and the Assistant Administrator/Director of Nursing meet twice a month as a decision-making body for nursing services as well as a planning and communications forum. Separate meetings to address product line development occur independently of these operational meetings. An adjunct organizational structure is now defined for the functioning of nursing services activities (Fig. 12–3). This structure was designed to consolidate all nursing support functions under one administrative manager who was then able to coordinate centralized nursing services and provide support to all the nursing units across divisional lines of organization. Nursing committees, such as standards, quality assurance, education, and retention and recruitment, continue to meet with a conscious effort to include members from each division. Joint Commission on Accreditation of Health care Organizations (JCAHO) and Commission on Accreditation of Rehabilitation Facilities (CARF) visited the Mount Vernon Hospital in 1987 and a 3-year accreditation was received for both. Because the JCAHO reviewed all hospitals within our system over one visit we were able to compare results in a product line versus nonproduct line organization. Those areas in nursing services that were noted as strong as well as those requiring improvement were identified the same in all the hospitals of the system, thus showing little or no difference in the implementation of JCAHO standards by organizational structure.

What are the relative advantages and disadvantages to being a nursing unit director in a product line system?

Advantages

1. Nursing unit directors, as all other departmental directors, answer directly to their respective assistant administrator without an additional layer of management, a process proving to be cost-effective with the ability to strengthen the lines of communication.
2. Nursing unit directors are being identified as leaders among the coordinating teams established to plan and implement product line development. Their clinical expertise in their respective service, their strength in knowing the relationships and roles of each department in the hospital, and their organizational abilities are being given more visibility resulting in more hospital-wide recognition.
3. Nursing unit directors are allowed more freedom to make changes that are needed for their units/services and the process of decision making has been decentralized and streamlined.
4. As a professional group, the unit directors are learning to think beyond patient care to financial management, the business environment, reimbursement, service area needs, and marketing efforts. They are feeling more control over activities leading to better patient outcomes and are recognizing and sharing with their staff the essential contribution that nursing care makes to the establishment and delivery of a product.
5. Greater interdisciplinary communication between department directors

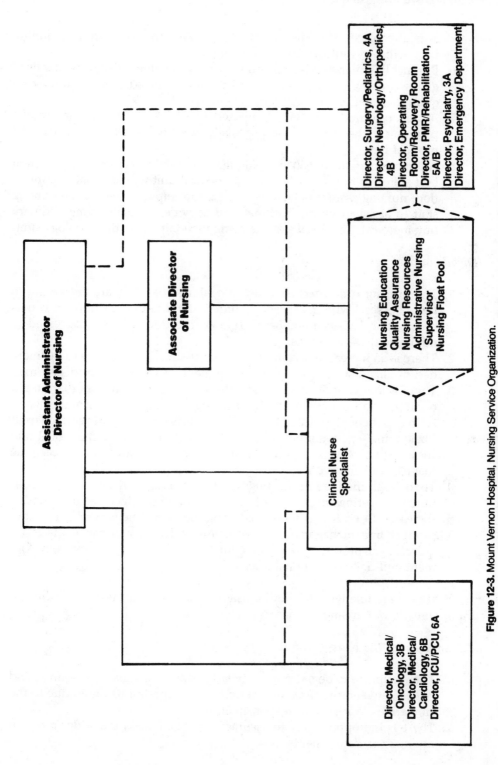

Figure 12-3. Mount Vernon Hospital, Nursing Service Organization.
———— : Direct reporting relationship ; —— —— : A functional nursing practice relationship ; ⁎ : *Nursing council: Nursing practice/standards. (Reprinted by permission of Mount Vernon Hospital, Fairfax Hospital System, Fairfax, Virginia. 910R0187.041, 6/87)*

is taking place. Multidisciplinary teams for product/program planning has increased mutual problem solving.

6. Product line management is cutting across functional departmental lines giving nursing the ability to access the individuals from whom they require information or cooperation.

7. Added resources are being projected for the 1988 budget for product planning if the department's specialty has been selected as a focused product line.

8. Autonomy is allowed in determining the nursing care delivery system best suited to the specialty. On one medical unit with a geriatric population, nursing assistants were requested and implemented by the nursing staff to assist in lifting, bathing, and activities of daily living. Primary nursing, with an all RN staff, is being maintained on the oncology unit.

Disadvantages

1. The nursing unit directors can feel at times that they are answering to two "bosses" who may respond differently due to their nursing versus nonnursing background. Better role clarification is being addressed to minimize these concerns.

2. There is an increased accountability for the unit directors due to the more decentralized style of making management and patient care decisions.

3. There is less cohesiveness among the nursing unit directors than might occur in a traditional setting, thus causing nursing in general at the hospital to experience a sense of loss for the professional support received from "belonging" to a defined nursing structure. In 1988, professional and social activities were planned for the nursing unit directors to overcome this lack of cohesiveness.

4. There is an increase in meetings for the nursing unit directors, such as nursing meetings in addition to divisional and product line meetings.

5. Increased flexibility is demanded of all the department managers under product line management. Negotiation with other departments is required over product line components as well as new program development and daily operational issues.

What are the relative advantages/disadvantages for the Assistant Administrator/Director of Nursing Services?

Advantages for the Nurse Executive

1. There appears to be more widespread support for nursing resources and issues between the three operational assistant administrators due to the similarities in roles and responsibilities.

2. There is the opportunity to assume responsibilities for a wider range of nonnursing departments.

3. There is the additional professional growth in gaining the ability to plan and implement hospital-wide program changes.
4. Future career options are expanded.
5. There is an increase in the autonomy for decision making relative to product lines.
6. There appear to be fewer divisional barriers between the assistant administrators and increased teamwork.
7. There is an opportunity to preceptor MHA administrative residents in addition to MSN graduate students.

Disadvantages for the Nurse Executive

1. The public in general and physicians still view the "traditional" director of nursing role and thus correspondence, phone calls, and so forth are directed to the director of nursing for patient care issues. Often these concerns are inherent to all nursing units and thus must be handled by the Assistant Administrator/Director of Nursing. Where possible, they are delegated to the appropriate Assistant Administrator.
2. Agency accreditation designates the Director of Nursing responsible for nursing services' standards and the Assistant Administrator responsible for each specific nursing department.
3. It takes constant evaluation and improved flexibility to determine what must remain centralized for efficiency, productivity, and practice reasons, and what can be fully decentralized to the unit level for independent decision making.
4. There is a sense of wearing "two hats" (i.e., does the Assistant Administrator/Director of Nursing defend division budgets first or those of *all* nursing units?)
5. There is an increase in the number of meetings. The Assistant Administrator/Director of Nursing is expected to attend all meetings required of the assistant administrator level as well as those requiring nursing executive attendance.
6. More time is needed to monitor the trends of professional nursing issues as well as those topics pertaining to product line and nonnursing department management.

In conclusion, MVH and its managers have grown and developed throughout the implementation of a product line structure. Future changes will be determined by an evaluation after 1 year of the functioning of the MVH product-line structure. At that time, the administrative team will seek formal input from the department directors as to their satisfaction/dissatisfaction with the current system. The administrator of the hospital and each assistant administrator will also give input. In addition, the appropriate placement of each department under its respective Division will be examined. Planned changes will occur based on these evaluations and recommendations.

BIOGRAPHICAL SKETCH

Patricia J. Graham, RN, MSN, is currently the Assistant Administrator/Director of Nursing at Mount Vernon Hospital, an affiliate of Fairfax Hospital System, Fairfax, Virginia. She has been at Mount Vernon Hospital for 1 year having held prior nursing administrative positions, most recently as a Vice-President, Nursing in a hospital with a traditional organizational structure. She received her master's degree from the University of Minnesota, Minneapolis, Minnesota.

CASE 12-2

Delineation of Nursing Services in a Community Health Agency
Jean Cross

The purpose of this case study is to look at the delivery of nursing care in a public health agency over a 10-year period. During the 1970s, public health agencies as well as other organizations that provided nursing care were discussing the pros and cons of team versus primary care nursing. The concept of team nursing was first instituted in the Montgomery Country Health Department in 1967, and has since continued in various forms in parts of the agency. In 1976, faculty from the Community Health Graduate Program of the University of Maryland School of Nursing joined nurse administrators of the Health Department to examine the organization of service delivery. Questions raised then are still relevant today and include: Does the type of service delivery affect the quality or effectiveness of care? What exactly do community health nurses do that has an impact on a client's health status? Is there a difference in client satisfaction? In nurse job satisfaction? What type of delivery is more efficient? Is there a cost difference? Is there a difference as measured by nursing standards?

Before the study, nurse administrators expressed belief in these advantages of team nursing:

1. The service to clients is not disrupted by staff turnover or by unfilled positions.
2. Staff expertise can be utilized better. For example, experienced staff can be assigned to high-risk families, whereas new staff can work with routine cases.

I wish to express appreciation to the people who contributed to the projects discussed in this review. Cynthia Northrop, a nurse attorney, previous member of University of Maryland faculty now living in New York, NY and Judith Strasser, Assistant Professor, collaborated with the Montgomery County Health Department nurse managers. The leadership and enthusiasm of Shirley A. Bederman, Chief Nurse, Montgomery County Health Department and Mary Virginia Ruth, Chairperson for Graduate Programs in Community Health, Maternal/Child Health and Primary Care Nursing, University of Maryland, made the projects possible and warrant special appreciation.

3. Staff members share knowledge and resource information among themselves.
4. There is increased opportunity for peer review and support.

Conversely, nurse administrators said they believed that these are the advantages of primary case management nursing:

1. When an individual nurse assumes the case manager role for families, there is less fragmentation and greater continuity of care.
2. More time can be given to client care when one nurse is familiar with the family and does not need to spend time conferring with other team members about care.
3. The individual nurse gains the feeling of job satisfaction upon completion of the work.

Nurse administrators and the graduate faculty have had a long association as a result of ongoing student affiliations. In agreeing to collaborate each group had its own interests as well as shared objectives. The administrators wanted to describe and verify staff and resource utilization. The faculty wanted to do research relevant to everyday service problems. It was a collaborative project from start to finish, from defining its purpose to putting its conclusions into effect.

After initial discussions in 1979 and early 1980, it was decided that to explore the question of the relationship of service delivery patterns and client outcomes, it was first necessary to describe how service was being delivered in the agency at that time.

Before this time, the community health nurses had participated in a state nurse reporting system. The data gathered were based on service activities, the location where service was administered, and the program to which the service was directed. The nursing administrators believed that the information they were receiving through the state reporting system did not fully meet their planning or budget needs. As a result, they decided to stop using the state system. This decision gave them the incentive to support the investigation as an effort to develop a different method of gathering nursing data. They hoped that investigating the time the nurses spent in different activities would provide a basis for comparing different service delivery systems and support planning and budget preparation. It could also dispel myths about how much time was used in different nursing activities.

In 1980, the Montgomery County Health Department was a complex, multiservice organization with a budget of more than $18 million. It had 647 positions, including 175 full-time and 25 part-time nurses serving a population of 600,000. One hundred nine community health nurses participated in the study. The participants were assigned to six health centers located in different areas of the 500-square-mile county. The community health nurses provided well-care services to individuals, families, and community groups. Each center had child and adolescent immunization and family-planning clinics. Five centers had maternity clinics, and one center also provided sick care to eligible children. Health Department personnel also provided health services to the public school system, public day-care centers, and parochial schools, for a total of 225 schools and centers. Nurses also made home visits for health promotion and disease prevention; they did not provide sick care.

Community health nursing services were organized in a variety of ways among the six centers, primarily at the discretion of the administrative nursing supervisor. Three centers used a team nursing approach, with two teams of five to nine professional nurses each. The clients served by each team were assigned according to the number and complexity of the families, geographic boundaries, or alphabetical order by family names. The other three centers used an individual primary case management nursing approach, with clients assigned by census tract or geographic boundary. One of these centers grouped the nurses to provide coverage for each other on some activities.

The organization of delivery of nursing service in the six centers was also influenced by the special needs of the local population, for example, single-parent families or ethnic groups. Another factor was population density. The experience level of the staff and the leadership style and experience of the administrative nursing supervisor were also factors.

The time study, which was conducted for one week, gathered the following information: descriptive facts on the participants, categories of nursing activities, and client information. Confidentiality on all client and participant information was maintained.

The seven categories of nursing activities chosen for this study were determined on the basis of the experience of the nurses involved and on whether the activities might help to demonstrate differences based on the type of service delivery. Results found were: (1) client contact (34 percent of the total time in all centers) included four subcategories: face-to-face individual, or group; telephone to or on behalf of client; and letter to client; (2) recording-related activities (25 percent), included professional recording and record review, conversion to problem-oriented recording format, and completing forms; (3) work planning (16 percent), defined as activities that a nurse performed in arranging how and by whom services were to be provided, included nurse alone and nurse with supervisor, team, other work group, or peers; (4) professional growth (19 percent), consisted of planned evaluation, conferences with supervisor, in-service education, and staff and department meetings; (5) case discussion (9 percent), included discussions the nurse had for case-management purposes with peers, supervisors, team members, or other professional staff; (6) travel (4 percent); and (7) supervision of paraprofessionals (3 percent).

The percentage of time related to the associated program was as follows: school health (30 percent); child/adolescent health (25 percent); family planning (19 percent); maternal health (8 percent); adult health (3 percent); tuberculosis (3 percent); children's specialty (2 percent); mental health (2 percent); communicable diseases (1 percent); and other, not attributable to a given purpose (17 percent).

Studying how community nurses spent their time in different activities provided information applicable to administration. For example, in some program areas more time was spent in client contact than in other categories, whereas in others, record-related activities required a greater percentage of time. Could changes in documentation of services increase the time available for direct client care? The study dispelled the myth that community health nurses spend 50 percent of their time in record-related activities. Another interesting and unexpected finding was that the way nursing services were organized in the centers—team or primary/case management—made little difference in the time spent in the categories of activities. Two of the centers that were the closest in the percentage of time spent in the same categories of activities had different service–delivery styles, and one center was urban, whereas the other was more rural. This implied that other factors or a group of factors influenced the efficiency of service delivery (Cross, Northrop, & Strasser, 1983).

One year later, in 1981, the study was repeated. During the interval between studies, there was a major reorganization of the agency that directly affected the provision of nursing services. A new, separate Division of School Health Services was formed. Previously, the nurses that provided school health services had been assigned to the six health centers. A total of 63 community health nurses, full-time and part-time supervisors, and staff were assigned to the new division. Another change was the closing of one of the area's health centers with the staff and clients divided between two of the other centers.

The second time study used the same structure and work plans as the first study including collaboration with the University of Maryland. This time all nurses in the agency participated. A second instrument was developed to record the activities of supervisors and program coordinators/specialists. Again, the instrument used for nurses providing direct client care applied the same variables as in the 1980 study, except that aspects of the nursing process were added.

Because of the organizational changes, it was neither possible nor advisable to compare the studies. Again, the second study was primarily valuable for assessing the time nurses were spending in various service activities. These were percentages of total time spent in each category: client contact (41 percent), record-related activities (25 percent), case discussion (13 percent), work planning (10 percent), supervision of paraprofessionals (2 percent), professional development (4 percent), and travel (4 percent). There was an increase in the amount of time spent in direct client contact and case discussion and a decrease in the work planning and professional development categories. The percentages of time attributed to aspects of the nursing process were as follows: initial assessment (16 percent), data update (19 percent), planning (19 percent), implementation (38 percent), and evaluation (8 percent).

These were the categories of activities and the percentage of time supervisors and program coordinators/specialists spent on them: (1) administration (55 percent), including work planning, setting priorities, communications, data collection, personnel matters, departmental and interagency meetings, monitoring contracts and nonnursing activities; (2) program development (16 percent), including meeting with community representatives, developing resource materials, and presenting in-service education; (3) supervision (21 percent), including case discussion, case review, record review, site visits, scheduled conferences, staff meetings, orientation, and supervision of paraprofessionals. The other two categories were (4) travel (5 percent) and (5) professional development (2 percent).

The two time studies provided baseline data for administrative purposes and demonstrated that the way the nursing services were organized did not greatly affect the provision of nursing care.

Any time study is limited, because it does not define all aspects that are required for the allocation of resources. It was not useful to predict care needs of clients; an intensity classification system is needed for this prediction. Together, the time study and classification data could be used to calculate nursing time required for specific care activities. Results could then be converted to full-time equivalencies of nurses needed for budgeting purposes and to compare needs among competing programs or service areas.

During the time the studies were being conducted, the agency was under pressure to increase its accountability and justify the cost of traditional services. Department officials had a difficult time explaining to the agency's funding source, the elected Montgomery County Council, exactly what community health nurses did in measurable terms that council members could understand and compare with other services. Additional questions raised by nurses centered on the results of nursing care. It was not possible to use the time study to answer questions about the outcome of nursing care, but combined with two other efforts a beginning was made. The first additional effort was an in-service, "A Model For Evaluating A Community Health Agency," presented by a nurse consultant from the Division of Nursing, U.S. Department of Health and Human Services (Morris, 1981). The model provided direction to nurse administrators to determine if the nursing health-care services had an impact on health status of families and cost of services rendered. The second effort, by two county nurse administrators, was to use the time study and patient records to determine the correlation between family complexity (one measure of demand for services) and the amount of nursing time devoted to that family. These three efforts were nursing's first steps to be fiscally accountable to the County Council.

Other activities designed to explore demand, outcomes, workload measures, and productivity in health care have been undertaken by nurses in the Montgomery County Health Department in subsequent years. Some have been in collaboration with the University of Maryland; for instance, a 1983 research project titled "Family Health Promotion Activities in Community Health Nursing Services." It used the national typology of disease prevention and health promotion activities as defined in *Promoting Health/Preventing Disease: Objectives for the Nation* in evaluating outcomes of community health nurses' services (U.S. Dept. of Health and Human Services, 1980). The research findings were presented to staff members and aided them in discussing their own practice. It also assisted in delineating health promotion activities of community health nurses.

Also in the early 1980s, one nursing supervisor examined and tested the use of a patient classification system in her service area. This system had been developed by the Visiting Nurse Association of Omaha, Nebraska, under contract to the Division of Nursing, federal Department of Health and Human Services (Simmons, 1980). The nursing supervisor used the client classification system as a standardized list of nursing diagnoses in the county department's problem-oriented records. This client classification system was found to be too cumbersome and not comprehensive for our well-care agency, as many of the nursing diagnoses were more appropriate to home-health sick-care situations. The project was valuable, however, as it clarified the need to standardize and sharpen the terminology used by nurses to define clients' problems in department records.

County efforts continue to increase rationality in planning and allocating resources. For instance, in the Division of School Health Services, a needs and complexity assessment based on demographic and population service requirements was conducted annually from 1983 to 1986 to determine allocation of resources among units. Record and data information collection was refined and streamlined annually to add to efficiency and effectiveness.

Under the current organization, nurses are assigned to three different divisions: school health, family health, and licensure, regulatory and special health services. This program management model stimulates competition for nurse positions and funding among the divisions.

Currently, efforts are being directed toward defining nursing workload measures to compare programs based on client health needs data. Each program is viewed as a product line. The tension between the pros and cons of team versus primary care management assignments continues. In one division of the Health Department, all nursing services are being reorganized into teams for greater uniformity and comparability of service provision among the area centers. In the other two divisions, both case management and team assignments are used.

These are current administrative goals: using the workload requirements to set efficiency measures, using the program requirements to make resource decisions among competing programs, and assessing client outcomes based on program goals. Nursing administrators need to have the strength, vision, and a sense of humor to work toward these goals. Progress is slow and sometimes circuitous but the overall direction is toward increased fiscal accountability and clearer delineation of nursing services.

BIOGRAPHICAL SKETCH

Jean Cross, MPH, RN, is Director of Dennis Avenue Health Center, Montgomery County Maryland Health Department. During the period of the time of the projects in this case study, she was the Director of Staff Development for the

Health Department. She received a master of Public Health from Johns Hopkins University, School of Hygiene and Public Health and her BSN from the University of Denver.

REFERENCES

Cross, J., Northrop, C., and Strasser J. (1983). How community health nurses spend their time: A study report. *Nursing and Health Care, 4*(6), 314–317.

Morris, M. (1981). A model for evaluating a community health agency. *Community Health Nursing.* New York: National League for Nursing, pp. 16–36.

Promoting Health/Preventing Disease: Objectives for the Nation. Fall, 1980. U.S. Department of Health and Human Services, Public Health Service.

Simmons, D. (June, 1980). Visiting Nurse Association of Omaha, Omaha Nebraska, *A Classification Scheme for Client Problems in Community Health-Nursing.* U.S. Department of Health and Human Services, Public Health Services, DHHS Publication No. H.R.A. 80–16.

13

Professional Development

Brenda S. Cherry

The why, how, and when of professional development of nurse–clinicians are questions frequently addressed in the nursing literature. They have been approached from an issue, strategy, and evaluation focus and based on varied definitions and assumptions of professionalism, education, and clinical practice. Although some approaches are reality-based, many are ideal types and perceived by administrators as not feasible. Consequently, those seeking guidance or insights from the literature are often forced to rely on their own knowledge, experience, intuition, and trial and error.

This chapter provides those responsible for professional development of the nurse clinician information needed to make informed decisions about administering professional development programs. It is based on the following assumptions: nurse clinicians need continuing professional development throughout their careers; professional development needs exceed those that can be accomplished through self-instruction; institutions are responsible for providing nurse-clinicians opportunities for professional development; and the commitment to professional development must be shared by employer and employee.

Professional development in this chapter is conceptualized broadly as any organized program that facilitates maintenance and enhancement of nursing competence in providing quality patient care. It includes those cognitive, psychomotor, and affective abilities needed for direct patient care as well as those needed to manage resources and persons providing care, collaborate with other health and allied health disciplines, and generate nursing care data.

PURPOSES OF PROFESSIONAL DEVELOPMENT PROGRAMS

One reality faced by nursing administrators is the disparity in clinical competence among nurse clinicians. Whether attributed to formal education, experience, disposition, or innate ability, differences in level of clinical ability and performance exist, making assessment of the target population an essential foundation. After educational needs have been accurately identified and documented, effective planning, implementation, and evaluation can proceed.

Education and training programs in service agencies must address the learning needs of new and continuing nurse employees. Many also provide offerings for nurses in the community.

New Nurse Employees

Orientation, a program offering common to all programs, is a critical factor in professional development. It is often cited as one of the most important variables in agency attrition rates and general socialization into the nursing profession. The quality and effectiveness of orientation programs is as variable as the service agencies in which they are offered. Their goals also vary, from a basic orientation to organizational structure, policies, and procedures, to clarification of mutual expectations, assessment of competence and learning needs, and establishment of plans for career development.

Different organizational structures are used to achieve orientation goals. The traditional approach is a structured centralized program with an introduction to support units and the nursing unit where the employee will work. More progressive approaches reflect a decentralized or a combination of centralized and decentralized structures. These approaches delegate all or some responsibility and authority for orientation to managers and staff of designated units. Designated units may or may not include the unit where the employee will work. The efficiency and effectiveness of these approaches, as well as the ideal goal(s) of orientation programs, are current nursing issues. Research supports the decentralized and centralized/decentralized combination as structures having the greatest potential for efficiency and effectiveness.

McCloskey and McCain (1987) explored satisfaction, commitment, and professionalism of 320 nurses newly employed in a large metropolitan hospital. Their findings indicate that all nurses, new graduates and experienced clinicians, entered a new employment agency with expectations of career development, participation in decision making, and other job rewards. They also found that organizational satisfaction, commitment, and professionalism decreased for all nurses in the study during the first 6 months of employment. Researchers attributed these decreases to discrepancies between initial expectations and actual experiences. One purpose of orientation programs is to inform nurses of the realities and expectations of nursing practice within respective institutions and to plan for career development based on assessment of professional needs. A successful orientation program provides a better fit between new employee expectations and institutional opportunities for fulfillment.

Preceptor and Intern Programs

A recent innovation is preceptor and intern programs. Usually part of a decentralized approach, both are useful for new graduates and experienced nurses.

Preceptor programs couple a new nurse employee with an experienced employee (one-to-one) who is responsible for orientation to the agency and nursing unit. Objectives for education and training of the new employee are based on mutual identification of professional needs. The preceptor has responsibility for education and training of the new employee and patient care, usually a reduced load. The support provided the new employee in this type of program is a great asset.

Intern programs may incorporate use of preceptors. Their structure reflects a decentralized approach to education and training and facilitates individualization of curriculum planning and implementation. They are usually designed for 3 months to 1 year of education and training with reduced patient care loads.

Continuing Nurse Employees

There are many changes within an agency that necessitate continuous updating of nurse clinicians' education and training. Within the agency, they may range from changes in equipment to changes in acuity level of patient populations. External changes effecting nurse's educational needs range from those in the general demographics of the patient population to changes in nurse practice acts. Two of the most basic and generalized reasons for professional development, however, are attainment and maintenance of clinical competence. Clinical competence is defined relative to standards of care for designated patient populations. Throughout a nurse's career clinical competence must be reestablished as one moves from student to nurse clinician, from one clinical area to another, one agency to another, or up a clinical ladder. In-service programs and continuing education programs are commonly used to assist in these transitions. Goals of professional development during these transitions are not only to facilitate orientation to an agency and its policies, procedures, and use of technological innovations, but also to support organizational commitment and job satisfaction.

Identifying and meeting the general professional developmental needs of the experienced nurse clinician has been less well developed by service agencies. Many issues surface when this topic is addressed: mandatory versus voluntary continuing education; nurse's motivation for participation, sources of education and training; teaching strategies; and payment by employer or employee. The underlying theme in these issues is who is responsible for career development—the nurse clinician, her employer, or both? The answer remains unresolved.

Professional socialization is recognized as a goal of most orientation programs for new graduates, but is often neglected in planning for professional development of experienced clinicians. Professional commitment and motivation to continually improve one's ability to provide quality patient care needs to be sustained and enhanced throughout a nurse's career. One alternative is to include role development in professional development department goals (O'Connor, 1980; Dolphin, 1983; Rosenfield, 1986). Professional growth may also be supported through counseling and recognition in the performance evaluation system. Studies in job satisfaction support that career development is one contributing factor.

Sources of education and training external to a nurse's employer include correspondence schools, governmental agencies, television, professional organizations, and varied institutions. It may be in the form of workshops, seminars, conferences, independent studies/learning modules, or formal courses. College or university semester/quarter hours, continuing education units (CEUs), or no credit may be offered for participation (Boshier & Peters, 1980; Axford, 1980).

NURSES AS ADULT LEARNERS

When planning educational and training programs for nurses, the instructor needs a firm foundation in both learning theory and adult learning characteristics. They also need to know if the content to be learned involves primarily psychomotor skills, cognitive understanding, or affective values and feelings.

Content

In designing a curriculum, the instructor needs to consider characteristics of both the content and the learner. Objectives focus on content to be learned or behaviors indicating learning that has been achieved.

Objectives can be broadly classified according to the taxonomy of Bloom, (1956) of educational objectives: cognitive, affective, and psychomotor. Cognitive objectives address behaviors depicting intellectual skills and abilities including knowledge, understanding, application, analysis, synthesis, and evaluation. An example of a cognitive objective for the evaluation level is:

> On October 19, 1988, each student in Nurs 800 will critique three research articles utilizing Cherry's five principles of research critiques.

Affective objectives are based on behaviors that demonstrate changes in sensitivity, attitudes, and values. This domain of objectives includes receiving, responding, valuing, organization, and characterization by a value. An example of an affective objective for valuing is:

> At the conclusion of the seminar on values clarification, each student will verbally judge the relevancy of seminar content to his/her current job responsibilities.

The third domain of objectives is the psychomotor. These objectives address motor skills and manipulative behaviors. Psychomotor behaviors are divided into four levels: observing, imitating, practicing, and adapting. An example of a psychomotor objective for adapting is:

> On Tuesday, May 18, 1988 each student in Nurs 561 will demonstrate, in selected simulated situations, body mechanics appropriate to the effective delivery of a formal speech.

Educational objectives should encompass three components, the learner, the behavioral change sought, and the content related to the behavioral change. Targeted behavioral changes in the learner must be based on knowledge of the learner's baseline behavior.

Learning Theories

Learning theory is a subfield of psychology. This broad subject has two competing main streams of theory: neo-behaviorist and Gestalt.

Neo-behaviorists are the current researchers using Skinner's principles of stimulus–response as the basis of learning. Neo-behaviorists believe "learning is a more or less permanent change of behavior that occurs as a result of practice. Key concepts are stimuli and responses. The process of learning can be understood by studying the relationship of processions of stimuli and responses and what occurs between them that results in desirable behaviors" (Bigge, 1976, p. 86).

Educators with a behaviorist orientation base their teaching efforts on the manipulation of external variables or stimuli to elicit a desired response from the learner. Members of this school of thought advocate control of the learning situation by the teacher, view students as passive receptors for stimuli, do not consider purposive or goal activities of students, do not recognize the value of past experiences and their influence on learning, and recognize extrinsic motivation as the compelling force in learning (Bigge, 1976).

This theoretical approach is useful for nursing instructors designing training programs to use new equipment or other psychomotor skills such as new procedures. It stresses the importance of presenting each step and requiring return demonstrations. Learning experiences using this approach are standardized and each learner goes through the same experience.

Gestalt theorists offer a contrasting view of how people learn. "Learning is a process of developing new insights or modifying old ones . . . learning is a purposive, explorative, imaginative, and creative enterprise" (Bigge, 1976, p. 95).

Gestalt educators believe learning occurs through goal insight, continuity of life space, and experiences facilitating learning. The prior experiences and knowledge of students are utilized as an integral part of the teaching–learning process. Their view of the student is that he or she is active, motivated by intrinsic and extrinsic factors, learns by discovery and problem solving, learns best in an environment that enhances his or her self-esteem and provides for his or her comfort (Knowles, 1984, 1978; Axford, 1980).

This theoretical approach leads the educator to examine individual differences among learners and to allow for flexibility in designing learning experiences.

Cognitive Style

One important way that people vary, regardless of age, is learning style or cognitive style. This has been called a theory of learning how to learn.

Helping people to gain insight into their cognitive patterns, methodological preferences, strengths and weaknesses, and to overcome blocks to learning effectiveness is the key to helping people learn. (Smith & Haverkamp, 1977, p. 4)

Ostmoe and colleagues (1984) indicate that style determines the "conditions under which a person is most likely to learn and the amount of structure required
for learning to occur" (p. 27). Assessment of cognitive style helps the adult educator to plan more effective teaching–learning strategies. Dolphin and Holtzclaw
(1983) state that "the need for diversity in teaching strategies becomes more
apparent when a combination of several divergent cognitive style emerges
within the same group of learners" (p. 68). Instructors also need to be aware of
their own cognitive style. Research shows that instructors tend to primarily use
the style they prefer. Thus, assessing both the instructor's and the student's
cognitive style and providing a variety of learning strategies connotes a particular philosophy of teaching in which instruction is viewed as an active two-way
communication process involving the direct and indirect exchange of knowledge, skill and affect (Ostmoe et al., 1984).

Adult Learning Theory

Another characteristic of nurses is that they are all adults. In her classic article
on the differences between adults and youth, Jane Zahn (1967) states that many
differences are related to age and they play a significant role in how adults learn.
She delineates some of these differences as (1) a physical decline in speed of
performance, reaction time, sight and hearing; (2) psychological changes in values, goals, responsibilities, self-image, and quantity of experiences; and (3)
cognitive–intellectual changes in stability of learning abilities when time limits
are controlled.

Physically, as Jane Zahn mentioned, the reaction time of adults is slower
and both sight and hearing may need to be augmented due to aging. This may
be relevant to planning training programs. Although cognitive abilities do not
decline with age, the educator must consider the need for additional reaction
time when planning learning activities. The difficulty encountered when re-
learning a procedure or content, cognitive dissonance, may also necessitate additional time for a learning activity.

Psychological differences between children and adults are due to developmental stage and differences in life experiences. The earliest developmental theories did not address adults. The three major adult developmental theories are
Havighurst's life cycle theory, Erickson's successive developmental crises, and
Buhler's biological clock theory. Havighurst alerts the educator of adults to consider chronological-related dominant concerns (tasks) that are based on biological development, personal and social expectations. Erikson separates the developmental needs of adulthood into three stages: young adult (18 to 29 years),
adults (30 to 65 years), and senior adults (30 to 65 years). Thus, adults in different stages may have different motivation in choosing learning experiences.
Buhler directs the instructor to consider that adults, unlike children, choose

learning experiences for pragmatic applications rather than undifferentiated future use. Adults use a present orientation in evaluating learning experiences.

Malcolm Knowles is the leading adult learning theorist. His primary concept is learning for adults should be based on "androgogy" rather than "pedagogy," which was originally developed for teaching children. Following are the five assumptions of androgogy.

1. Adult learners are self-directed.
2. Adults are a resource for their own learning (experience).
3. Adults have learning needs based on social development roles (readiness).
4. Adults need immediacy of application (time perspective).
5. Adults have a problem centered orientation to learning. (Knowles, 1984, p. 116)

For adults, unlike children, learning experiences are often based on personal choice. Adults seek learning experiences to augment what they already know (Knowles, 1978, 1980). They may be motivated by external forces, such as occupational obsolescence, changing societal roles, economic advancement, or the knowledge explosion (Hiemstra, 1976). They may also be motivated by internal desires such as professional growth, self-improvement, or social interaction (Boshier & Peters, 1980; Axford, 1980).

Any or all of these motives may apply to nurse clinicians and should be understood in planning flexible and relevant professional development programs (Schoen, 1979; O'Connor, 1979, 1980; Dolphin, 1983; Millonig, 1985). O'Connor surveyed nurses attending continuing education workshops and found they indicated maintaining professional currency and improving the ability to serve the public to be the primary reasons for participation. Other motivators, such as mandated continuing education for relicensure and acquisition of credentials, were also mentioned. These findings were consistent with those of other researchers (Clark & Dickinson, 1976; Tibbles, 1977; Millonig, 1985).

The application of concepts from Gestalt learning theory, cognitive style research, and adult learning theory should be used together in designing individualized learning experiences for nurses. This is most applicable when content focuses on cognitive and affective objectives.

The Learning Experience

A final factor to consider in planning a learning experience for nurses is the environment. Knowles (1984) states that an environment that facilitates physical comfort, privacy, informality, and lack of distractions promotes learning. He also identifies the quality and amount of interaction between educator and learner as a crucial factor in success of learning efforts by adults. An atmosphere of respect, trust, mutual helpfulness, freedom of expression, and acceptance of differences promotes learning. The environment is important regardless of content being presented and teaching strategy chosen.

Teaching strategies available to the instructor include independent reading or programmed learning modules, one-to-one coaching as in a preceptorship, informal unit in-services led by peers, or formal classes using lectures, audio visuals, role playing, discussion, and other interactive strategies with varying group sizes. Choice depends on resources, learning theory perspective, domain of learning objectives, learner characteristics, institutional goals, and demand.

Important points for the educator to consider in planning adult learning experiences are (1) creating a physical environment conducive to learning, (2) adjustments based on adult characteristics, and (3) the interpersonal aspect of learning is an important environmental factor.

CENTRALIZATION VERSUS DECENTRALIZATION OF PROFESSIONAL DEVELOPMENT DEPARTMENTS

Organizational structures of professional development programs have traditionally been based on structure of the parent institution and available resources. Consideration of the target population's learning needs in determining source and locus of responsibility for professional development is a more recent phenomenon. Impetus for this consideration has been from two general areas, management literature and adult learning and development literature.

Management Literature

A centralized department is currently the dominant organizational structure for professional development units. Given the bureaucratic nature of health care organizations, this is not surprising. Centralization is more congruent with bureaucratic systems. Understanding scientific management theory (F. W. Taylor) serves as a basis for implementing the ideal type bureaucratic system and illuminates centralization's assets and limitations. This theory emphasizes planning, standardizing, and improving human effort at the operative level to maximize output with minimum input. Time and motion studies are performed to identify the most efficient way to perform a task and then performance expectations are standardized using policies and procedures. Workers who are best suited to perform the specific task are selected and trained to follow the standardized procedures. Workers are assumed to receive job satisfaction and be motivated by economic rewards from increased output (Mitchell, 1982).

The advantages of a centralized department are (1) use of fewer human resources, thus decreasing planning and coordination time; (2) increased control of curriculum; and (3) decreased up front cost. These advantages, however, must be considered in terms of their long-term effects in achieving the goals of education and training.

Decentralization, the dispersement of functions, authority, and power, is more consistent with the human relations theory of management that advocates the importance of social and psychological factors in determining organizational structure. This theory facilitates a more open system of organization, one that is continually adapting to change in its environment and achieves a steady state or dynamic balance of changes (Perrow, 1986). There is a current trend toward decentralization of professional development in health care delivery agencies. This reflects a growing awareness that a change in organizational structure is needed to accommodate the many rapid changes that are occurring in health care. Professional development units have been taxed by demands for education and training of clinicians in the many technological and managerial changes taking place.

Current Practice

Orientation of new employees has traditionally been a two-step process: centralized formal classes and decentralized informal introduction to the job. Harper Grace Hospitals in Detroit, Michigan, however, report they have a successful decentralized program. All new graduates are assigned to "orientation units," designated medical–surgical patient care units, where nurse preceptors permanently assigned to the units are responsible for their orientation. Each is described as a half-way house for new graduate nurses that bridges the gap between the idealistic world of formal education and the realities of the clinical setting. Application of critical thinking and problem solving in practical settings are the primary objectives for orientees.

Orientations are structured to provide classroom and supervised experiences in all areas of nursing care. The new graduate follows the work schedule of his or her preceptor, including evenings and nights, after the classroom portion of the orientation is completed. Orientation is individualized based on needs of the orientee and evaluation is based on behavioral objectives. Preceptors write weekly critical incidents and provide feedback through conferences. Orientation is completed when mutually agreed on objectives are met, no specific time limits are set.

This program is primarily designated for new graduates. Staff nurses, however, can use the orientation units to enhance skills and obtain supervised experience with certain types of patients. Educators found that this program not only reduced attrition rates for new graduates, but promoted quality and innovative nursing care by all nurses (Lee & Raleigh, 1983).

Many other health care organizations are also decentralizing their professional development departments and learning to involve nurse clinicians. With support from nursing educators, nurse clinicians are presenting in-service classes to their peers and acting as preceptors for new graduates, new experienced employees, and nurses assuming new jobs due to lateral transfers and promotions. In fact, in her research, Benner (1984) found the most effective instructors were those who had recently had similar learning experiences. Thus, a staff nurse with 2 years experience is better suited to be a preceptor of a new graduate than an expert nurse with 10 years of experience. The expert solves clinical problems based on guidelines developed through experience. The new graduate solves clinical problems based on comparing what is observed with the knowledge learned in school and common sense.

No organizational structure can assure accomplishment of objectives, but literature clearly supports structure as a factor in program success (Rufo, 1981; Lee & Raleigh, 1983; Kasprisin & Young, 1985; Goodall, 1985). Shamian and Lemieux (1984) did a comparative study of centralized and decentralized new nurse employee orientations. The preceptor method was primarily based on a decentralized approach with only one central session. The formal method was based on two central education and training sessions. Although no significant difference in knowledge was found between the groups immediately after the program, the preceptor group demonstrated greater retention after 3 months. Shamian and Lemieux surmise that benefits of the decentralized preceptor method appear to emerge after a lapse of time, which makes it "more conducive to reinforcement and internalization of material than the formal model" (p. 89).

Whether or not the professional development unit is centralized or decentralized should be based on institutional resources, philosophy and theory of learning, program goals, and nature of target populations. Although there is an increasing trend toward decentralization, a move in this direction should be considered carefully (Moloney, 1986). A combination of the centralized and decentralized structure is a third option that may be viable and effective in many institutions.

CREATIVE LINKAGES BETWEEN SERVICE AND EDUCATION

Facilitating achievement of professional objectives is crucial to the development of nurse clinicians within specified agencies as well as to the entire nursing profession. Ultimately, this will only be achieved through collaboration between formal education and service. Both formal affiliations and collaborative endeavors are advocated as the key to strength of the nursing profession by the National Commission on Nursing and the National Institutes of Health, Committee on Nursing and Nursing Education (Grace, 1981; Styles, 1984; Walker, 1985). These relationships may range from informal networking between educators and clinicians to formal institutional mergers. The forms of relationships are limited only by the creativity and commitment of educators and clinicians.

Ideally, information emanating from such relationships should influence basic nursing education programs as well as professional development programs for clinicians. If this were the rule instead of the exception, perhaps the conflict in expectations and role confusion of new graduates would be diminished. Instead, Kramer's (1981) insights concerning "reality shock" of new graduates continues to be applicable and lines of effective communication between education and service remain inadequate (Baker and Hart, 1981; Rosenfeld, 1986).

According to Walker (1985) the desire to improve communication channels and collaborative efforts is the first step in achieving it. This must be coupled with what she describes as attitudes for partnership; these are a commitment to the total profession, realistic expectations, willingness to accept responsibility for helping each other, and flexibility. Although these prerequisite attitudes are believed to create a conducive mental set, they do not explain how bridges of communication and collaboration can actually be established.

Margretta Styles' (1984) framework for analyzing collaboration between education and service provides a useful background for developing and examining collaborative models. Her continuum of collaborative modes (Table 13–1) depicts stages of unity that reflect progressive frequency of interaction on topics of mutual interest, reciprocal advising, mutual approval before acting, and unified policies on selected issues (p. 22).

Barrell and Hamric (1986) describe how one school of nursing and the associated university medical center developed a collaborative model that did not incorporate a unified structure. Their model created consultative links between counterparts in each organization at the levels of dean and director, assistant dean and education director, and department chair and clinical director (p. 497). The impetus for the links included the need to strengthen course content in the formal and continuing education curricula, enhance clinical research, promote joint discussions on health care issues, and unify the voice of nursing within the university (p. 498).

Engstrom (1984) elaborates on the need for collaboration to enhance nursing research. She believes collaborative research projects are needed to maximize limited resources, apply research to clinical practice, investigate complex research questions, and acquaint clinicians with the research process (p. 76).

Literature abounds with articles advocating increased collaboration between education and service (Grace, 1981; Blazeck et al., 1982; Gresham, 1983; Styles, 1984; Wooley, 1984). All of the major professional nursing organizations, the National League for Nursing, American Nurses' Association, American Academy of Nursing, and American Association of Colleges of Nursing, have presented position statements supporting collaboration. Conflicts and adversarial stances between education and service, however, continue. Kramer (1981) attributes this to differences institutional goals and products, abdication of responsibility for collaboration with service by nurse educators, and the unclear, unrealistic expectations of nursing service. She points out the primary barrier to collaboration is that "the product of nursing service is care . . . and the product of nursing education is an educated individual" (p. 645). Although the argument can be made that these products do not need to be incongruent, differ-

TABLE 13–1. STAGES OF UNITY

Stage 1	No relationship
Stage 2	Communication independent functions
Stage 3	Consultation
Stage 4	Consent
Stage 5	Unified policy joint functions
Stage 6	Unified structure

From Styles, M., 1984, pp. 21–23.

ences in philosophies and priorities continue to be powerful contraints. Little actual collaboration beyond Styles' stage 2 exists.

Efforts to bridge the gap between service and educational organizations, thus promoting professional interaction, have increased. Unification and affiliative models, such as those described by Grace (1981) are being examined for feasibility by more institutions. Unified institutions now have National League for Nursing accredited programs. Creation of advisory boards between education and service institutions have increased. Adjunct faculty–staff appointments are more common in both service and educational institutions. Individual consultation, faculty practice, and guest lectures are evidence of increased interaction between nurse–clinicians and educators. Problems are not rare, but enough success is documented to be encouraging. Perhaps the most common successful efforts in this area are preceptorships and extern/internships.

Collaborative Teaching

Some formal nursing educational programs now use nurses in service agencies as preceptors. A preceptor is a nurse–clinician who serves in a dual role of clinician and educator. In a collaborative role, he or she works on a one-to-one basis with nursing students and assumes part of the responsibility for their education and training (Williamson & Therrien, 1978; Turnbull, 1983; Moloney, 1986). By serving as a positive role model, providing support, encouragement, learning opportunities, and progressively less supervision, the preceptor fosters self-confidence, accountability, and independence in a reality-based setting.

Other advantages of preceptorships are related to general enhancement of the nursing profession. By gaining a clearer understanding of the education process, establishing closer relationships and communication lines between educators and clinical staff, sharing ideas and insights, and assuming responsibility for future colleagues, the preceptor contributes to the total profession and develops an increasing sense of self-worth (Williamson & Therrien, 1978; Lee & Raleigh, 1983; Shamian & Lemieux, 1984).

This model, however, also has limitations. Nursing service administrators and educators must negotiate means for the resources necessary to support preceptorships. Education, training, flexibility in scheduling, salary differentials, and other rewards for increased workload are a few of the variables that will affect success of the preceptorship program (Lee & Raleigh 1983; Wieczorek, Weissman, & Devereux, 1985). Regardless of the reward system some clinicians may not want to participate. Assuming that all qualified nurse–clinicians should be interested in becoming preceptors and using administrative pressure to convince them to do so is a mistake that will jeopardize the success of any program.

Although not truly collaborative, internships and externships do enhance communication between service and education and promote socialization of new nurses into practicing clinicians. Internships and externships lengthen traditional orientation programs adding more formal classes and a preceptorship. The former is focused on nurse–clinicians, primarily new graduates learning to be staff nurses and employees preparing for specialized practice. The latter is targeted for nursing students. Students meeting selected criteria are employed during summers, evenings, and weekends, with the expectation that they will work in that agency/institution after graduation and completion of the registered nurse examination. Both usually have goals related to reduction of orientation time/cost, stress, and attrition, while increasing motivation, organizational commitment, and productivity. Each may differ in organizational structure, design, curriculum, and length. Both are often highlighted in recruitment and marketing efforts.

Mentoring, a system in which an experienced adult befriends and guides a less experienced adult, can also be viewed as a collaborative effort to promote professional development (Fagan & Fagan, 1983). Mentors may be in education or service and are part of the "patron system . . . conceptualized as a continuum of sponsorship activities that can assist a person to advance within a given organization or profession" (Campbell & Heider, 1986, p. 110). This collaborative effort is less widely used than others previously mentioned, but is receiving increased attention and advocacy. Hunt and Michael (1983) indicate that the career advice, education, and social support provided by mentors assists proteges to develop confidence to take professional risks, which accelerates career growth.

Contract courses are an additional collaborative effort. They provide college/university credit that may lead to a degree or certification at the undergraduate or graduate level. Courses are taught by college/university faculty and offered within or near the designated health care institution/agency. The education institution contracts with the service institution to offer specified courses, within a selected time frame, to a certain number of nurses. Efforts to establish contract courses would appear to indicate some mutual valuing of these programs.

Outreach continuing education programs may be offered by service institutions or schools of nursing. Some offerings may be by contract, at the work site. The majority are offered at the home institution and open to attendance by others for a fee. Increasingly both research days and continuing education programs are being offered through joint sponsorship. Often this is evidence of a beginning collaborative relationship between service and educational institutions.

Professional development of nurse clinicians is a more complex endeavor than is commonly recognized. Understanding the varied factors that contribute to success or failure of these programs helps place this complexity in perspective. Adult educators and program planners responsible for professional development are faced with constantly changing education and training needs of clinicians who may or may not be motivated to participate in any form of continuing education. Program planners are responsible for identifying learning needs, designing programs to meet them, and motivating clinicians to attend.

Establishing relevance is generally accepted as a key element in motivating voluntary attendance and participation in continuing education/professional development programs. Relevance must be considered from the viewpoints of the learner, service agency, and educational institution. Each must perceive the learning experience to enhance competence in the delivery and improvement of patient care.

Responsibility for improving patient care through professional development must be shared by education and service. Collaboration between these areas is necessary and models that promote this effort should be given careful consideration.

Strategies for implementing professional develoment programs are based on knowledge of adults and how they learn, cognitive styles, domains of learning, and target populations. They must be varied and flexible to accommodate constantly changing education and training needs of nurse clinicians.

BIOGRAPHICAL SKETCH

Brenda S. Cherry, PhD, RN, is the Dean of the College of Nursing, University of Massachusetts, Boston. Brenda received her BSN degree in 1968 from North Carolina A&T State University, MSN from the College of Nursing, University of Nebraska Medical Center in 1977, and PhD from the University of Nebraska—Lincoln in 1981. Her work experiences include staff nurse and charge positions in the U.S. Army Nurse Corp, civil service and private health agencies. Since 1977, she has held positions as nurse educator and educational administrator in baccalaureate and master's degree nursing programs. At the time of writing this chapter she was Associate Dean for Academic Programs and Associate Professor, School of Nursing, George Mason University. Her participation in professional organizations include ANA, NLN, Sigma Theta Tau, Virginia Nurses Association, Virginia Society of Professional Nurses, and the Virginia Association of Colleges of Nursing. The professional service activities include membership on advisory boards and committees, participation in continuing education programs, and consultation with educational and health related organizations. Brenda has recently been selected to the editorial board of *Pediatric Nursing.*

SUGGESTED READINGS

Professional Development Programs

American Nurses Association. (1984). *Standards of Continuing Education.* Kansas City, MO: American Nurses Association.

Butterfield, S. (1985). Professional nursing education: What is its purpose? *Journal of Nursing Education, 24*(3), 99–103.

Fogelsong, O. (1983). The impact of a staff development offering on nursing practice. *The Journal of Continuing Education in Nursing, 14*(6), 12–15.

Gerstein, M., & Amos, M. (1986). Implementation and evaluation of adult career development programs in organizations. *The Journal of Career Development, 12*(3), 210–217.

Oliver, S. (1984). The effects of continuing education on the clinical behavior of nurses. *The Journal of Continuing Education in Nursing. 15*(4), 130–134.

Smallegan, M. (1981). Continuing education: How do you build a program? *The Journal of Continuing Education in Nursing, 12*(3), 12–15.

Welch, D. (1980). The real issues behind providing continuing education in nursing. *The Journal of Continuing Education in Nursing, 11*(3), 17–21.

Zebelman, E., Davis, D., & Larson, E. (1983). Helping staff nurses use learning modules. *Nursing and Health Care, 4*(4), 198–199.

Adult Education Theory

Betz, C. (1984). Methods utilized in nursing continuing education programs. *The Journal of Continuing Education in Nursing, 15*(2), 39–44.

deTornyay, R., & Thompson, M. (1982). *Strategies for Teaching Nursing,* 2nd ed. New York: John Wiley and Sons.

Garity, J. (1985; March-April). Learning styles: Basis for creative teaching and learning. *Nurse Educator,* pp. 12–15.

Hayter, J. (1983). Educational taxonomics revisited. *Journal of Nursing Education, 22*(8), 339–342.

Havighurst, R. (1980, November). Life-span developmental psychology and education. *Educational Researcher,* pp. 3–8.

Houle, C. (1978). *The Design of Education.* San Francisco: Jossey Bass.

Kennedy, M. (1983). Designing and implementing successful CE programs. *The Journal of Continuing Education in Nursing, 14*(1), 16–20.

Knowles, M.S. (1984). *Andragogy in Action: Applying Modern Principles of Adult Learning.* San Francisco: Jossey-Bass.

O'Connor, A. (1982). Staff development: The problems of motivation. *The Journal of Continuing Education in Nursing, 13*(2), 10–14.

Trammell, D. (1984). Educational preparation: Its effects on selection and degree of involvement in continuing education activities. *The Journal of Continuing Education in Nursing, 15*(6), 223–226.

Yonge, G. (1985). Andragogy and pedagogy: Two ways of accompaniment. *Adult Education Quarterly, 35*(3), 160–167.

Zebelman, E., Davis, D., & Larson, E. (1983). Helping staff nurses use learning modules. *Nursing and Health Care, 4,* 198–199.

Centralization Versus Decentralization

Lesher, D., & Bomberger, A. (1983). The roving inservice/an innovative approach to learning. *The Journal of Continuing Education in Nursing, 14*(3), 19–22.

Koontz, H., O'Donnell, C., & Weihrich, H. (1984). *Management.* New York: McGraw-Hill.

Creative Linkages of Service Delivery and Schools of Nursing to Increase Professional Development

Marcus, M., Swent, K., Valadez, A., et al. (1986). Community care practicums ready students for new levels of practice. *Nursing and Health Care, 7*(7), 377–380.

Riddell, D., & Hubalik, K. (1981). Bridging the gap: Responsibility of education or service? In McCloskey, J. & Grace, H. (eds.): *Current Issues in Nursing*. Boston, MA: Blackwell Scientific Publications, pp. 621–626.

Squires, R. (1980). Statewide continuing education for nurses increases accessibility to university resources. *The Journal of Continuing Education in Nursing*, 11(4), 46–49.

Wasch, S. (1980, February). The role of baccalaureate faculty in continuing education. *Nursing Outlook*, pp. 116–120.

REFERENCES

Axford, R. (1980). *Adult Education: The Open Door to Life Long Learning*. Indiana: The A.C. Halldin Publishing Co.

Baker, N., & Hart, C. (1981). Nurses in action. *Nursing and Health Care*, 11(3), 130–32, 168–169.

Barrell, L., & Hamric, A. (1986). Education and service: A collaborative model to improve patient care. *Nursing and Health Care*, 7(9), 497–503.

Benner, P. (1984). *From Novice to Expert: Excellence and Power in Clinical Nursing Practice*. Menlo Park, CA: Addison-Wesley.

Bigge, M.L. (1976). *Learning Theories for Teachers*, 3rd ed. New York: Harper & Row.

Blazeck, A., Selekman, J., Timpe, M., & Wolfe, Z. (1982). Unification: Nursing education and nursing practice. *Nursing and Health Care*, 3,18–24.

Bloom, B.S. (1956). *Taxonomy of Educational Objectives*. New York: David McKay Co.

Boshier, R., & Peters, J. (1980). Adult needs, interests and motives. In Klevins, C. (ed.): *Materials and Methods*. New York: Klevens Pub., pp. 197–211.

Campbell, H., & Heider, N. (1986). Do nurses need mentors. *Image: The Journal of Nursing Scholarship*, 18(3), 110–113.

Clark, K., & Dickinson, G. (1976). Self-directed and other directed continuing education: A study of nurses participation. *The Journal of Continuing Education in Nursing*, 7(4), 16–24.

Dolphin, N.W. (1983). Why do nurses come to continuing education programs? *The Journal of Continuing Education in Nursing*, 14(4), 8–16.

Dolphin, P., & Holtzclaw, B. (1983). *Continuing Education in Nursing: Strategies for Lifelong Learning*. Reston, VA, Reston Publishing.

Engstrom, J. (1984). University, agency, and collaborative models for nursing research: An overview. *Image: The Journal of Nursing Scholarship*, 16(3), 76–80.

Fagan, M., & Fagan, P. (1983). Mentoring among nurses. *Nursing and Health Care*, 4(2), 77–84.

Goodall, C. (1985). Applying aspects of educational psychology to the practice of nurse teaching. *Nurse Education Today*, 5, 263–266.

Grace, H. (1981). Unification reunification; reconcililation or collaboration— Bridging the education/service gap. In McCloskey, J. & Grace, H. (eds.): *Cur-*

rent Issues in Nursing. Boston, MA: Blackwell Scientific Publications, pp. 626–643.

Gresham, M. (1983). Joint appointments. In Hamric, A.B., & Sposs, J. (eds.): *The Clinical Nurse Specialist in Theory and Practice.* New York: Grune and Stratton.

Hiemstra, R. (1976). *Lifelong Learning.* Lincoln, NE: Professional Publications.

Hunt, D., & Michael, C. (1983). Mentorship: A career training development tool. *Academy of Management Review, 8,* 475–485.

Kasprisin, A., & Young, W. (1985). Nurse internship program reduces turnover, raises commitment. *Nursing and Health Care, 6*(3), 137–140.

Knowles, M. (1978). *The Adult Learner: A Neglected Species,* 2nd ed. Houston: Gulf Publishing.

Knowles, M. (1980). *The Modern Practice of Adult Education.* Chicago: Follett Publishing Co.

Knowles, M. (1984). *Andragogy in Action: Applying Modern Principles of Adult Learning.* San Francisco: Jossey-Bass, pp. 417–422.

Kramer, M. (1981). Why does reality shock continue? In McCloskey, J., & Grace, H. (eds.): *Current Issues in Nursing.* Boston, MA: Blackwell Scientific Publications, pp. 644–653.

Lee, G., & Raleigh, E. (1983, January). A half-way house for the new graduate. *Nursing Management,* pp. 43–45.

McCloskey, J., & McCain, B. (1987). Satisfaction, commitment and professionalism of newly employed nurses. *Image: Journal of Nursing Scholarship, 19*(1), 20–27.

Millonig, V. (1985). Motivational orientation toward learning after graduation. *Nursing Administration Quarterly, 9*(4), 79–86.

Mitchell, T. (1982). Motivation: A new direction for theory, research, and practice. *Academy of Management Review, 7*(1), 80–88.

Moloney, M. (1986). *Professionalization of Nursing: Current Issues and Trends.* Philadelphia: J.B. Lippincott.

O'Connor, A. (1980, September-October). The continuing nurse learner: Who and why. *Nurse Educator,* pp. 24–27.

O'Connor, A. (1979). Reasons nurses participate in continuing education. *Nursing Research, 28*(6), 354–359.

Ostmoe, P., Hoozer, H., Scheffel, A., & Crowell, C. (1984). Learning style preferences and selection of learning strategies: Consideration and implications for nurse educators. *Journal of Nursing Education, 23*(1), 27–30.

Perrow, C. (1986). *Complex Organizations,* 3rd ed. New York: Random House.

Rosenfeld, P. (1986). Nursing and professionalization: On the road to recovery. *Nursing and Health Care, 7*(9), 485–488.

Rufo, K. (1981). Guidelines for inservice education for registered nurses. *The Journal of Continuing Education in Nursing, 12*(1), 26–33.

Schoen, D. (1979). Lifelong learning: How some participants see it. *The Journal of Continuing Education in Nursing, 10*(2), 3–13.

Shamian, J., & Lemieux, S. (1984). An evaluation of the preceptor model versus the formal teaching model. *The Journal of Continuing Education in Nursing, 15*(3), 86–89.

Smith, R., & Haverkamp, K. (1977). Toward a theory of learning how to learn. *Adult Education, 28*(1), 3–21.

Styles, M. (1984). Reflections on collaboration and unification. *Image: The Journal of Nursing Scholarship, 16*(1), 21–23.

Tibbles, L. (1977). Theories of adult education: Implications for developing a philosophy for continuing education in nursing. *Journal of Continuing Education in Nursing, 8*(4), 25–28.

Turnbull, E. (1983, January). Rewards in nursing: The case of nurse preceptors. *The Journals of Nursing Administration,* pp. 10–13.

Wieczorek, R., Weissman, G., & Devereux, P. (1985). Clinical career pathway: The Mount Sinai experience. *Nursing and Health Care, 6*(3), 143–145.

Williamson, J., & Therrien, B. (1978). The nurse preceptor. In Williamson, J. (ed.): *Current Perspectives in Nursing Education: The Changing Scene,* Vol. 11. St. Louis: C.V. Mosby.

Wooley, A. (1984). The bridge course: Transition to professional practice. *Nurse Educator, 9*(4), 15–19.

Walker, D. (1985). Nursing education and service: The payoffs of partnership. *Nursing and Health Care, 6*(4), 189–191.

Zahn, J. (1967, Winter). Differences between adults and youth affecting learning. *Adult Education,* pp. 67–77.

APPLICATION 13-1

Guidelines for Establishing a Clinical Nursing Research Program in a Medical Center Teaching Hospital
Margaret R. Dear

A priority for the nursing profession is the generation of a new clinical knowledge through scientific endeavor. Currently, many hospital nursing divisions are addressing this need through the establishment of clinical nursing research programs. This is especially true in medical center teaching hospitals where it is expected that nursing be part of the research mission. This application discusses the major considerations to be addressed when a hospital nursing division initiates a research program.

Initially, the purpose of the research program must be identified along with the expected outcomes and impact. These must articulate with the general philosophy of the nursing division and the parent institution. The Director of Nursing and his or her management team may delineate the purpose, or delegate it to

Note: This article was prepared on the authors' personal time and was not part of her official responsibilities with nor should it be attributed to the National Institutes of Health.

a task force, research committee, or the department responsible for the research program (usually education or quality assurance).

GOALS AND OBJECTIVES

Purposes vary depending on the needs and resources of a particular hospital nursing organization. Decisions need to be congruent with the priorities of the nursing division. The first decision is whether the purpose is to facilitate research, conduct research, use research methods and findings, or a combination of these. The second decision is the focus of the research program. Shall it be administrative studies in line with hospital priorities, patient care studies in line with clinical priorities, or any significant investigation chosen by the investigators, or a mixture. If the Division has particular centers of excellence, the program may be focused or targeted to those areas. If the Division is facing a problem, such as evaluation of new graduates' performance, initial studies could focus on that issue. Examination of departmental goals and articulation with them allows for a realistic developmental process. A third priority is, who will lead and carry out the program? In any case, basic decisions need to be made and a firm plan and timetable established with the support of administration.

If administrative support is weak or lacking, no type of research program can succeed. Enthusiasm and commitment is necessary throughout the nursing division from staff nurses to middle managers and nurse executives. Without vigorous encouragement the program will not get off the ground, much less thrive.

SUFFICIENT FINANCIAL RESOURCES

A major concern centers on budget for the program. Is there a designated budget for this effort, or is the program to be absorbed as part of educational or other administrative cost centers? Administrative commitment must go beyond ideology. If there is an identified budget, then this must include all necessary resources: personnel, typing, duplication, printing, data entry, and data processing. If there is no identified budget, then decisions must be made concerning the source and level of support for the research program. Who will supply the secretarial services and pick up other costs of carrying out a project? Where is the slack in another budget for appropriate support? If services are not provided, nurses will end up doing their own secretarial work, either during duty hours or on their own time. Research will become an added task at high personal cost rather than a new dimension of nursing work. At this cost, the likelihood of nurses completing studies and applying results is small. These issues, then, are vital to the success of the research program and, therefore, worthy of frank, open and honest consideration by nurse administrators in defining what their organization's nursing research effort should be.

LEADERSHIP OF THE PROGRAM

Ideally, the program director should be a doctorally prepared nurse with considerable experience in clinical nursing research. Many hospitals, however, do not have such personnel on staff and may not have the moneys to recruit such a person. Other alternatives are available. For example, it may be possible to arrange part-time employment, periodic consultation, or even a joint appointment with a nurse researcher at a nearby school of nursing. The hospital nurse responsible for the research program should possess a master's degree, or be committed to learning more about research through formal courses, reading, and substantive support from an outside nurse researcher. Goals must be in line with the level of preparation of the hospital nurses responsible for the research program. Emphasis is placed here on development of realistic and clear goals for development of the program.

FACILITATING RESEARCH: PROPOSAL REVIEW

Protocols for review of research proposals are the first step in program development taken by most hospital nursing research programs. A committee or other organizational subunit must be designated to carry out this important work. The committee, once identified, should design a standard format, outlining content, attachment of instruments, and so on; therefore, any investigator understands what a proposal should contain before submitting it. The proposal should be similar or identical in form to what will be required for submission for review by the institutional review board (IRB) that reviews all medical research. Guidelines should be provided so that nurses understand the review process and time frame to expect a reply. A resource person from the committee or a research consultant should be available to answer questions, provide information, and facilitate the investigator's movement through the process.

The research review process will not only act as an educational experience for new investigators, but also for committee members. Nurses on the research committee should have criteria available to assist them in evaluating proposals. Ideally, they should also have a research consultant sit in on reviews. Criteria should be established in advance and should address each section of the research proposal. Several samples are available in the literature. Questions should address relevance of the problem to nursing, research methodology, protection of human subjects, and feasibility and cost to the hospital when the study is conducted. For example, some questions to be answered include:

1. Are the research purpose, problem, or questions stated clearly?
2. Has the relevant literature been reviewed and incorporated into the proposal?
3. Is there a guiding framework for the study?
4. Have hypotheses been formulated? If so, are the variables clearly identified and measurable?

5. Is the study design appropriate to the research problem?
6. Have the study subjects been identified and eligibility criteria developed? If sampling is to occur, has the process been described?
7. Have the study variables and their measures been described? Have the psychometric properties of the instruments been fully addressed?
8. How, where, and by whom will data be collected? Are hosptial staff required to assist in this study, and if so, what is the effect of their participation?
9. What is the plan for data analysis? Is it appropriate for answering the research questions?
10. Are there ethical issues present that need to be addressed?
11. Is the informed consent form prepared in accord with IRB guidelines? Have risk/benefit ratio and related issues been identified if present?

After nursing research committee approval, the proposal is reviewed by the IRB, if there is one, and also undergoes administrative review by hospital officials. One must bear in mind that the review must include the scientific aspect, the protection of human subjects, and the administrative endorsement. They are all of central importance in hospital research studies. Supports need to be in place to help staff nurses, clinical specialists, and administrators reach these standards, if in-house research is one purpose of the program. Administrative endorsement is sought to assure that participation is economically feasible and the hospital's concern for patients and its image are not jeopardized or harmed by the study.

The latter area is one that is not always addressed in nursing reviews. At times nurses are reluctant to understand that a hospital administration or nursing administration may not be willing to support a particular nursing study with their patients or staff. For example, hospital administrators may be reluctant to allow some patient populations to be studied, or to permit research on certain topics that may be viewed as especially sensitive, poorly timed, or of questionable scientific interest. Administrators may be skeptical about the expertise of novice nurse researchers. For all of these reasons, the question of administrative endorsement is central to the success of an individual study, and, indeed, to the viability of the research program itself. If support is weak or initially guarded, it may be best to postpone the initiation of the research study.

RESEARCH UTILIZATION: EDUCATION FOR RESEARCH

Because nurses vary widely in their research preparation, many are not aware of the relevance of research methods as findings to their practice. In-service education is needed to promote acceptance of the program and integration of research into practice. The research program should include an introductory course in nursing research for staff who wish to have such a learning experience. The course should be taught by a doctorally prepared nurse researcher and should be structured to include the basis of the scientific process with examples drawn from nursing practice research. Emphasis should be on understanding the logic of the research process and its applications to nursing procedure. The curriculum should include experiential learning such as participation in the research committee's critique of a proposal or review of research studies to apply to a current clinical problem on their unit. Certainly some active participation in the research program should be a desired outcome of the course.

Other educational activities of the research program should be less formal. Unit-based nursing research journal clubs, in which members take turns presenting studies, may generate interest among staff. A "brown bag research seminar" is another valuable tool. In this activity, a nurse investigator informally presents her study, discusses the process and the findings, and responds to questions during a lunch break. These and other educational offerings help hospital nursing staff gain knowledge of research and feel more comfortable in discussions of it. Attending research days sponsored by local universities or chapters of Sigma Theta Tau is another informal learning opportunity.

CONDUCTING NURSING RESEARCH

When the program has begun, nurses will wish to carry out independent research projects either singly or in groups. To assist them, the head of the research program needs to carry out an assessment of the investigators' interest, knowledge, skill, and commitment to offer help in the area most needed. The investigators may wish to also use nurse researchers from outside the organization in discussions of significance and relevance of nursing studies.

Developing the position of nurse researcher within the nursing division, the nurse researcher and nurse executive must address the following questions: What is the purpose of the program? Is the nurse researcher to support and facilitate the research of others, or is she expected to carry out her own research, perhaps involving staff in the process? Some nurse researchers seek to combine these activities. Clarification of these points is necessary to allow the program to begin with mutual understanding of role expectations.

Nurses with all levels of educational preparation can conduct research if expert advice and consultation are available to them. Although beginning investigators may have abundant energy and enthusiasm for research, these must be balanced by rigor and quality of research design and process. Nurse administrators need to be aware of this central point so that their research programs may be characterized by strength and growth potential.

ACCEPTANCE OF THE RESEARCH PROGRAM

Resistance to change is always an issue in establishing innovative programs in nursing. The resistance may be overt or covert, may be short-lived or permanently established. Persons responsible for the establishment of the research program should be prepared to deal with resistance to change from the beginning. Nurses and administrators who oppose a research program may cite short staffing and recruitment problems as reasons for not supporting a research effort. The advantages for recruitment and retention of an active research program, no matter how small, counter the short-staffing argument. There may always be divided opinions concerning the overall value of a research program. Although its worth may be identified, there may be concern that research activities draw nurses' energies away from the real needs for development in practice, quality assurance, staff education, primary nursing, and other areas where staff are engaged in ongoing work. The question of resistance must be addressed, for a fledgling research program to take root and grow. Timing, then, becomes an important factor in starting the program. Choosing a time when the nursing division is relatively stable helps assure a good start for the program.

Staff physicians are likely to question the establishment of a program, particularly if there is a staff shortage. Informing physicians during the planning phase, responding to questions and concerns, and seeking their support helps in securing access to patients later. Physicians who are unfamiliar with nursing research may be skeptical or hesitant at first. Physicians, however, will respond favorably if the program is well thought out, has reasonable goals, and has sufficient research expertise available to it.

EVALUATION OF THE RESEARCH PROGRAM

One of the early considerations for the research program is measurement of outcomes. Evaluation should address all the objectives of the program and emphasize measuring quality of the work, rather than a simple count of activities in progress. For example, there is no "right" number of research studies for any hospital to use as a standard for its own nursing research activities. Rather, the nursing division should build slowly, insisting on significance and quality in the studies supported. Criteria for measuring success might include:

1. There is a measurable impact on practice, no matter how small. This may be apparent as the outcome of two or three research application projects directed toward one practice area or nursing problem.
2. Nursing staff are aware of the existence of the program, its priorities, personnel and resources, and staff make use of the program appropriately.
3. Nurses who wish to carry out research in the hosptial contact resource persons and receive information about the review process.

These and other simple criteria, set forth in advance and periodically evaluated, help to assure that the program is well known in the organization, available for those who need it, and influencing nursing care to some degree.

The establishment of a nursing research program in a hospital nursing division is an exciting, challenging venture. It requires faith and trust on the parts of both administration and nursing staff. There must be some outlay of departmental resources to support the program, even one that is relatively modest in size and scope. Physicians, administrators, and some nurses need to be persuaded that the program is worthwhile and necessary. There may be controversy over aspects of the program, particularly as it grows in complexity. The challenges of this activity parallel the challenge the profession faces in trying to place its research agenda squarely in the mainstream of scientific inquiry.

Yet, the reward of successful establishment of a program is very great. Nursing staff expect medical center teaching hospitals to be in the forefront in medical and nursing care; they also expect that scientific research is ongoing in such hospitals. Nursing must be a part of such research.

Although the effort may be great and the required energy may be considerable, the rewards in terms of staff development, interest, and participation are also great. The future of nursing research depends on the opening up of clinical research opportunities for nurse investigators. With careful attention to structure, process, and outcome, the establishment of a nursing research program will advance this process.

BIOGRAPHICAL SKETCH

Margaret R. Dear holds a bachelor's degree in nursing from St. John's University, New York City. Her graduate degrees in Nursing and Sociology are from the Catholic University, Washington, D.C. Dr Dear has served on the faculties of Georgetown University and Johns Hopkins University. She was Director of Nursing Research at Johns Hopkins Hospital from 1980 to 1984. At the writing of this application she served as Senior Nurse Scientist and Director, Nursing Research and Education, at the National Institutes of Health, Clinical Center Nursing Department. Her research interests center on phychosocial issues in illness, on care delivery systems in nursing, and in particular, on research design. She is currently Professor, and Director of Nursing Research & Faculty Development at George Mason University, School of Nursing.

14

PERFORMANCE APPRAISAL

R. Douglas First

The performance appraisal is one of the most important functions in the employee relations process. Appraisal documents show how the health care agency views the employee's performance and provide the basis for the formal periodic supervisor–employee interviews about mutual expectations and achievement. Also, the employer can use the process to assess staffing levels, training needs, and employees to promote, counsel, or terminate. Compensation adjustments, requirements to analyze certain positions, and labor relations conditions can also be ascertained by careful analysis of performance appraisal data. Although the performance appraisal process must not be the sole criteria for personnel decisions, it should be one of the organization's principal tools in human resource management. Figure 14–1 illustrates how evaluation using performance appraisal fits into human resource management.

The intent of this chapter is to present an overview of the performance appraisal (PA) system. It covers the reasons PAs are performed, steps in the PA process, and common validation problems. The suggested readings at the end of the chapter permit further exploration of areas of interest in greater detail.

Various systems for evaluating performance have been used over the last 100 years. Performance appraisal started when factories began to specialize the work force and develop a management hierarchy. One of the earliest and simplest means to recognize performance was for the foreman to hang a flag over the work bench of the employee having the highest productivity for the previous day. Early this century, Frank and Lillian Gilbreth added an additional level of sophistication through the development of time and motion studies to prepare work standards to measure expectations and distribute resources. The third major advancement came during World War II when the military developed trait-oriented appraisals to identify potential leaders for accelerated promotion. One outcome of the civil rights movement of the last 20 years has been that PA methods have become more objective. As a result, most of today's performance

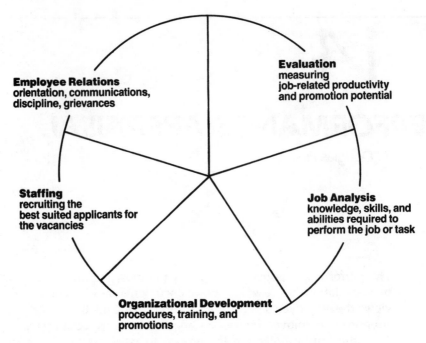

Figure 14-1. Functions of human resource management.

appraisal processes are oriented to measure job-related performance rather than subjective criteria.

PURPOSES OF THE PERFORMANCE APPRAISAL

Performance appraisals assist the individual employee, the supervisor, and management. The principal use is usually to determine salary adjustments. However, PAs may also be used by management for promotion or demotion/termination decisions, training, transfers, manpower requirements, and developmental needs. For the employee, the PA is a means to obtain feedback on his or her performance and contribution to the organization.

All too often, organizations embark on a performance appraisal program without first deciding what it is they want to accomplish. To do so would be like hiring an assortment of nurses, technicians, and clerks and then deciding what health services to provide. To be effective, conserve effort, and not create ill-feelings, the PA must be consistent with management's goals and policies. For example, if hospital policy is to promote nurses based primarily on senority and to encourage group cohesiveness, it would be a waste of effort and probably counterproductive to have a PA program that requires supervisors to rank the nurses in order of productivity. In this case, all management really needs to know is whether a nurse's performance is satisfactory or unsatisfactory.

Inappropriate use of the PA often causes the whole process to be suspect or abandoned. For example, a performance appraisal instrument designed to assess only satisfactory work for continued employment within a prescribed salary range would probably not be precise enough to identify junior personnel for a "fast track" promotion program. Another inappropriate use of the PA is to try to use the same instrument for all personnel in the organization. Senior administrators perform different types of functions and have responsibilities that do not exist in lesser positions. Just as a hospital chooses from a myriad of sophisticated instruments for measuring specific bodily functions, each known for its capabilities and limitations, management should select appraisal instuments that are appropriate for the positions to be assessed and for the desired use of information gathered. The more common uses of the PA are compensation adjustments, job productivity, staffing, organizational development, and training.

Compensation

Salary adjustments based on performance should be directly correlated to the contribution of the employee and overall productivity of the work unit. For example, has a nurse been able to handle the prescribed patient load and resolve problems with minimal conflict and intervention by the hospital's central administration? If the "prescribed patient load" is fair and equitable, and the expected performance and responsibility have been determined ahead of time, the appraisal instrument can measure the degree to which the nurse fulfilled or exceeded the norm. The more productive nurse should receive the higher salary increase.

Job Productivity

Job-related, productivity-oriented PAs of observable job behavior are becoming an accepted model. These appraisals permit both management and the employee to see how well the specific job has been performed over a given period of time. The terms *job-related* and *productivity-oriented* mean that the questions of ratings are oriented to the job. For example, "Does this nurse demonstrate a knowledge and practice of handling controlled substances?" The responses might be: (1) not applicable to job, (2) requires some assistance, (3) satisfactorily performs job, (4) exceeds expectations, and (5) outstanding. If handling controlled substances is not part of the job, there is an appropriate "not applicable" response. If it is part of the job, the supervisor can observe the performance and measure (rate) the nurse based on some objective criteria or perception of satisfactory performance.

Trait-oriented evaluation scores are more effective in evaluating promotability and individual training needs. Trait questions are oriented to the employee rather than the job or productivity. A typical question might be, "Does this nurse express an active interest in performing functions of greater responsibility?" The responses might be: (1) not observed, (2) assumes only those responsibilities required of the position, (3) will assume greater responsibilities when so directed, (4) willingly assumes greater responsibilities when the need arises, and (5) routinely seeks out challenges and greater responsibilities. Although this question does not address how competently the nurse performs the duties of greater responsibility, management is able to identify nurses for supervisory training and encourage them to seek promotion.

Staffing, Organizational Development, and Training

Determining manpower requirements and employee development needs are corporate assessments made after reviewing all PAs. For example, if a number of nurses in a particular unit are unable to handle their prescribed patient load, this may be an indication that more nurses are required. This manpower requirement would be translated into staffing needs for particular skills. A development need to impove employee relations might be indicated by an exceptional number of PAs that note employees could not get along with their supervisors. Although training needs tend to be individual and job-related, *development* is oriented toward the overall upgrading of the work force to be more effective.

Personnel actions, such as termination, promotion, or transfer, are frequently indicated and documented on the PA. An appraisal instrument, used by a knowledgeable supervisor, should be able to distinguish between the high performer who has minimal growth potential and the employee who should be promoted to a position of greater responsibility. On the other hand, demotion, transfer, and termination are the result of the PA indicating that the employee is either unable or unwilling to do the work. *Unable* relates to competency to perform tasks or assume responsibilities. A nurse may be a very willing worker, but simply unable to move patients without assistance or lack knowledge of the equipment being used. *Unwilling* is a behavior modification problem. A nurse may be fully competent to do the job; however, personal problems or lack of motivation may cause the nurse to fall below expected performance norms. The appraisal instrument and the supervisor must be discriminating enough to identify the cause of unsatisfactory performance. Failure to document properly unsatifactory performance on the PA has often placed the organization in the untenable position of having to retain personnel who otherwise should have been removed from the job.

COMPONENTS OF THE PERFORMANCE APPRAISAL

The PA is an ongoing program that is cyclic in nature. The program should be directly related to the function of every member of the organization. The PA program starts when an employee is first hired and ends when the employee leaves. Figure 14–2 is a graphic description of the program.

Goals, Position Descriptions and Work Standards

Responsibilities, duties, functions, and similar elements are associated with every job. They may be set forth in a formal position description or verbally described to the new employee. For example, a nurse's position description

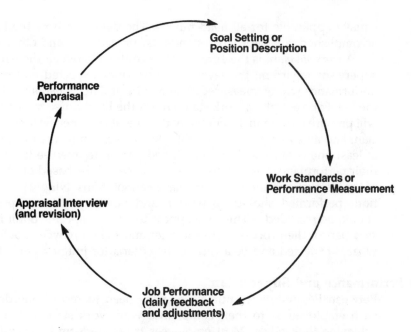

Figure 14-2. Components of performance appraisal program.

might contain the duty to oversee a shift in the unit and supervise personnel. In addition, work standards specify the quantity and quality expected for each of the duties. The work standard would state the anticipated number of patients, the probable number of assistants, the level of responsibility, and the expected quality of care.

Professionals, project managers, and persons in supervisory positions perform functions that extend over a period of time or are outcome oriented. At the beginning of each PA period, the employee and the supervisor reach a consensus as to the expected accomplishments by listing *goals* for job functions. For example, the nursing coordinator might set a goal with a nurse that documentation errors would be reduced from three to two per week within 6 months. At the end of the period the results are measured and discrepancies noted. The PA is the formal means through which goals are evaluated and is the starting point for the next goal. This is sometimes referred to as management by objectives (MBO).

Functional, ongoing jobs that are part of overall operations are usually defined in a *position description* (PD). These PDs set forth five or six general functions, tasks, or responsibilities expected of the incumbent. For example, one of the responsibilities of a head nurse might be, "Prescribes and oversees the work of all LPNs, technicians, and other personnel assigned to the unit." Notice that the statement does not go into great detail as to exactly what work is prescribed or how it will be accomplished. The PD is purposely kept general so that it is equally applicable for all head nurses. The details of how the function will be accomplished is left for work standards, procedures, and other documents.

A *work standard* is the agreement or contract between the employee and the supervisor regarding the level of performance expected and how satisfactory performance will be measured. The work standard is usually related directly to the PD. For example, a work standard for the head nurse might be, "Incumbent will prepare written instructions, both general and specific for each LPN, technician, and aide assigned to the unit. During each shift, the incumbent will make at least one contact with each assigned person to oversee their work and note their performance. Satisfactory performance will be based on the completeness of the instructions and the performance annotations. Ninety percent of the functions performed should be written and ninety percent of possible contacts should be recorded." This may appear to be very specific but it is a very necessary part of the process. Both the rater and the employee should know exactly what is expected and be aware of the criteria for judging performance.

Job Performance and Supervision

Between PA interviews nurse managers need to record anecdotal records on each employee as to their compliance with work standards and progress in achieving their goals. Most employees try to perform their assigned jobs in a manner they perceive as competent and productive. Sometimes their perceptions of job requirements do not coincide with those of their supervisor. In these instances, the supervisor must counsel the employee, train the person in the correct procedures, or take the appropriate action to ensure that functions are performed in accordance with organizational policies and the work conducted in a manner to achieve the expected outcome.

Feedback, both positive and corrective, should be a normal part of the daily supervisor–employee relationship. Employees must identify job problems to their supervisor; likewise, supervisors must inform employees when employee performance requires improvement. For example, if the laundry always delivers daily linens late, that data should be reported to the head nurse. Similarly, if a patient's bed linens are soiled, the head nurse should notify the LPN responsible for having the linens changed. Day-to-day interactions similar to those mentioned not only enhance productivity, but also alleviate surprises at the formal PA interview.

Appraisal Interview

Employees want to know how well they are performing their job. To know this they need feedback about how others perceive their endeavors. They also need to validate their own perceptions as to their contribution to the organization. The PA interview provides an excellent opportunity for management and employees to formally provide this feedback. The interview also provides opportunity for an employee to point out job stresses and to suggest ways the supervisor could improve work conditions.

A PA interview should have no surprises. It should be a summing up of the employee's performance over the entire period being evaluated. The competent supervisor should have provided daily feedback to the employee, both complimentary and constructive. In a similar manner, the employee should have kept the supervisor informed of his or her performance concerns and aspirations. If organizational priorities or policies have changed, the appraisal interview is not the place for the employee to find out about them.

The supervisor who prepares the appraisal is usually the management representative designated to conduct the interview. Sometimes the interview is done by an employee relations specialist, a committee of supervisors, or one of the senior managers. In whatever manner it is conducted, the PA interview should be a formal meeting in which the parties know the purpose and the agenda. Occasionally, the interview by the supervisor is cursory and only conducted because it is expected by the organization. Such encounters are usually frustrating for both parties because important career-affecting decisions are being discussed without proper preparation and communication.

Some supervisors or employees find the appraisal interview to be a confronting and threatening experience. It becomes a "show and sell" function. When the employee comes into the office, he or she finds the completed performance appraisal form in the center of the table. The employee is then asked to read the form and invited to ask questions or comment. The supervisor has to "sell" the evaluation to the employee. Even if the appraisal form is not absolutely final, the employee is placed in the position of having to challenge the PA and the supervisor having to defend it.

When the PA is either outstanding or unsatisfactory, both parties have probably discussed the work performance during the year and the evaluation is readily accepted. With the majority of personnel in the work unit, however, those who have worked hard to perform their duties efficiently and effectively and believe they have done everything satisfactorily, have probably had less feedback. Being presented with a ranked-performance appraisal rating of "average" may be a shock to their ego and self-perception. Even if they accept the rating, it will provide little to make them feel that they have made a contribution to the organization and that it is recognized and appreciated.

The best PA interviews are conducted before the completion of the rating form. They use a problem-solving approach. This does not suggest any less formality or preparation for the interview. Rather, both parties discuss the duties and responsibilities in the position description, the work standards, the relative weight given to each duty, and how well the employee fulfilled his or her assignments. If goal setting is a part of the system, the discussion is oriented to how closely last year's goals were met and to the development of next year's goals. If the PA contains trait-oriented questions, these can be discussed in relation to job requirements and promotion potential. Other issues, about which the supervisor may not be aware, may be introduced and considered. After the interview, the supervisor completes the PA rating form and may further discuss the rating with the employee. Even if another formal interview is not done, the employee needs to see what was written and have an opportunity to formally comment. This approach to performance appraisal makes the interview a discussion between two colleagues rather than a confrontation between two adversaries.

METHODS TO EVALUATE PERFORMANCE

Organizations have tended to develop a formal process for evaluating performance. This has three benefits: (1) a standardized form is less expensive to administer, (2) common work standards encourage consistency, and (3) a prescribed process lessens supervisor bias and resulting complaints and lawsuits. Most PA instruments involve ranking, checklists, rating scales or narrative descriptions as data collection devices.

The objective of the PA form is to identify those behavioral elements of job performance or those employee traits that are deemed critical by management, and then to measure the elements. The important words here are *identify* and *measure*. Therein lies the problem. Few jobs are exactly alike and the quantification of employee traits is very subjective. Furthermore, various evaluators have different perceptions of quality performance and ideas about what makes one employee better than another. For example, one head nurse may perceive that the primary function of a staff nurse is to oversee or provide the treatment of a patient in accordance with the physician's instructions. Another head nurse may believe that the principal function is to ensure the patient's well-being. On the other hand, if hospital management is interested in evaluating a trait such as a nurse's "loyalty," the appraisal becomes very subjective and difficult to define. The PA instrument attempts to control subjectivity by standardizing the questions and the evaluation process.

Ranking

The PA instrument that is the simplest, cheapest, and easiest to administer is based on the supervisor ranking all personnel in a given group. To be equitable, all employees should be performing the same general function or be in the same job classification. The strength of this method is that management achieves a score or rank order that can be readily converted to compute salary increases. That is, those employees with the highest ranking receive the largest salary increases. A weakness of this method is that it presumes that there is a measurable difference between the employees being evaluated. This may lead to supervisory frustration and employee hostility. Another weakness is that a work unit may become competitive and workgroup members may sabotage others to raise their own rank. The following are two ranking techniques:

The *straight ranking* PA uses selected factors and requires the supervisor to rank from high-to-low all employees in the work unit. A typical ranking question might be, "In productivity, nurse ranks (number) out of (number) nurses with similar duties and responsibilities." Or, "In dependability, nurse ranks (number) out of (number) of all personnel evaluated in the work unit." This appraisal technique is very effective when there is a great deal of supervisory interaction with employees and the variable (item) is measurable.

The *forced distribution* PA allocates a certain percentage of the work force to each group to achieve a bell-shaped distribution; that is, 5 percent outstanding, 20 percent above average, 50 percent satisfactory, 20 percent acceptable, and 5 percent unsatisfactory. Although this format tends to soften the harsh ranking of each employee, it still has the same strengths and shortcomings of the straight ranking method. Studies have found that most conscientious workers perceive themselves to be above average. Thus, evaluating 75 percent of employees as satisfactory (average) or below may have an adverse effect on motivation to be productive and on commitment to remain with the organization.

Checklists

The checklist PA is used to achieve a profile of the employee based on selected characteristics, traits, or behaviors. Lists are prepared by specialists that select words and phrases that minimize rater bias and are job-related. The head nurse can then check off the item that most closely describes staff personnel under his or her supervision. Each item has a "Yes" or "No" evaluation scale. The shortcoming of this approach is that it assumes that yes or no responses adequately identify the employee with the item and that the supervisor has good observation skills. Inasmuch as the checklist produces an employee profile that may be compared to a desired standard, the checklist is most useful for assessing training and promotion.

The *simple checklist* is composed of numerous words or phrases describing various employee behaviors or traits. There may be several checklists on the PA. The rater is asked to check all those that describe the employee on each checklist. Descriptors are often clustered to represent different aspects of one dimension of behavior. Table 14–1 illustrates one checklist for assertive behavior and another for work group behavior.

The *weighted checklist* tends to arrange choices in order of perceived desirability or assigns a "hidden" prioritized value to each item used in totaling the score. After the rater completes the checklist, those items checked are multiplied

TABLE 14-1. SIMPLE CHECKLISTS.

Please check the items on each of the lists that seem to describe the employee

A (Assertive)	B (Work Group Behavior)
_____ Confrontive	_____ Tries to reconcile differences
_____ Aggressive	_____ Works best by self
_____ Arrogant	_____ Helps others complete assignments
_____ Take charge	_____ Assumes more responsibility
_____ Follower	_____ Respects feelings of others
_____ Confident	_____ Discusses work with group
_____ Deference	_____ Protective of territory
_____ Leader	_____ Signs own work

TABLE 14-2. WEIGHTED CHECKLIST

Please check three items that best describe the employee

		(Hidden weight)
_____	Person I would expect to take charge in an emergency	(10)
_____	Does what is expected of the job	(5)
_____	Limits work to his/her position description	(3)
_____	Anxious to assume greater responsibility	(9)
_____	Seeks short-cuts	(4)
_____	Seeks new and better ways to do the job	(8)
_____	Occasionally does more than is expected	(6)

by their respective weights and totaled for a cumulative score that describes a particular profile. Table 14–2 illustrates a weighted checklist for initiative.

The *forced checklist* requires the rater to read a number of pairs of words or phrases and select the most appropriate item describing the employee from each pair. Sometimes there are all possible pairs of a set of characteristics. Another variation is a checklist requiring the rating of the degree to which an employee demonstrates a characteristic using two extreme descriptions. The purpose for changing combinations and forced selections is to describe the employee's true performance or strength in certain characteristics and to be able to compare employees on the same selections. Table 14–3 shows examples of the forced checklist to evaluate work attitude.

Rating Scale

The most common PA is the rating scale. In general, a phrase or sentence describes a situation and the employee is evaluated on a scale as to how he or she fits the model. Figure 14–3 is a simple Likert-type scale for rating performance. The evaluator marks the evaluation along a continuum.

TABLE 14-3. FORCED CHECKLIST

In each of the sets below choose the items that are
the most and least descriptive of the employee

Most Descriptive	Least Descriptive	Item
_____	_____	Talks easily to patients
_____	_____	Does not talk to patients when checking charts
_____	_____	Knows patients' first names
_____	_____	Prefers to work the night shift
_____	_____	Always on time for duty
_____	_____	Stays after shift to finish paper work and other details
_____	_____	Satisfactory attendance
_____	_____	Sometimes hard to find at the work station

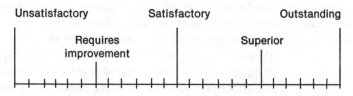

Figure 14-3. Likert rating scale.

The rating scale method is highly dependent on the observational skills of the evaluator. Individual understanding of the job and perceptions of behaviors that demonstrate characteristics will vary. For example, to evaluate initiative on the part of a home health nurse, the rater must have a good comprehension of the expected norm or work standard before the employee can be rated. If the work requires only visiting assigned patients and carrying out physician's orders, initiative may simply be keeping up with daily work. The rater must also have a knowledge of what is required to care for patients in the home, the outcomes expected, and the consequences of error to differentiate between several home health care nurses performing similar tasks. Another problem may be length. If the scale tries to measure all relevant behaviors, it is likely to become time-consuming and cumbersome.

A typical rating scale is professionally prepared and uses carefully selected job-related questions or statements that have been judged important for determining successful job performance or predictive of future success. A more sophisticated instrument is the behavioral anchored rating scale (BARS) in which a question is asked and discrete responses to the question are provided. Table 14–4 is an example.

Narrative Description

The narrative description instrument describes an employee's performance or characteristics and is particularly useful in assessing training needs, promotability, labor relations conditions, employee development, and manpower requirements. Appraisal instruments frequently require the supervisor to write narrative statements describing their perceptions of how the job was performed or

TABLE 14-4. BARS MODEL

Does this nurse maintain self-control during periods of extreme stress?			
Never	Sometimes	Usually	Always
[ ]	[ ]	[ ]	[ ]

descriptions of events that occurred during the reporting period. Although such instruments are an excellent means to achieve an in-depth and general assessment of the employee, they are time-consuming and depend heavily on the writing and analytical skills of the supervisor. They also may not result in comparable data for determining compensation changes.

The *essay PA* asks certain general questions and then requires the supervisor to comment on how well the employee appears to relate to each question. For example, "How effectively could this nurse supervise a 24-patient unit?" The supervisor matches his or her perceptions of the skills required to manage a 24-patient unit against the observed behavior of the nurse being evaluated. A short paragraph is written as to why the supervisor believes the nurse can or cannot handle this responsibility. If several qualified observers make a similar valid assessment of the employee, the essay performance appraisal becomes an excellent way for management to identify which persons have supervisory potential or which persons require additional training. This type of appraisal may only be appropriate if the observation of current duties is predictive of future performance in a different job.

The *critical incident PA* requires summary statements, both positive and negative, regarding the employee's performance in accomplishing specific tasks or responsibilities. Table 14-5 shows two examples.

The critical incident method requires the supervisor to maintain a logbook and record of events as they occur. This process overcomes evaluator subjectivity through the straightforward reporting of events. The critical incident method, however, has two human shortcomings: (1) employees become anxious when they know their supervisor is keeping a log of their behavior and (2) supervisors are hesitant to report activity that might reflect negatively on their own supervisory skills.

The *field review* evaluation is conducted by a third party, often a staff specialist whose sole function is to prepare evaluations. The supervisor, employee, and co-workers are interviewed and comments regarding the employee's performance or character traits are melded into a summary. Because the field review writer is independent of the work unit, he or she is apt to be more candid, less biased in the evaluation, and more reflective of overall organizational norms. On the negative side, the field review method is the most costly and time-consuming of all PA techniques.

TABLE 14-5. CRITICAL INCIDENT NOTATIONS

01/25/88. Nurse demonstrated initiative and knowledge of narcotics when she noted that a patient was allergic to the prescribed medication. Nurse notified the physician and clinical pharmacist.

02/15/88. Nurse required considerable supervisory assistance to calm down patient who believed that his mail was being withheld. Nurse's admonition of patient only made matters worse.

A management by objective (MBO) PA system is oriented to how well the employee has performed the agreed-upon tasks or how successful the employee has been in accomplishing goals set for the period. At the commencement of the reporting period, the supervisor and employee make an agreement or contract regarding job-related performance, usually containing four to eight items. The performance appraisal at the end of the period is a rating scale as to how successfully the employee has performed each item. For example, the charge nurse of the unit might have an objective to conduct a 1-hour class on hospital procedures each week for all the nurses in the ward. The rater would describe how successfully he or she completed the training quantitatively and qualitatively.

VALIDITY AND RELIABILITY

The validity and reliability of performance appraisal instruments have proved to be a continual problem. If compensation, promotion, and other important personnel decisions are contingent on the outcome of the PA, then the instrument must be an accurate assessment that gives consistent results. For example, a thermometer used with proper procedure will consistently measure the accurate Fahrenheit temperature of all patients, whether a nurse's aide, Liscensed Professional Nurse, or Registered Nurse takes the temperature. Although one can never expect cognitive measurement to approach this degree of validity and reliability, objective accuracy and impartial consistency should be the goal. Other important concerns are rater bias and human interaction that may invalidate even the most objective instrument.

Validity

Validity deals with accuracy. Does the appraisal instrument measure that which it is supposed to measure? For example, if there is an interest in identifying the most productive nurses, do the questions and rating scales cause these persons to get the highest ratings? Developing a valid appraisal instrument requires a direct correlation between the position description, work standards, and evaluation questions or rating scale. If the answer to a question cannot be justified as indicative of present or future job success, then the question is not valid.

Construct validity is related to how accurately the instrument can measure the variable that the evaluator perceives to be important. As individuals, we may have different perceptions as to reality or truth (the "construct") of a variable. For example, the patient load may be a work standard in evaluating a nurse in an ambulatory care clinic. Ten different evaluators might have ten different ideas about what constitutes a normal patient load. At one extreme is the raw number of case contacts without regard to the severity or type of problem presented. At the other extreme is concern only for the type of patient without regard for the number of cases handled. To be a valid instrument, the performance appraisal must measure the proper balance between the quantity of cases and the type of patients. If you agree that in many instances consensus about this criterion is impossible, then you can appreciate how difficult the process is to achieve construct validity.

Measurement deficiency occurs when some critical elements that influence the appraisal question or item are not considered. For example, when evaluating the productivity of a primary nurse on a medical unit, a hospital should have an interest in both the quality and quantity of work. A nurse should process a new physician's orders expeditiously, but not so fast as to overlook critical indices. Not to consider both factors fully, probably in separate questions, would be a measurement deficiency in the appraisal instrument.

Measurement contamination occurs when irrelevant information is allowed to influence the "construct." Each employee modifies the position to some extent due to style, interests, or special competencies or shortcomings. This overall modification is also reflected in the performance of specific tasks. For example, a nurse might have exceptionally neat handwriting; however, if data are put directly into the computer, handwriting has only marginal importance. If the evaluator includes handwriting in the construct of patient care documentation, this is measurement contamination.

Reliability

Reliability deals with consistency. Will the appraisal instrument produce the same results everytime if completed by several evaluators observing the same behavior or traits? Or, will the same evaluator give the same ratings for the same behavior or traits every time if the appraisal instrument is completed on several occasions? For instance, in studying the reliability of patient satisfaction with nursing care, the head nurse notices a significant difference in evaluations based on the variable of patient room assignment. For example, patients assigned to private rooms may evaluate nursing care significantly higher or lower than those assigned to semiprivate rooms, even when the patients have the same nurse and medical diagnosis. Assuming that all patients receive the same nursing care, patients should have answered the question, "Was the primary nurse always prepared to answer your questions?" in the same way. The fact that there may have been a significant variation of responses between patients in private and semiprivate rooms raises a question about the reliability of the instrument to assess satisfaction with nursing care. Furthermore, it would also be expected that a "reliable" instrument would impel individual patients evaluating the same nurse several times over a 6-week period, to rate the nurse identically each time. When selecting, using, or reviewing results no matter which performance appraisal instrument is used, one must always be aware of this reliability factor.

Human interaction and its related bias is probably the greatest barrier encountered when trying to validate a PA program. The *halo effect* occurs when the rater allows one highly evaluated item to influence inappropriately a high evaluation in other areas. For example, a nurse who always has an exceptionally neat and energetic appearance might also be rated high in job competency even though her nursing skills are only average. Conversely, the *horn effect* occurs when one low evaluation causes all the other appraisal items to have a lower mark. Sometimes a very recent event may unduly influence either a higher or lower mark, causing the *recency effect*.

A common shortcoming is the *generalization effect* when a nurse is evaluated based on the whole unit's performance instead of her own. This is a more likely occurrence on a "problem unit" or a "star unit" and may result in overly harsh ratings for everyone as a form of discipline or overly generous ratings for everyone as a reward. Another human bias problem is *self-reflection*; a head nurse will rate all the staff high to show how good his or her own performance is. Sometimes, the supervisor, not wanting to create ill will within a work unit, will exhibit a bias for *central tendency* and rate everyone at about the central midpoint. One way to avoid these errors is to constantly check and remind yourself that appraisal to evaluate individuals must be based on job-related criteria over the time period being examined. A moment's reflection looking at all the appraisals on a unit and reviewing these potential errors should assist in minimizing bias.

The PA program is a significant tool for human resource management. A well-designed instrument should be capable of identifying productivity, promotion potential, training needs, staffing requirements, and organizational changes. There are several critical features of the PA program; it must contain questions that will consistently measure that which it is supposed to measure, it should encourage evaluator objectivity, and it should be relatively easy to administer and analyze. The most imortant part of the PA program to an employee is the interview. Here, the supervisor and the employee meet to review past performance and set future goals and performance criteria. During this meeting each need to communicate their expectations, frustrations, and validate the employee's contribution to the organization mission and strategic plans. The outcome affects employee morale and commitment to the organization.

BIOGRAPHICAL SKETCH

Douglas First is a Senior Research Associate focusing on manpower issues in the Office of Institutional Planning and Research at George Mason University. He was previously Director of Personnel at George Mason University for 8 years. He also spent a number of years in manpower planning and administration for the federal government. Dr First is also a lecturer in the Public Affairs Department where he teaches the course, Public Personnel Administration. As an undergraduate, Dr First attended Miami University and received his doctorate from George Washington University. Dr First's dissertation dealt with systematic variance or rater bias in performance appraisals.

SUGGESTED READINGS

Beck, R.A. (Ed.). (1986). *Performance Assessment*. Baltimore: Johns Hopkins University Press.

Bernadin, H.J., & Beatty, R.W. (1984). *Performance Appraisal: Assessing Human Behavior at Work*. Boston: Kent Publishing.

Blanchard, K. & Johnson, S. (1982). *The One-Minute Manager.* New York: Berkley Books, Inc.

Campbell, J.P., Lawler, D.E.E., III., & Weick, K.E. (1970). *Managerial Behavior, Performance and Effectiveness.* New York: McGraw-Hill.

Cocheu, T. (1986, September). Performance Appraisal: A Case in Points. *Personnel Journal,* pp. 48–55.

Cummings, L.L. & Schwab, D.P. (1973). *Performance in Organizations: Determinants and Appraisal.* Glenview: IL: Scott, Foresman and Co.

Drucker, P.F. (1974). *The Practice of Management.* New York: Harper & Row.

Fottler, M., Hernandaz, R., & Joener, C. (Eds.). (1988). *Strategic Management of Human Resources in Health Sciences Organizations.* New York: John Wiley & Sons.

Jernigan, D.K., & Pepper Young, A. (1983). *Standards, Job Descriptions and Performance Evaluations for Nursing Practice.* East Norwalk, CT: Appleton & Lange.

Jernigan, D.K. (1988). *Human Resource Management in Nursing.* E. Norwalk, CT: Appleton & Lange.

Latham, G., & Wexley, K. (1981). *Increasing Productivity Through Performance Appraisal.* Reading, MA: Addison Wesley.

McGregor, D. (1957, May-June). An uneasy look at performance appraisal. *Harvard Business Review,* pp. 89–94.

Vroom, V.H. (1960). *Some Personality Determinants of the Effects of Participation.* Englewood Cliffs, NJ: Prentice-Hall.

CASE 14-1

Goal Setting by Staff Nurses in a Community Hospital
Susan Simms

The employee evaluation system at The Arlington Hospital in the mid-seventies consisted of a single sheet with performance areas (e.g., quality of work, gets along well with peers) and a five-level Likert scale check-off, with three being "average." There were then four drawn lines for "comments." As the new nursing administrator, I felt that one way to get to know my staff's strengths and weaknesses quickly was to see their prior evaluations. What I actually found was that everyone who reported directly to me was above average or superior (the highest rating) and that few, if any comments were made. My curiosity led me to look at head nurse and staff evaluations, and they too read the same. No one could have described any individual as different from any other by reading and comparing evaluations. In addition, I found that every member of the hospital staff, from all departments and at all levels, was evaluated using the same tool. The wording of the scale (from poor to superior) with average as the mean value seemed to convey a negative connotation to what should have been acceptable performance. No one wants to be thought of as average. It seemed that this evaluation system was accomplishing nothing and that evaluators were "keeping the peace" by marking everybody above average or superior.

Nursing position performance descriptions were woefully inadequate as well, and as the Joint Commission on Hospital Accreditation was recommending criteria-based job descriptions, the time seemed right to begin a change process to upgrade the entire system.

The communication system we were developing within the nursing division was fairly unique in 1978 (Fig. 14–4) and a project of this magnitude seemed an excellent way to test the structure. We were certainly correct in that assumption,

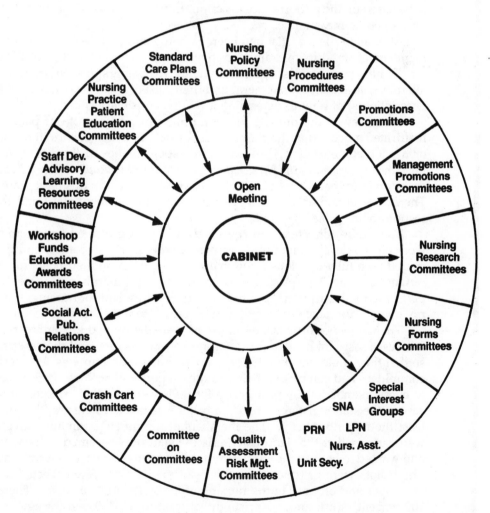

Figure 14-4. Communication system nursing division. *(Used by permission of Arlington Hospital, Arlington, Virginia.)*

as this project has been significantly shaped by the committee structure. Step one was to have the nursing administrative cabinet discuss the issue and to look at possible problems, current theories, and a range of methodologies. Individual topics were assigned to each of us, and we accepted the responsibility of doing a literature search with presentation of viable ideas to the group. Members also agreed to collect copies of various job descriptions (or performance descriptions as we now know them) from our "sources" at other hospitals and even at non-health care work sites. What we were looking for was a model that would enable us to describe acceptable performance that was broad enough in scope to be used among professionals of varying levels of competency working in the same position. We also determined that we wanted our performance appraisal system to be based on the performance description, so that it was critical that the criteria developed be measurable.

After all of the material had been gathered and reviewed by each of us, the members of the nursing administrative cabinet determined the basic elements for the new position description—a one to two paragraph *summary statement* of job role, a *qualifications* statement, and then a list of *performance reponsibilities* and description(s) of how to determine if that responsibility is met.

We reviewed the nursing division philosophy as part of our planning and reaffirmed a belief that the nurse is responsible to many publics in fulfilling his or her job commitment. These include responsibilities to *the patient, to self, to the nursing division, to the physician, to peers* and to *the hospital*. The performance description for each level of staff would be written using this basic framework. There was an additional public identified for management staff, and that was responsibility *to the community*.

The clinical directors and the head nurses each formed subcommittees to work on the development of performance criteria and outcomes, and then presented each fully developed performance description to their peers for their input and critique. This process took approximately 1 month, and three "model" performance descriptions resulted (as the vice president for nursing, I too wrote my own performance description, with input from the hospital administrator).

The model performance descriptions were distributed to volunteer subcommittees of assistant head nurses, staff nurses, instructors, and clinical specialists, so that they could develop their own performance descriptions. When the subcommittees had completed their work, each performance description was given to every member of the peer group for review and written critique, and in the case of the staff registered nurses, a ballot was taken, to ensure "buy-in" by at least the majority of staff. The members of the nursing administrative cabinet were surprised at the rigorous criteria the staff nurse seemed to have accepted and wanted to be sure the subcommittee had been realistic in determining them. The ballots were distributed by the head nurses and were collected in sealed envelopes and brought to the nursing office by the unit secretary. There was a 100 percent return and, surprisingly, at least to us, 100 percent agreement on the performance criteria (Table 14-6).

TABLE 14-6. STAFF NURSE JOB DESCRIPTION

Summary

The professional primary nurse is responsible for assisting the patients under his or her care to reach an optimum level of wellness and comfort. To this end, he or she uses the nursing process in conjunction with the patient, patient's family, physician, and other members of the health care team.

Qualifications

Graduated from an accredited school of nursing and eligible for or possessing current registration in the State of Virginia. After probationary period, will have successfully completed the required skill list or basic exam for the specific area.

Performance Responsibility	The Responsibility is Met When
A. To Patient	
1. Patient's total care needs are assessed at regular intervals and an adequate plan of care is developed based upon this assessment.	• It is documented or observed that the professional nurse uses simple physical assessment skills to include inspection, palpitation, percussion, and auscultation combined with a knowledge of altered physiology to determine patient needs and changes in patient status. • Documentation exists that the professional nurse provides an ongoing assessment of patients' psychological, spiritual, and nursing needs. • Documentation exists that the assessment obtained is then translated into specific nursing diagnoses that form the basis for the nursing care plan.
2. Plan of care is continually updated and revised.	• Documentation exists that the interventions in the nursing care plan are continued or revised based on documented outcomes.
3. Nursing care provided is directed toward maximum self-care abilities and patient safety.	• Documented evidence exists that the nurse promotes patient independence within the limits of their ability to include: basic hygiene, ROM and ambulatory, daily nutritional intake, proper means of elimination, rest, activity, and privacy. • Documentation exists regarding risk management needs and adequate measures for ensuring that patient safety have been implemented. • Documentation that the nurse administers treatments and medications as prescribed by the M.D., assesses patient's response to same, notifies physician of response to therapy, and documents same on the appropriate patient's record.

(continued)

TABLE 14-6 *(Continued)*

4. Patient teaching is directed toward achieving maximum self-care abilities.

- Patient's knowledge base is appropriately assessed and documented before teaching.
- Patient and other caretakers are actively involved with planning, implementing, and evaluating teaching.
- Patient and/or caretaker is able to properly demonstrate administration of his or her medications before discharge.
- Patient and/or caretaker can demonstrate procedures necessary for patient's self-care before discharge.
- Patient and/or caretaker can verbalize or write the cause and effect of his or her altered health state within his or her knowledge base before discharge.
- Coordination with activities of other disciplines exists in patient's care.

5. Ensures that the patient receives adequate support posthospitalization.

- Documentation exists that the patient and current support system has been evaluated for effectiveness based on his or her current self-care needs, primary caretaker capabilities, environmental status posthospitalization, and financial status.

6. Patient/family demonstrates ability to meet self-care needs after hospitalization.

- Documentation exists on the patient's record. The patient/family demonstrates the ability to meet goals.
- Discharge notes include all self-care capabilities and deficits and how family/patient plans to meet these deficits.

B. To Physician

1. Patient care regimen is discussed with physician at regular intervals to achieve maximum benefits to patients. Physician orders are carried out appropriately.

- Documentation exists that patient care regimen has been discussed and updated with doctor and patient.
- Documentation exists that the medical therapeutic regimen is implemented thoroughly and correctly.

2. Communication is on a professional level.

- Evidence exists that interaction with physicians is done in a professional and competent manner.

3. Attending physician is notified of significant changes in patient condition.

- Documentation exists that the attending physician is notified of all significant changes in a patient's condition in a timely manner.

C. To Peers

1. Maintains and promotes appropriate interactions with peers.

- Evidence exists that appropriate coping mechanisms are employed in times of stress with peers and that tact and good judgment are employed.

2. Standards of professional practice are maintained by self and peers.

- Inappropriate and/or nonprofessional behavior is recognized in peers and addressed with peer in an attempt to solve problem. If the problem cannot be solved, presents necessary documentation to management.

3. Assists peers in the performance of their daily activities.

- Evidence exists that the individual provides active assistance and support to peers.

4. To be a professional role model.

- Evidence exists that the individual actively problem solves to resolve conflict on unit or in-house.
- Participates freely in unit staff meeting.
- The professional nurse strives for membership in a professional organization.
- The professional nurse seeks to have active input in nursing committees within the hospital.

D. To Self

1. Participates in continuing education to maintain and expand clinical skills.

- Documentation exists of attendance at continuing education programs.
- Evidence exists that the individual uses this new information in their clinical practice.
- Evidence exists that the individual shares this new information with peers.

2. Seeks and promotes personal satisfaction within professional role.

- The individual periodically evaluates self based on goals set in annual evaluation and discusses progress with head nurse.

3. Maintains punctuality and attendance.

- Periodic review of time and attendance records demonstrates them to be within hospital guidelines.

E. To Nursing Division

1. Recognizes and uses appropriate chain of command and goals.

- Head nurse and assistant head nurse are informed of concerns and events.

2. Assumes responsibility for charge role in absence of head nurse or assistant head nurse.

- Prioritizes, delegates, and problem solves unit management for the shift.
- Notifies supervisor of appropriate information.
- Completes the function of charge nurse determined by each unit.

F. To Hospital

1. Functions within limits and/or guidelines established by hospital and nursing division policy.

- Evidence exists that actions are within nursing division and hospital policy guidelines.

2. Maintains the standards of hospitality extended by employees to all guests of the hospital, including patients, visitors, physicians, and co-workers.

- Hospitality standards are demonstrated on a consistent basis. (Refer to Administration Policy–Guest Relations 8-104.)

Used by permission of Arlington Hospital, Arlington, Virginia.

The personnel department worked with Nursing throughout this process, to ensure that the performance descriptions met (or exceeded) both the standards for our entire organization and legal affirmative action standards, and that the format could be adapted should other departments/divisions wish to convert.

By April 1978, we had a new performance description for every job role in the nursing division. We then began to work on the development of a performance evaluation system based on our belief that the one in use seemed ineffective. There was much discussion at the open meeting concerning the reasons for evaluation, what our own goals for the evaluation process should be, subjectivity versus objectivity, and of course, format. We started out again to review the literature and to tap sources, both in and out of health care, for examples of evaluation tools that might be helpful. We gathered copies of over 30 different evaluation forms.

We returned to the nursing division philosophy, and determined that our performance evaluation must include, in addition to information regarding the employee's actual work performance, a mechanism to provide assistance with both personal and professional growth. The subcommittee recommended a descriptive narrative based on the outcome statements in the performance descriptions as the first portion of the evaluation and then a listing of goals to be achieved, with activities to be undertaken to reach those goals, and reasonable time frames within which to achieve them. The last portion would be comments from the individual being evaluated.

The concept was accepted at the open meeting, and the implementation process began. The evaluators had many questions. First, head nurses wanted to know how they could remember and describe incidents that had happened during a full year? That question led to the development of a process of anecdotal note keeping and quarterly review of progress toward goals. There was a lot of concern regarding the time required to "write everything down." Using a checklist is a quicker process. We did calculate the time spent was about ten times greater, but concluded that the product was worth the effort, and in our view, led to greater staff satisfaction and increased communication of expectations between managers and staff. Additional concerns were voiced regarding variation in personal standards and values—did the management group have similar enough individual philosophies to be able to administer consistent standards? A subcommittee of head nurses worked on this issue, and then agreed on definitions for five levels of performances. Other questions centered around whether the management group felt they had the skills necessary to actually write a narrative. They were unsure they could be clear, concise, and to the point. A training program was designed and implemented for the use of this new system. The assistant directors of nursing and vice president taught the various course components. Communication, interviewing, and evaluation skills were included. This program was a part of a more extensive management development program (Simms, 1982).

The narrative evaluations were attached to the old evaluation forms along with a copy of the job description. There was no impact on the payroll or personnel systems as there was, as yet, no merit (or pay for performance) plan in place. It would be less than candid not to admit that some of the early efforts were little better, in terms of providing a picture of an individual employee, than were those done using the old check-off system. We did persevere, and each evaluation was read, counter-signed, and critiqued by the responsible assistant director of nursing and by myself. The ability to do evaluations properly became an important part of the performance description/evaluation of all members of the management team (assistant head nurse to associate director of nursing).

Nursing had been using the narrative system for about 4 years when the hospital administrative team and the Board of Trustees determined that the hospital should introduce a pay-for-performance system, and change the hospital-wide evaluation system to one that was more objective and descriptive of performance. The director of personnel felt that the system that nursing was using, with some modifications, was adaptable hospital-wide. We did need to add a new rating scale that was used as an overall indicator of performance, and is shared with the employee at the close of the evaluation interview (to allow for a free-flow of dialogue between manager and employee).

The administrative council did look at the advisability of requiring a bell-curve distribution system for each division, but decided not to "force" the curve by placing restrictions on numbers for each category worker. However, an expectation of "usually" having a normal curve hospital-wide was disseminated. Quarterly and yearly reports do show that nursing regularly fails within the bell-curve norms. We did determine, however, that since "average" had such negative connotations, we would not include it as a rating category. The scale included exemplary, superior, commendable, fair, and unacceptable. These descriptors and definitions appear on the front of every evaluation, so both evaluators and employees clearly understand what each rating means. In developing the merit pay "grid" (another subject entirely), we determined that a "fair" rating would carry with it a minimum wage increase, to maintain the acceptability of commendable as a good evaluation. We also built in a greater range of percentage increase the evaluator could give to employees in the commendable rating category.

This type of system is not without its complications. Now that evaluations led to numerical ratings and to actual salary determination, many of our head nurses and assistant head nurses felt more uncomfortable with the system and how comparisons were made unit to unit as well as intraunit. We encouraged the head nurse group to interact with their peers and to develop a system that was workable and comfortable to them. Some of the head nurses developed numerical systems, weighting each performance category by importance. After determining the highest possible total score, ranges were then developed for each rating value. Other head nurses were satisfied that they could look at their staff as a group, at any point in time, and rate them against the criteria fairly and competently.

Another issue that came to light was the question of evaluating staff nurses who were new graduates, novices, intermediates, and experts as described by Benner (1984). The head nurse group decided that they could not expect the same productivity and expertise from each of these groups and determined that the narrative evaluation would look at the nurse in relation to both length of time in nursing and educational degree. We also decided that the rating would be done using the same rating scale, as new graduates can range from unacceptable to exemplary in their performance at their own level, just as nurse experts can perform along that same continuum at any given time.

In 1980, we felt that a component was missing from the evaluation process as it had developed thus far, and we began discussing the role of the professional in monitoring and evaluating their own behavior and productivity. The nursing administrative cabinet brought this issue to the head nurse group, and they too, felt it was important for the staff to be active in the evaluation of their own practice and growth needs. In the early 1980s we developed our self-evaluation form with seven questions for short answers and suggested goals. This form is given to the employee three to four weeks before the evaluation interview is to take place, and is meant to have the nurse think about the issues raised by each question, in preparation for the interview. Initially, response to the self-evaluation was not overwhelmingly positive, particularly from experienced staff members.

We did find that the evaluation interviews became more interactive when the self-evaluation was used. Comments such as "working with MDs," "helping others," "the challenge and rewards," "the salary," "the people I work with" have been among the answers to the questions. Going back over self-evaluation forms of nurses who have been employed here 6 or more years, it is possible to see great personal and professional growth in each individual merely by reading the response to the questions.

For nursing management, another interesting finding was the descriptions of job stressors. These descriptions documented breakdowns in both intradepartmental and interdepartmental procedures and in interpersonal cooperation. Head nurses were often able to intervene and resolve many of these issues. Head nurses were also able to identify staff–staff problems that would never have been voiced in a group setting but were hinted at or actually described in the self-evaluation. Other problems were recognized when the assistant directors reviewed a batch of self-evaluations from one unit at one time. They could then alert the head nurses to unit problems, and help them develop strategies to work through the issues with the staff. As you may have already suspected, "short-staffing" was listed most often as a stressor with the suggested solution being "Hire more staff." Today I am happy to report that even when short staffing is listed as a stressor, suggested solutions are far more creative. Indeed, we have implemented many of the suggestions that have come to us through the self-evaluation process—while giving credit to the originator.

Over time, individual head nurses have added their own questions to the tool, enabling them to better maintain their records and files. Our staff development and quality assurance programs have become decentralized, and records are maintained at the unit level. Examples of additions on some units are date of CPR recertification, intravenous medication certification, nasogastic certification, in-services attended, in-services given, infection control updates, membership in professional organizations, hospital committee memberships, quality assurance project involvement, and special projects such as diabetes resource nurse for the unit, involvement in the health fair, and speaking to school groups. A committee is currently working on revising the self-evaluation form to incorporate suggestions.

Innovations continue to occur as different units work to refine the appraisal system. One such attempt is peer evaluation. This process was begun by the head nurse of our pediatric/young adult unit, with specific policies and guidelines developed for staff participation. Word of the success of this innovation spread rapidly on the nursing grapevine, and soon other staff and managers on other units were asking for copies of the guidelines and for permission to add this process. Currently, five of 15 nursing units are using a peer review process. It is a difficult time-consuming methodology, but one that has certainly demonstrated its worth to participants. Preparation for an evaluation is not taken lightly, and is a true learning experience for the entire peer group, as well as for the individual being evaluated. Because of the trust and skills necessary for peer evaluation, staff need to be committed for the process to be worthwhile, therefore, we do not require peer evaluation.

Recently, the nursing administrative cabinet became interested in program evaluation of our performance appraisal system. We chose to do two studies in collaboration with Dr. Jackie Dieneman (of George Mason University, and an advisory member of our Research Committee). The first study developed a tool to evaluate retrospectively our goal setting process. The second study examined staff nurse and head nurse satisfaction with our system and its component parts using a questionnaire. Although specific results of these studies will be reported elsewhere we can share some general information with you.

The key findings of the retrospective study are listed in Table 14–7. Administrative action as a result of the study has been:

1. Discussion of follow-up on goal achievement by head nurses at the open meeting. A decision to require notation of goal achievement from the previous year at the beginning of the written narrative.
2. Review of the standardization of narratives to follow the performance criteria outline and importance of head nurse signatures at the open meeting.
3. Plans by the assistant directors to note if weaknesses are noted in narratives and if trends indicate that specific head nurses need support in developing the ability to confront sensitive issues.
4. Commendation to all evaluators for carrying out the overall PA process efficiently and effectively.

The second study indicated generally high satisfaction with some differences that logically related to the perspective of the respondent as a receiver or

TABLE 14-7. KEY FINDING RETROSPECTIVE PA REVIEW

Completion of Performance Evaluation Process

	(n = 89)
Action sheet	100%
Face sheet	42%
Narrative evaluation	100%
Plan for improvement	95%
Signature HN & staff	93%
Self-evaluation	93%

Narrative Evaluation by HN

	(n = 89)
Organized by job description	85%
Strengths described	98%
Weaknesses described	65%
'85 goals mentioned	29%
Note if '85 goals achieved	29%
Note why '85 goals achieved	12%
Note if '85 goals achieved on time	18%
Signed by HN	56%

Goals in Plan for Improvement

Wrote goals not related to work	10%
Discussed achievement of last year's goals	12%

1. Areas for improvement in process of performance evaluation:
   a. Completing face sheet
   b. Narrative evaluation   organization by job description
                              discussion of weaknesses
                              Head nurse signing
                              Follow-up on last year's goals
   c. Plan for improvement   Setting time frames for completion.

2. Areas especially well done:
   a. Narrative evaluation discussing nurse's strengths.
   b. Setting measurable, operationalized activities to achieve goals.
   c. Balancing goals for job improvement and career development.

evaluator. A few specific items such as those relating to design of self-evaluation forms indicated need for revision.

The performance appraisal system at The Arlington Hospital has been evolving since 1978. The major strength of the system lies in the fact that it is always "in process." It is dynamic and never stagnant. As described, the current product is considerably different from the original effort. The soundness of the framework allows elements to be changed without necessitating a major restructuring of the concept. Because staff have participated fully in the development process, they "own" the system and emphasize a formative career development viewpoint rather than a summative, static view. As our nurses have become more autonomous in their practice, evaluation has assumed a vital role in dictating and measuring professional growth.

BIOGRAPHICAL SKETCH

Susan Simms, RN, MPS, CNAA, served for 10 years as the Vice President for Nursing at The Arlington Hospital. A 350-bed voluntary hospital in Northern Virginia offering a broad range of services, The Arlington Hospital enjoys a reputation for the provision of quality patient care. The Nursing Division was included among the 41 in the country that were cited as "magnet hospitals," places where nursing turnover is low and satisfaction high. Active in many professional associations, Sue Simms lectures locally and nationally, and has served as clinical preceptor for students in Nursing Administration at Marymount, George Mason, and Catholic Universities. She is currently the Nursing Administrator at Fresno Community Hospital.

REFERENCES

Benner, P. (1984). *From Novice to Expert.* Reading, MA: Addison-Wesley.

Simms, S. (1982). A new approach to the development of a head nurse management course. *Nursing Leadership, 5* (1), 23–26.

15

Program Evaluation

Wayne P. Thomas

Research and program evaluation are inquiry activities whose characteristics, techniques, and intents are discrete. Nonetheless, the distinctions among these activities are sometimes blurred and frequently not recognized by professional practitioners in many disciplines. One way to differentiate between program evaluation and research is that research is typically conclusion-oriented, whereas evaluation is typically decision-oriented. Intents for using knowledge differ. Researchers investigate phenomena to understand and draw conclusions about the phenomena. Evaluators usually try to investigate phenomena to provide information to decision makers for purposes of program modification (as in quality assurance efforts) or program continuation or termination.

Additional distinctions between evaluation and research note that research attempts to find "truth" in the sense that researchers typically attempt to show that there are differences between groups or relationships between variables. Evaluators, on the other hand, attempt to assess the worth of these differences or relationships to various interested parties. Finally, researchers are interested in drawing conclusions in ways that are maximally generalizable to other similar groups or situations (e.g., effective therapies for heart disease in any geographical area), whereas evaluators are interested in drawing conclusions in ways that are context-specific (e.g., needed improvements in one hospital's services and care of cardiac patients).

Research and development (R & D) activities represent a third researchlike endeavor that might be conducted in health care settings. In R&D the emphasis is on developing and validating procedures, processes, and products for use in a professional area of endeavor (Borg & Gall, 1983, p. 772). Activity leads not only to the development of new products, but, in contrast to research, it provides for the testing, refinement, and readying for use of these new products, processes, or procedures.

A nursing example may clarify the distinctions between research, evaluation, and R & D. An R & D project is a company's effort to develop, field-test, and perfect an improved dressing for wounds. Such a project would certainly make use of *research* studies previously completed on the physiology of skin integrity, but the primary emphasis in this *R & D* effort is on the development and refinement of the medical product, rather than on finding out how skin integrity normally works. If several competing dressings have been developed, a comparison of their relative worth and value to patients who need this medical product could be conducted as an *evaluation* study.

Some generalizations of these points and examples are that:

1. The purposes of the research study are to generate new knowledge that can be used in future research or in R & D efforts and also to find the most plausible answers to specific hypotheses regarding differences between groups and relationships among variables.
2. R & D projects are used to develop and refine promising processes or products with the intent of releasing these for professional use at the completion of the R & D project.
3. Evaluation studies are conducted to provide information for decision making regarding programs and program operation by managers and administrators.

EVALUATION: A CLOSER LOOK

Evaluation is the systematic attempt to assess worth and value for decision-making purposes. The degree of worth of programs or curricula in nursing, education, or in governmental agencies is largely determined by the value systems of the evaluators and evaluatees rather than by any immutable guidelines of logic or laws of nature. It follows, then, that program evaluation should be capable of assuming a number of forms, depending on the values of those who have interests in the program. These forms manifest themselves as evaluation paradigms and models, each with different intents and emphases. A number of these are discussed later in this chapter.

A second point, derived from the definition of evaluation, is that the techniques and methods of evaluation and research overlap. Many of the techniques of data collection, data analysis, and data interpretation, which are taught in graduate courses emphasizing quantitative and qualitative research methods, are the same. Thus, evaluators may use interviews, on-site observation, evaluation designs that attempt to control for the effects of extraneous variables, and statistical analysis methods just as researchers do. There are, however, some techniques of evaluation that do not come from research but rather from the inquiry traditions of the law or of the investigative reporter. These are discussed shortly.

Third, as evaluations are decision-driven, they are inextricably caught up and influenced by the politics surrounding the decision-making process. Thus, many evaluators (and the persons who hire them) find that they can better "inform and improve the operations of the social system" (Cronbach et al., 1980) if they have substantial amounts of experience, not only in evaluation methods but also in those factors that involve the political aspects of decision making in that area.

Here, a distinction emerges between the internal and the external evaluator. The internal evaluator is a permanent member of an organization's staff who performs evaluations for and is accountable to the organizational managers. This person is usually experienced in the politics and the workings of the evaluated programs. An external evaluator is usually a person who is brought in as a consultant when upper level managers desire an evaluative point of view from outside of the politics and culture of the organization or when the evaluation task is too politically "hot" for internal evaluators.

A fourth point derived from the definition of evaluation is that evaluations may be funded in situations in which research studies might not. Funding decision makers in an organization tend to favor efforts whose results help them make better decisions and justify their actions, creating or aiding advocacy for their positions. This may be problematic where evaluation, research, and R & D compete for funding from the same limited sources.

In summary, program evaluations attempt to satisfy "many masters." The successful evaluator has to be well versed in the politics and culture of the organization being evaluated, be knowledgeable concerning all of the traditions, paradigms, and techniques of the various approaches to evaluation and research, and be able to diagnose the evaluative needs of a particular situation and select compatible data collection, data analysis, and question-framing strategies. Finally, the successful evaluator must be able to synthesize all of these into a feasible plan for evaluative data collection and analysis—which is unique to the particular characteristics and context of the program being evaluated. Table 15-1 is an overview of program evaluation purposes, focus of measurement, methods, evaluators, and reports.

Today, evaluation is a well-entrenched part of many organizations. The federal government alone spends several hundred million dollars each year for evaluation (Borg & Gall, 1983, p. 733). Industry and foundations add substantially to this total. Many universities have programs and coursework leading to degrees in evaluation methodology.

Development of the Field of Evaluation

Although the need for evaluation of curricula and programs in nursing and other human services is not new, the existence of a body of practitioners calling themselves evaluators as opposed to researchers is quite new. The most important developments in the methods and theory of program evaluation have occurred in the past 20 years.

During the first quarter of the century, epidemiologic studies, which gathered data on human morbidity and mortality, were the earliest empirical work that led to more formal evaluations later in the third quarter of the century (Coursey, 1977). Especially during the 1930s, researchers in psychology, sociol-

TABLE 15–1. PROGRAM EVALUATION

Purposes

Program improvement: Formative evaluation
Judgment program impact: Summative evaluation
Monitor performance using standards: Quality assurance

Focus of Measurement

Resources for program: Structure of people, equipment, setting.
Judgments of process performance by evaluator.
Information for administrative decisions.
Concerns and issues of all stakeholders (those with an interest in the program).
Goals and objectives of program.
Intended and unintended program outcomes.

Methods of Measurement

Empirical research designs with statistical analysis.
Pencil and paper tests.
Criterion measure checklists or screens.
Normative comparison of program to others.
Surveys for attitudes, satisfaction, goal attainment, etc.
Review of documents, policies, procedure manuals, etc.
Cost analysis for effectiveness, benefits, feasibility, etc.
Interviews of individuals or focus groups.
On-site observation.
Adversarial investigative evaluation.

Evaluator

External consultant, preferably expert in evaluation and service.
External accreditation visitor(s).
Internal position, preferably full-time expert in evaluation. May be part of program staff or central department.
Committee may have internal program members and others.

Report

Written document with judgments and recommendations.
Oral briefing with pictures, graphics, and executive summary.
Periodic meetings of managers and evaluator(s).

---

ogy, and education began to apply the empirical techniques of their disciplines to the assessment of governmental and industrial programs intended to benefit the recipients of these services.

World War II stimulated great interest in questions of the relative effectiveness of one method of training over another as Europe and the United States attempted to train citizens to become soldiers in the shortest possible time. The testing movement also expanded enormously as military psychologists sought ways to better match the abilities of recruits with the jobs that were necessary in a wartime environment. At that time, the primary organizing factors for evaluation were differences among individuals as measured by standardized tests, as well as the concepts of scientific inquiry and industrial production (Tyack, 1974).

Both before and after World War II, evaluators began to focus less on the description of the program and more on the degree to which the program had attained specific goals. In education, Ralph Tyler (1969) proposed that programs should have major goals, specific objectives, and measurable outcomes, and that every attempt should be made to attribute changes in outcomes to program characteristics. He also saw preprogram and postprogram measurements as the primary means of determining the degree explicit program goals had been met. Finally, Tyler introduced the notion that evaluation should provide continuous feedback to program implementors, managers, and administrators, and should function as a means of professionals being accountable to themselves and to the recipients of their services. Many identify this objective-based approach to evaluation as the beginning of the separation of evaluation and research.

After the launching of Sputnik in 1957 and during the period of expansion of government expenditure for human services during the 1960s Great Society programs, many came to the conclusion that an objective-based approach was inadequate to meet the evaluation needs of large government programs carried out in a wide variety of local settings. Evaluators and program administrators began to realize that the nature and quality of decisions might be a more important focus. Other evaluation theorists, among them Michael Scriven and Lee J. Cronbach, proposed new organizing frameworks. For example, it was proposed that decisions that needed to be made by a program administrator should help determine the types of data to be collected and the types of data analysis to be performed. These decision–facilitative evaluation approaches are well represented in modern evaluation models (Popham, 1988). Evaluators, such as Robert Stake, proposed that the concerns and issues of the persons affected by the program, including the recipients and implementors of the program services, might be the most valid focus for an evaluation. Thus, evaluations based on the concerns, values, and issues important to the "stakeholding audiences" came into vogue under the label of "responsive evaluation" (Guba & Lincoln, 1981).

This process of the development of new organizing frameworks for evaluations continues at present. During the 1970s, the number of evaluation models became so large that there were efforts to classify them by their primary organizing concept and to list their most important features along with attendant advantages and disadvantages. This led evaluators to engage in a practice humorously referred to by Popham as "model meddling" (i.e., combining features of different evaluation models into new combinations), followed inevitably by "model muddling" (Popham, 1975).

MAJOR CHARACTERISTICS OF EVALUATION MODELS

There are several important characteristics commonly associated with the various evaluation models. Choices regarding each of these tends to determine many of the characteristics of the evaluation design that is employed.

Qualitative and Quantitative Evaluation

For many, the distinctions between evaluation approaches may be divided into a qualitative versus quantitative dichotomy. These approaches are generally described as differing from each other in one or more of the following ways:

1. Disciplinary tradition of inquiry technique.
2. Organizing factor of the evaluation.
3. Type of evaluative question identified.
4. Type of data collected.
5. Methods and intent of data collection.
6. Techniques of data analysis.

Most of the quantitative evaluation techniques come from the scientific or empiricist tradition, taking an approach that tries to connect evaluative outcomes with program characteristics in a cause-and-effect relationship. The physical sciences and social sciences, such as psychology and sociology, have been primary contributors to these techniques. Typically, questions of differences between groups or relationships among variables are addressed. Data are gathered by surveys, tests, or other objective measures and both descriptive and inferential statistics are often used in the data analyses.

Smith (1986, p. 38) has defined qualitative evaluation as an approach that "involves the long-term and first-hand study of a case by the investigator for the purposes of understanding and describing human action in the context of that case." Smith describes "field methods" that are used to collect data. These include direct observation of action in its natural context, clinical interviews to elicit the multiple meanings of participants in that case, and collection of documents. Data analysis and reporting may consist of words, pictures, and displays rather than formal models or statistical findings.

Quantitative approaches to evaluation are generally touted by their supporters for their objectivity, efficiency in data collection and analysis, and their causal orientation in attempts to link program features with measured program outcomes. Quantitative evaluation studies are generally replicable and satisfy the same specifications for reasonable internal validity as do research studies. In addition, reliability or consistency of measurement is usually a strength of this type of evaluation.

On the other hand, qualitative evaluations emphasize the context in which the evaluated program occurs, the complete description of the program phenomena, and the eliciting of the values of program participants, managers, and recipients of program services. Qualitative techniques are powerful when used to monitor the ongoing processes of a program being evaluated. Validity of measurement (measuring appropriate variables and constructs) is a strength of this type of evaluation.

Many evaluations have features that might qualify as both qualitative and quantitative in nature. Most evaluation questions and situations are sufficiently complex to benefit from the multiple perspectives offered by these evaluation approaches despite fundamentally different assumptions, operational guidelines, and organizing paradigms.

Goals, Objectives, and Criteria for Attainment

Goals, objectives, and the specification of criteria that define the level of attainment are commonly encountered features. Goals are generally distinguished from objectives in that goals are broadly stated and are concerned with terminal or long-term outcomes of a program. For example, a health care staff's intention to "improve the quality of health care for hospital patients" is a common goal. For measurement, it is necessary to restate that goal in more specific, operational terms and to specify significant points in the short term that are necessary but not sufficient for the eventual goal attainment. This restatement is an objective.

Objectives are frequently stated without an indication of how they might be met. For the evaluator, an objective accompanied by a statement of the behaviors to be observed when the objective is attained and a description of the circumstances that might accompany the attainment of the objective would be useful in conducting the evaluation. Such behavioral objectives were in vogue during the 1960s, especially among evaluators of curricula. Since then, the disadvantages of such minutely specific statements of behaviors (e.g., fragmentation of the program evaluated) have become apparent.

Many evaluators now feel that setting of performance standards should be done only after there is sufficient operational experience with the program to justify the otherwise arbitrary statements of performance expectations. A widely accepted modern view of specifically stated behavioral objectives is that they should not be imposed by the evaluator or the program managers at the beginning of the program, but should evolve through program experience and by means of negotiations with interested parties, if they are to be used at all.

Formative and Summative Evaluation

The distinction between formative and summative evaluation, as propounded by Michael Scriven (1967), is another feature differentiating evaluation models. Scriven distinguished between evaluation activities for the purpose of improvement of the program evaluated (formative evaluation) and evaluation for the purpose of assessing and judging the program (summative evaluation).

Summative evaluation attempts to provide policy makers or decision makers with information as to how well a program has worked during some period of operation. Summative evaluators are most interested in assessing the impact of a program and thus, they measure outcomes and the intended and unintended effects of the program, on its recipients and implementors. When most people think of program evaluation, they think of the activities of summative evaluation that provide information for decision makers who need to make a "go or no-go" decision for continuing, modifying, or terminating a program. Formative evaluation is used for ongoing revision.

Process and Product Evaluation

Several evaluation models focus separately on the processes of a program, those procedures and characteristics that enable it to work, and the products or outcome impacts of the program on those whom it serves. These are studied as they are embedded in the context of the program.

Process evaluation (or structure and process evaluation) focuses evaluative attention on factors such as procedures, logistics, and adequacy of staff and facility performance that support and facilitate the long-term accomplishment of a program's goals. The strategies and techniques used by staff members to enable program goals to be met are considered in evaluation activities that focus on the *structure and processes* of program implementation and operation. Information received in process evaluation activities is only one source of formative evaluation. Short-term product or program impact information is another source. This distinguishes process evaluation from formative evaluation.

Similarly, product evaluation offers evidence of program impact to the summative evaluator who is interested in providing information to decision makers as to how well a mature or fully developed program has worked in practice. Product evaluation can be distinguished from summative evaluation in that it may be done in short-term or long-term time frames. Short-term product information can be used as a means of formative evaluation or quality assurance, a set of procedures that seeks to assure that program procedures and services maintain a consistently acceptable quality during the operation of the program.

In summary, each of these major features may appear in many combinations in the various models for evaluation. By the early 1980s, more than 40 evaluation models had been described in the literature (Guba & Lincoln, 1981, p. 11). The evaluative "truth" that emerges from such an effort is viewed through the "lens" of the perspective emphasized by the particular model used. It is important to note that the same program might be evaluated as "successful" or "worthwhile" using one model and as "unsuccessful" when another model was used. The difference between these two conclusions may lie in the factors emphasized by a particular model guiding the evaluation.

EVALUATION MODELS: PARADIGMS FOR EVALUATION

The purpose of the various evaluation models is to establish one or more primary evaluative intents and to provide procedural guidelines to carry out those intents in specific situations. Thus, these models offer the evaluator a framework within which to work. The needs of each evaluative situation, however, are unique and a slavish devotion to procedures of any one evaluation model is likely to lead to lackluster evaluations that may only partly address important program features, processes, and outcomes.

Major Classes of Evaluation Models

Popham (1988) and others have described several major classes of evaluation models grouped by their primary organizing factors. The classes of models may have different labels depending on the authors (see Worthen & Sanders, 1987), but there seems to be general agreement on the nature of the categories. Popham's (1988, p. 24) list includes the following:

1. Goal-attainment models.
2. Judgmental models emphasizing inputs.
3. Judgmental models emphasizing outputs.
4. Decision–facilitative models.
5. Naturalistic models.
6. Efficiency models.

Within each of these classes, there are one or more specific evaluation models developed by evaluation theorists. Table 15–2 is a summary of prominent theorists and models by their organizing factors.

Goal Attainment Models. As the category name implies, each of these models is organized around the examination of the degree to which the pre-specified goals and objectives of a program have been met. This simple and rational approach appeals to the "first-plan-it-then-do-it" inclinations of many managers, and leads naturally to management-by-objectives (MBO) and other similar management styles. It sets up a natural framework for monitoring progress toward the attainment of goals, and it is easy to explain to staff members.

The fundamental underlying assumptions of this class of models seem to be that: (1) it is possible to state all important goals and objectives before the pro-

TABLE 15–2. PROMINENT PROGRAM EVALUATION THEORISTS AND THEIR MODELS

Goal Attainment

Tyler: Goals and objectives attained

Judgment

Accreditation: Structure of inputs, process, outcomes
Stake: Countenance description and judgment of outcomes
Scriven: Goal-free description of intended and unintended outcomes

Decision–facilitative

Provus: Discrepancy identification through periodic evaluation of standard achievement
Quality assurance: Periodic monitoring of standards
Stufflebeam: CIPP description of context, inputs, process, and products
Waltz: Nursing education program evaluation

Naturalistic

Guba: Naturalistic or holistic description
Stake: Responsive evaluation
Eisner: Connoisseurship description by an internal expert

Efficiency

Cost–benefit analysis
Cost effectiveness analysis
PERT: Program evaluation and review technique
CPM: Critical path analysis

gram begins; (2) it is possible to derive standards for comparing objectives and measured performance; (3) if most or all of the individual objectives have been met, then the program goals have been met and the program is a success.

Two Judgmental Models: Inputs and Outputs. Judgmental models emphasizing inputs organize the evaluation around the program's input features, such as the professional qualifications of the program service providers (e.g., number of nurses possessing advanced degrees) as well as the quality of the facilities or equipment used to provide services. This approach to evaluation is most familiar to those who have participated in evaluations for purposes of institutional accreditation by professional associations such as the Joint Commission on Accreditation of Healthcare Organizations (JCAHO). The JCAHO promotes general goals for outputs but focuses its primary attention on the inputs (or structure) and processes by which professional staff provide their services to clients. For example, JCAHO might encourage the improvement of patient care as a general output goal while providing explicit guidelines for equipment use, staff training, and procedural correctness, which are inputs (structure) and processes.

The underlying assumption of this class of evaluation models seems to be that the provision of superior equipment, training, and facilities will result in superior performance in delivery of program services. Detractors of this evaluation approach point out that inputs, such as those mentioned, may be necessary to the attainment of desired outcomes but are not, in themselves, sufficient for those outcomes to occur.

It is for this reason that JCAHO and other accreditation models have become increasingly attentive to program outcomes. Most models still collect information on program inputs (structure) and processes, but they use this information in attempts to link program procedures to specific program outcomes, either informally or from a definite causal perspective.

Judgmental models emphasizing outputs represent one of the ways evaluators attempt to link program inputs with documentation and assessment of program effects. Evaluation theorists, such as Robert Stake and Michael Scriven, have contributed important evaluation concepts to these models. Scriven's contributions include the concepts of formative and summative evaluation (as discussed previously) and the notion of goal-free evaluation (Guba & Lincoln, 1981).

In goal-free evaluation, the evaluator avoids any knowledge of the intended program goals and instead closely observes and describes the program as implemented to make inferences about the effects of the program. This deliberate search for serendipitous or unintended program outcomes, including those with both positive and negative implications, is an important contribution. It is this author's opinion that unintended outcomes are often of more interest.

Stake (1967) described a system using evaluation that was one of the first to focus on evaluative descriptions and judgments of program effects. He referred to these as two "countenances" defining a complete act of evaluation (Guba & Lincoln, 1981, p. 13), and this became known as the countenance model. Each countenance was applied to three stages of a program: the program antecedents or conditions at the beginning of the program, the program transactions or processes and procedures, and the program outcomes.

Some underlying assumptions of the judgmental models that emphasize outputs are: (1) the informed evaluator is best able to make valid judgments regarding program success; (2) differences in the value systems of program service providers and program recipients are not important; and (3) evaluations should be primarily focused on outcomes with attention given to how both intended and unintended outcomes were achieved.

Decision–Facilitative Models. The decision–facilitative approach to evaluation forms a fourth category. Each of these models is focused on the need to provide pertinent and appropriate information to decision makers regarding the program for decisions to modify or terminate the program. Thus, the decision-facilitative evaluators generally view themselves almost as facilitators of information flow to management rather than as independent judges of the program's merit.

As one might imagine, this view of evaluation is popular with managers, most of whom are interested in better program evaluative information and retaining program control. This view of evaluation also fits nicely into the concept of administrative accountability in that information is packaged by the evaluator in forms referring to program features and costs. This class of evaluation models is quite important because of its frequent use by local, state, and federal agencies or their funding dependents who are the primary evaluation funding source.

The discrepancy and the content, input, process, product (CIPP) models are two well-known decision–facilitative models. The discrepancy model, developed by Malcolm Provus (1971), compares standards with performance in each stage of a program. At each stage, the evaluator reports the discrepancies between standard and performance so that program decision makers can revise the standard or performance. The first stage, the *design stage*, identifies program objectives, specifications, and required resources. In the *installation stage*, the evaluator compares the program as designed with the program as actually installed and run. In the *process stage*, the evaluator examines enabling objectives (those whose attainment enables program goals to be met) for discrepancies between plans and performance. Finally, the *product stage* examines discrepancies between the program objectives and final performances. An optional fifth *ranking stage* calls for a comparison with other programs with similar goals in a cost–benefit analysis.

Stufflebeam's (et al. 1971) CIPP model specifies four different evaluation types in a program. *Context* evaluation establishes and documents the setting in which the program takes place. These activities lead to the statement of objectives for the program. *Input* evaluation provides information on the allocation of resources necessary for program objectives to be met. *Process* evaluation allows the evaluator to monitor the operation of the program for modification as necessary to meet program objectives and goals. Finally, in *product* evaluation, the evaluator assesses the attainment of program objectives during as well as at the end of the program.

The underlying assumptions of this class of models are: (1) decision-making values should be determined primarily by the decision makers and not by the evaluator; (2) the most important information that the evaluator should collect as needed for decisions merit to be made by decision makers; and (3) the lines of authority and decision-making influence are clear and there is at least moderate consensus among decision makers on program priorities and intents.

Naturalistic Models. Guba and Lincoln (1981) and others have written about organizing an evaluation around the goal of "naturalism" in matters of evaluative question definition, data collection, and data analysis and interpretation. The term naturalistic has different meanings depending on the author. It is variously defined as studying phenomena that are not fragmented into variables, studying programs without controlling for extraneous influences, or studying outcomes without formal measurement or preconceived hypotheses or even questions.

Although naturalistic evaluation is frequently equated with qualitative evaluation, especially from an anthropological perspective, there are some distinctions between the two.

Many naturalistic evaluators use qualitative data collection and data analysis techniques but they may also use quantitative techniques to supplement or supplant the qualitative data. In this view, Guba (1987, p. 26) points out that any evaluator, collecting and analyzing qualitative or quantitative data, can use naturalistic techniques but that "thinking naturalistically" would appear to preclude this mixture of research, as ". . . the ontological, epistemological, and methodological assumptions of naturalism . . . are fundamentally at odds with those of positivism" (p. 31). Obviously, there is lack of agreement as to what constitutes naturalistic evaluation.

Guba and Lincoln are well-known proponents of the naturalistic evaluation. They have built upon the responsive evaluation theory of Robert Stake. In addition, Elliot Eisner's (1975) connoisseurship model presents evaluation naturalistically. Connoisseurs of phenomena would be steeped in the knowledge and nature of the thing to be evaluated and would form judgments in much the same way as an art critic forms judgments about a work of art.

Some fundamental assumptions of this form of evaluation are: (1) observation is the best means of collecting and analyzing evaluative information; (2) measuring precision is less important than intense focus on the attributes of the phenomena; and (3) the context in which the phenomena occur should form the setting of its study.

EFFICIENCY MODELS

Human service professions and agencies provide essential services that are frequently supported at least in part with public funds. In addition, privately funded agencies face enormous pressures to provide essential services at a high level of quality while satisfying stringent cost restraints imposed from outside or inside the organization. Thus, health care providers must be well versed in evaluative procedures that allow the comparison of quality of services with cost of services.

Cost Analysis Models

Cost–benefit analysis attempts to translate program features and outcomes into monetary terms so that the financial worth of each feature or benefit can be directly compared with its cost. Results may be used to evaluate one program or to *compare several programs with dissimilar goals.* For example, the cost of a training program for nurses might be calculated and compared with the benefits of costs saved in increased efficiency, in better care for patients, and in reduced waste of materials used in hospital care. A comparison of the dollar costs for the training with the estimated dollar value of the benefits would provide a measure of "return on investment" for nurse training.

Cost–benefit procedures may be difficult to implement in real life. For example, the monetary value of benefits, such as improved patient attitudes and increased willingness to patronize the hospital in the future, may be estimated only subjectively and with a probable wide range of uncertainty. Thus, different evaluators using different assumptions may arrive at quite different estimates of benefits and costs.

Cost–effectiveness analysis, the second type of cost analysis, converts program costs to monetary units as before, but in this case, program outcomes and benefits are expressed in their normal units. Results may be used to *compare* actual costs of alternative *programs with similar goals.* For example, an evaluator might be asked to determine which of two programs intended to reduce the number of in-hospital patient infections had been more successful. Let us assume that the first program, consisting of a $20,000 expenditure for new equipment and staff training, resulted in the reduction of the infection rate per patient from 0.20 infections per 100 patients to 0.10. If the same reduction in infection rate had already been achieved in other comparable areas of the hospital by means of additional training of health care staff regarding preventive measures at a cost of only $5,000, the choice with the best cost-per-unit-benefit ratio is apparent.

Obviously, both cost–benefits and cost–effectiveness analyses are useful only if the benefits of health care strategies and programs are known and measurable. In addition, the direct as well as the indirect costs over time of a program must be considered before the real cost impact of a program becomes apparent. For example, a medical procedure that is more cost–effective in the short term may cause greater expenditures and reduced patient benefits in the long term. Of course, there can be considerable difference of opinion on the existence and degree of indirect costs.

A third type of cost analysis, *cost–feasibility* analysis, is simply a process to determine if a certain program is affordable. In cost–feasibility analysis, the costs of planned programs are calculated before implementation and compared with available resources. This allows program managers to eliminate in the planning stage those programs whose costs are unacceptable or exceed available resources. The program alternatives that remain are deemed feasible based on their costs and are candidates for trial and for the use of cost–benefit or cost–effectiveness evaluation. For example, a hospital may consider the possibility of setting up an artificial heart research and development program, but may find that the start-up costs and the costs for required staff, space, and equipment resources exceed reasonably attainable financial resources.

Cost–utility analysis differs from other forms of cost analysis in that the utility of outcomes of the program are rated by persons who have an interest in the program. The utility of the program is usually rated using a numerical scale such as a 1 to 10 point scale with equal intervals between its units (Popham, 1988, p. 265). Levin (1975) further suggests that the ratings of the program judges can be aggregated so that the values of the raters who view the program from different perspectives can be combined to yield an overall program rating of utility or usefulness. These ratings are then compared with the program's cost so that cost-per-unit-benefit can be measured.

QUALITY ASSURANCE

A second program evaluative aspect of major importance to health care professionals is quality assurance. Quality assurance in nursing has been defined as "guaranteed excellence, the goal of which is to improve care and the role of which is to monitor the quality of that care" (Vail & Jacobs, 1986, p. 172). Coyne and Killien (1987, p. 26) define quality assurance as "a process that is directed toward evaluating the quality of patient care that is provided in a particular setting through setting standards for care and implementing mechanisms for ensuring that the standards are met."

Quality assurance is similar in intent to the concept of quality control from systems analysis theory. Quality control procedures attempt to determine the current level of quality in a program by sampling data or procedures and producing estimates of their overall quality from this sampling. Measures of typical performance can be readily derived from these samplings. Usually there is an expectation that performance will not be perfect, but that the failure rate should be minimized to an acceptable level. For example, employee absenteeism could be sampled over a 1-month period with the finding that the typical nurse missed 1.1 days per month and that 99 percent of all nurses missed three or fewer days. From these findings of typical absenteeism, managers may or may not decide to act to reduce absenteeism.

In health care situations, the concept of an acceptable failure rate becomes more difficult to use because human welfare or even lives are at stake. Thus, the framework for a quality assurance program, in contrast with a quality control program, is to set standards whose attainment would result in no serious failures that would adversely affect patient welfare in known ways.

These definitions provide descriptions of quality assurance that allow us to place it in the context of existing evaluation theory. These definitions also describe a form of evaluation that allows judgments to be made based on standards of practice or care. This calls to mind the accreditation model of evaluation that belongs to the class of evaluation models labeled "judgmental models emphasizing inputs" by Popham (1988).

Connections between the quality assurance programs and the conventional evaluation theory have become more obvious with recent JCAHO actions. The JCAHO has encouraged the augmentation of the auditing of compliance with predetermined standards by means of the development of program monitoring procedures that provide for the collection of process information (e.g., activities of the health care providers) and product information (i.e., the outcomes of the actions of health care providers) with a primary emphasis on formative evaluation (use of available data for purposes of program improvement).

In addition, it seems that one model of value for quality assurance systems may be the discrepancy evaluation model. The discrepancy model's five stages, discussed earlier, correspond nicely with recent descriptions of quality assurance programs as having three components: a value system, an appraisal system, and a response system (Coyne & Killien, 1987, p. 26). Table 15–3 gives an overall outline.

The first stage of Provus's model, the design stage, can be employed to document the characteristics of the program of health care services, elicit staff input to set standards for program performance in delivering these services, and identify the staff and equipment resources necessary for those standards to be met. During this stage, a value system emerges in which staff and organizational values are made specific in defining standards of patient care using a system that elicits staff opinions and degree of support for each program characteristic.

The second stage, installation, compares the plans for program procedure, equipment, and staff use in providing health care services with the characteristics of the health care program as actually delivered to patients. In this stage, the standards are the program plans, and the performances are the actual program procedures and services delivered. Discrepancies between these two are reported to managers or other decision makers for possible adjustments.

TABLE 15–3. QUALITY ASSURANCE USING THE DISCREPANCEY MODEL BY PROVUS

Stage 1: Design	Stage 2: Installation	Stage 3: Process	Stage 4: Product	Stage 5: Rank (optional)
Values and assumptions are compared with program plans	Program plans are compared with services delivered	Appraisal system results compared with response system actions	Goals and objectives are compared with intended and unintended outcomes	Program is compared with other similar programs

In the third stage, process, the appraisal system and the response system of the quality assurance program begin to operate. During this stage, evaluators formulate enabling objectives. Such information may be used to produce forms called screens to audit nurse behavior. This audit provides for the examination of the processes of the health care delivery system reflecting actual performance of the staff in delivering health care.

The product stage is last. Here outcomes are compared to goals and objectives. Unintended outcomes are also identified and evaluated as positive or negative. The response system provides feedback to the health care staff regarding any discrepancies (positive or negative) between standards set and corresponding performances measured. If performance has fallen below standards, an inquiry into the reasons for this discrepancy is called for with attendant adjustments in standards or in the level of performance. If performance has met or exceeded the standards, positive feedback or even rewards to the staff members will help to maintain high performance.

If a quality assurance program were to be implemented using the framework of the discrepancy evaluation model, the participation of persons with several different professional roles would be necessary to its success. The active participation of the unit-based staff in setting standards, in determining important areas for monitoring, and in providing assessment information regarding the degree to which program goals and enabling objectives are met is absolutely essential.

The success of the evaluation effort depends on the staff's understanding of its goals, and actively supporting its efforts. What is required is a type of health care quality circle, similar in intent to those promoted by Japanese managers in recent years to provide for higher levels of quality in manufacturing. In such an arrangement, nurses and other providers of health care would have direct access to management regarding any suggestion that they felt would improve the quality of patient services. Rewards would be attached to greater efficiency or improved levels of service.

A second participant is the evaluation specialist. This person may be an external evaluator hired as a consultant. The best situation, however, is an internal evaluator, a person who reports to managers and decision makers, and who is involved in evaluation issues from their inception. This person may or may not have a health care background. Such a person, however, should be expert in group dynamics, training skills, framing evaluation questions and designs appropriate to health care settings, data collection, data analysis, and the reporting and interpretation of findings.

Health care program managers also should have some evaluation training so that they can work knowledgeably with the evaluation specialist and the unit staff. Managers should be health care specialists and should be able to provide the intimate knowledge of health care issues, procedures, and processes that the evaluation specialist may lack.

A limitation on the success of present evaluation efforts in health care is that many evaluators are health care professionals pressed into service as evaluators without a substantial background in evaluation. As the JCAHO and other health care organizations promoting improved evaluation continue to press for more sophisticated evaluative efforts, health care professionals will no doubt recognize that program evaluation is an area worthy of concentrated study and specialization by health care professionals who support the highest professional standards and levels of performance possible for themselves, for the health care agencies whom they represent, and for the recipients of their services.

BIOGRAPHICAL SKETCH

Wayne Thomas is an associate professor of research and evaluation methodology in the Department of Education Leadership and Human Development at George Mason University in Fairfax, Virginia. His graduate degrees are in program evaluation and social science research methodology and he teaches doctoral courses in these areas. He has worked as a program evaluator in several educational agencies. In addition, he has extensive consulting experience in evaluation with federal, state, and local governments as well as with corporations and professional associations.

SUGGESTED READINGS

Quality Assurance

Bloch, D. (1977). Criteria standards, norms—Crucial terms in quality assurance. *The Journal of Nursing Administration, 7* (9), 20–30.

Carter, J. H., Hilliard, M., Castles, M. R., Stoll, L. D., & Cowan, A. (1972). *Standards of Nursing Care: A Guide for Evaluation.* New York: Springer Publishing.

Coyne, C., & Killien, K. (1987). A system for unit-based monitors of nursing care. *Journal of Nursing Administration, 17* (1), 26–32.

Hegyvary, S. T. (1980). An evaluator's perspective. *Nursing Research, 29* (2), 91–93.

Vail, J. D., & Jacobs, M. (1986). Quality assurance: The pieces of the puzzle. *Journal of the Association of Nurse Anesthetists, 54* (2), 171–176.

Willis, L. D., & Linwood, M. E. (Eds.). (1984). *Measuring the Quality of Care.* New York: Churchill Livingstone.

Evaluation Models

Hicks, L. L. (1985). Using benefit-cost and cost-effectiveness analysis in health-care resource allocation. *Nursing Economic$, 2* (2), 78–84.

Popham, W. J. (1988). *Educational Evaluation.* Englewood Cliffs, NJ: Prentice Hall.

Provus, M. M. (1971). *Discrepancy Evaluation.* Berkeley, CA: McCutchan Publishing.

Rossi, P. H., & Freeman, H. E. (1985). *Evaluation: A Systematic Approach.* **Beverly** Hills, CA: Sage Publishing.

Veney, J., & Kaluzny, A. (1984). *Evaluation and Decision Making for Health Services Programs.* Englewood Cliffs, NJ: Prentice Hall.

REFERENCES

Borg, W. R., & Gall, M. D. (1983). *Educational Research.* New York: Longman Press.

Coursey, R. D. (Ed.). (1977). *Program Evaluation for Mental Health.* New York: Grune & Stratton.

Coyne, C., & Killien, K. (1987). A system for unit-based monitors of quality of nursing care. *Journal of Nursing Administration, 17*(1), 26–32.

Cronbach, L. J., Ambron, S. R., Dornbush, S. M., Hess, R. D., et al. (1980). *Toward Reform of Program Evaluation.* San Francisco, CA: Jossey-Bass.

Eisner, E. W. (1975). The perceptive eye: Toward the reformation of educational evaluation. *Occasional papers of the Stanford evaluation consortium.* Stanford, CA: Stanford University.

Guba, E. G., & Lincoln, Y. S. (1981). *Effective Evaluation: Improving the Usefulness of Evaluation Results Through Responsive and Naturalistic Approaches.* San Francisco: Jossey-Bass.

Guba, E. G. (1987). What have we learned about naturalistic evaluation? *Evaluation Practice, 8,* 23–43.

Levin, H. M. (1975). Cost-effectiveness in evaluation research. In Guttentag, M. & Struening, E. (Eds.): *Handbook of Evaluation Research,* Vol. 2. Beverly Hills, CA: Sage Publications.

Popham, W. J. (1975). *Educational Evaluation.* Englewood Cliffs, NJ: Prentice-Hall.

Popham, W. J. (1988). *Educational Evaluation.* Englewood Cliffs, NJ: Prentice-Hall.

Provus, M. M. (1971). *Discrepancy Evaluation.* Berkeley, CA: McCutchan Publishing.

Scriven, M. (1967). The methodology of evaluation. *AERA Monograph Series in Curriculum Evaluation,* No. 1. Chicago: Rand McNally.

Smith, M. L. (1986). The whole is greater: Combining qualitative and quantitative approaches in evaluation studies. In Williams, D. D. (ed.): *Naturalistic Evaluation,* Vol. 30. New directions in program evaluation. San Francisco, CA: Jossey-Bass.

Stake, R. E. (1967). The countenance of education evaluation. *Teacher's College record, 68,* 523–540.

Stufflebeam, D. I., Foley, W. J., Gephart, W. J., Guba, E. G. (1971). *Educational Evaluation and Decision Making.* Itasca, IL: F. E. Peacock.

Tyack, D. B. (1974). *The One Best System: A History of American Urban Education.* Cambridge, MA: Harvard University Press.

Tyler, R. W. (1969). *Educational Evaluation: New Roles, New Means.* Chicago, IL: University of Chicago Press.

Vail, J. D., & Jacobs, M. (1986). Quality assurance: The pieces of the puzzle. *Journal of the Association of Nurse Anesthetists, 54* (2), 171–176.

Worthen, B. R., & Sanders, J. R. (1987). *Educational Evaluation: Theory and Practice.* Belmont, CA: Wadsworth Publishing.

CASE 15–1

Maintaining JCAHO Accreditation
Mary S. Tilbury

The Joint Commission is Coming. These words not infrequently result in frantic and frenzied activity on the part of nursing leadership. All too often the activity is accompanied by a sense of doom and feelings of inadequacy. Such responses are understandable when one considers that the JCAHO visit culminates in a summation conference open to any member of the staff, Board, or public interested in attending. No one likes to feel that they might look bad in front of people that they work with on a day-to-day basis. Thus, the challenge becomes—How can nursing leadership utilize the administrative process so that formal notification of a forthcoming visit is met with calm confidence and the outcome is accepted with a sense of pride and accomplishment? The primary purpose of this case application is to outline a process, with illustrations from our practice at The Alexandria Hospital, that can be effectively used by a nursing leadership team.

The ideal goal of a JCAHO visit is to have no formal recommendations for the nursing service department. On the other hand, occasionally, nursing leadership may anticipate problems and outline a course of action that cannot be completed before the next scheduled visit. For example, one of the most frequently cited deficiencies is the nursing documentation system. In 1981, at the Alexandria Hospital, the JCAHO nurse surveyor cited documentation as an area that required attention. The leadership team made a decision to develop a computerized documentation system based on the department's conceptual model for practice. This decision meant that the same deficiency would be found during the 1983 visit, but the surveyor, upon request, did note that a comprehensive plan had been adopted and was being implemented to address the problem. Indeed, the 1983 surveyor was used as a "consultant" to review the developing system against the standards. In 1986, the necessary elements were in place to achieve the goal and objectives set 5 years earlier. The administrative opportunity presented by the documentation deficiency had been rectified and a cutting edge system had been developed.

Preparation for the next JCAHO visit should begin at the conclusion of the summation conference of the current visit. The information gained at this time should be used in conjunction with planning, which is organized and systematic. Information forms the foundation upon which planning is built. The first source of information that the nurse executive should consult are publications by JCAHO.

The most meaningful Commission publication available for planning is the *Accreditation Manual for Hospitals*. This text contains all of the standards that apply to the majority of agencies where nursing is practiced. In a separate section, the manual contains the eight nursing service standards adopted by the JCAHO Board of Commissioners. There are also standards located elsewhere in the text that apply to areas such as special care units, psychiatric units, and ambulatory settings that nursing administrators may review and incorporate in the planning process. Nurse executives who have administrative responsibility for areas other than nursing will also need to have a working knowledge of the standards that govern those functions.

Due to the dynamic nature of the health care system and the diversity of its institutions, new standards are added and existing standards are revised on a continuing basis through a definitive process that is driven by technology, federal regulations, legal statutes, consumer actions, and health care provider input. Professional groups, like the American Association of Critical Care Nurses and the American Nurses' Association, in conjunction with a number of other professional organizations, review the proposed standards before they are adopted by the Board of Commissioners. It is at this point that the newly developed or revised standards become part of the JCAHO manual.

The manual is used to survey a variety of settings from 50-bed rural community facilities to 1000-bed urban teaching hospitals. This necessitates that the standards be written in general terms. The application of the standards varies with the setting, but it presents a challenge to all nursing service administrators.

In response to the concerns of nurse executives, to better understand how standards are applied in various settings, in 1983, the JCAHO published *A Guide to JCAHO Nursing Service Standards*. Here each of the eight nursing service standards are reviewed in terms of the goals and objectives the standard is designed to achieve, its required characteristics, answers to the questions most frequently asked about the standard and a "test" that can be self-administered to determine the nurse executives' level of comprehension. This publication has greatly improved communication between surveyors and administrators.

The Commission also publishes two additional informational items of use to nurse executives preparing for a survey. The *Hospital Survey Profile* is a self-assessment tool routinely forwarded to hospitals a few months before the survey to facilitate the identification of areas requiring attention. *Perspectives*, the official JCAHO newsletter, is a useful "keep current" resource. For example, the JCAHO announced in 1987 that it had set a goal to survey agencies on the basis of clinical standards/monitors by 1990. This reflects a major change in policy and should be closely monitored by nursing service administrators so that preparation for survey visits can be managed accordingly. The JCAHO visit leadership is a dynamic process, requiring continuous rather than episodic attention.

A second major source of information that helps nursing service administrators are the educational seminars sponsored by JCAHO. These offerings are particularly helpful to individuals who are new to nursing management. The nurse executive will determine who will benefit most from attending one of the seminars. Occasionally, when major revisions have been made in the standards, the chief nurse executive and selected members of her team may need to attend so that first-hand information can be obtained. If, after taking advantage of these information sources, a need for clarification still exists, the JCAHO provides a toll-free number for direct communication. The number is (800) 621-8007 or (800) 572-8089 for Illinois agencies.

In addition to publications, conferences, and direct communication, networking is always a good way to gather information about how others approach standard compliance and what experience has taught them about preparing for the survey. The primary purpose of networking is to gain additional information about areas being emphasized during the actual survey or preferences of the individual surveyors.

As the surveillance time approaches two additional opportunities, to further assess readiness, are available to the nursing administrator: presurvey conferences and hiring a consultant. State and local hospital associations now sponsor presurvey conferences for the agencies that are scheduled for upcoming visits. This provides the nurse executive and members of her team with an opportunity to meet the actual surveyor responsible for reviewing the nursing function. Recent changes in standards or points of general interest can also be discussed during the meeting. Nursing consultants are primarily used in special circumstances. Intensive problem-solving, turn around situations, or nurse executives who have assumed their duties and responsibilities just before a visit are particularly appropriate circumstances for consultant intervention.

The planning cited assists the nursing service administrator to do a comprehensive assessment of compliance with the standards before the visit. Hand in hand with information gathering the nursing department organizes to: (1) assess deficiencies, (2) devise plans to remove them, (3) implement changes, and (4) prepare for the actual visit. A variety of structural approaches can be taken to develop and implement the preparation plan. Several factors should be taken into consideration before developing an organizational design.

As with any matter internal to the department of nursing, the chief nurse executive is ultimately responsible for the visit's outcome. The role that he or she elects to play in the preparation activities of the visit is shaped by multiple factors. These factors must be thoroughly analyzed before any decisions regarding structure and delegation.

A nursing director who is new to the executive position should play a major role in the activities that surround the visit. On the other hand, the director who has occupied the position for a time may well elect to play a less active part in the functions outlined to prepare for the review. The director's leadership team may feel well prepared to assume responsibility for assessment, followed by consultation with the director for planned interventions, and implementation of changes and staff education for the visit. For example, the nursing director of a psychiatric facility engaged in merger discussions might want to delegate the preparation plan to a member of the nurse executive team. On the other hand, if the prior visit identified a number of administrative opportunities, even the busiest nurse executive will set this visit as a top priority.

The organizational structure will understandably be effected by any major ongoing project. In the example of the development of a computerized documentation system, the task force assigned responsibility for the project was released from other matters surrounding the upcoming visit.

In small organizations the nurse executive may accept first-line responsibility for planning and operational activities. In large complex agencies, primary responsibility may be delegated to a staff or line officer within the department to coordinate the function and keep the objectives and action plans approved by the executive group on target.

The first principle of any organizational plan is that form follows substance. The magnitude of the project—to prepare for JCAHO visit—will in large measure determine how you organize. Nursing departments who have been reviewed in the past without recommendations in years without major JCAHO charges may elect to only address continuing compliance.

As indicated earlier, JCAHO standards are constantly being reviewed and revised. It is important that "keep current" responsibility is specifically identified and delegated to one or more members of the nursing executive team, depending on the size and complexity of the agency. This delegation should result in continuing update, identification of need, and the development of action plans to address the implications of new or changing standards. In this way, the frantic activity that is so typical before a visit is avoided.

The final report of the JCAHO now highlights areas of developing need. If a nursing executive team is able to anticipate and initiate organizational change in these areas, the review team's expertise can be used to evaluate the plan and advance organizational readiness for the next visit. Another factor that may affect the structural organization adopted by the department for the visit are the developmental goals set for subordinates. Delegation of administrative responsibility for the visit may be appropriate to support professional growth of subordinates once expectations have been clearly identified at the executive level.

On the other hand, if various members of the executive team are at different developmental stages, then situational leadership strategies can be used. Different subunits of organization, and their leaders, can have very different expectations set regarding the visit. In the case where the director of maternal-child nursing has no prior experience with JCAHO reviews and only a year of experience with the agency, the chief nurse executive may wish to develop different expectations and support systems with the maternal-child director than the medical-surgical director who has been with the organization for 6 years and has experienced three major JCAHO reviews. Whatever the organizational approach adopted by the nursing executive team, the ultimate goal is to handle the visit and all activities related to it with skill.

At the Alexandria Hospital two different organizational approaches were used for visits in 1983 and 1986. The 1983 visit involved the achievement of three major objectives. These objectives were developed by the chief nurse executive 6 months after the completion of the 1981 survey, and they served as the group's primary organizational focus over the years.

First, an objective was set to rectify prior JCAHO recommendations. Seven deficiencies had been identified by the JCAH surveyor in 1981. These areas were addressed on a point-by-point basis and action plans developed to meet each. One of the seven objectives was related to the documentation deficiency cited, thus the action plan to develop a computerized system. The remaining six deficiencies were assigned to members of the executive team for resolution. These deficiencies generally related to policies and standards that needed development.

The second major objective was the continuing need to keep current regarding JCAHO standards. Shortly after the 1981 visit one member of the executive team was assigned responsibility for keeping up with JCAHO publications and also attended a JCAHO workshop on nursing standards 1 year before the scheduled survey.

The third major objective involved evaluation of continuing compliance with all aspects of the remaining JCAHO standards. This was assigned to the executive team member that had monitored the publications and attended the workshop. Her reports began approximately 8 months before the anticipated visit and were structured on a standard-by-standard basis. Networking among colleagues was also used as a resource in completing this aspect of the preparation cycle.

The executive group monitored the action plans developed for the areas of deficiency; formal reports were provided on publication review, internal evaluation, and the content of the JCAHO workshop. Four months before the survey the executive team felt that the department had attained the preparation objectives. The visit and the written report confirmed the conclusion—the only citation referred to the documentation problem and the steps that had been taken since the last visit to address it.

The next visit was 3 years later. The executive team had grown and developed over that time, both in its administrative maturity and in the autonomy of its members. The team no longer felt the need to centralize so much of the responsibility in an internal expert. The group set their plan and departmental goal was a citation-free visit 8 months before the survey.

Each clinical director accepted responsibility for the evaluation of her area against the three major objectives identified above.

The documentation system development was on track and progress reports from the committee's chairperson were reviewed by the chief nurse executive and the team on a regular basis. An analysis of continuing standard compliance was completed during two administrative retreats. Each director accepted responsibility of identifying problems and of developing and identifying action plans to rectify the deficiency before the anticipated visit.

The executive team again assigned the review of JCAHO publications and the attendance of the standards workshop to one member of the group, but in 1986 this individual was used as a consultant to the administrative group. Thus, the group had every reason to feel well-informed and competent in this area. Without a person with ongoing responsibility, updating of the group's knowledge of current standards should have begun at least 1 year before the visit.

The self-assessment process should be continuous rather than static. For example, an assessment cycle should be completed before the arrival of the *Hospital Survey Profile* and also after the *Profile* is filled out by the group or individual to whom it is assigned. In this way, a system of checks and balances is made as part of the process. Other sources of data should be included in the analysis. Special attention should be paid to standards that are new or those that have been revised.

As the time for the 1986 visit approached, two other decisions were made. First, one of the clinical directors was assigned to attend the presurvey conference sponsored by the Virginia Hospital Association and report back to the group. Second, the chief nurse executive delegated the responsibility for coordinating nurse surveyor activities during the actual survey to a clinical director who had a chief nurse executive career objective. When the surveyor arrived, this goal was explained and she welcomed the opportunity to contribute to the development plan. At the summation conference the goal set some months ago was realized—there were no recommendations for the Department of Nursing Service at The Alexandria Hospital.

Additional typing and clerical work may be required for the visit. The nurse executive should budget additional clerical resources for the fiscal year with a JCAHO visit. External resources, rather than additional full-time equivalents are a sound economical approach to address this need. There may be former clerical employees of the hospital who would like to earn extra income and who know the procedures used by the organization. If nursing consultants are used, financial resources must be planned for this as well.

Activities should include deadlines for each of the key steps. Executive group meetings should include deadline compliance reviews and further problem-solving when the unexpected develops. Continual updating assists the chief nurse executive to keep her superior informed.

When formal notification of the site visit is received, a general announcement should be made to all the staff. At this point, the impending visit should not be a surprise, but the staff will understandably be interested in all the preparation activities and what is expected of them during the survey process. Staff should be kept informed during the preparation cycle, and advised that if questioned by a surveyor, a straightforward, truthful response is all that is expected. Mock surveys and role playing are two educational approaches nurse managers may use to ease staff anxiety and create a climate of readiness.

During these final weeks reassure the staff that the department is well prepared for the survey. If there are any questions, issues or concerns that are outstanding, reserve them for the surveyor, who can assist the executive group in resolution. Above all, fully utilize the expertise of the surveyors. Your facility is paying for the site visit and the team members should be approached as if they were consultants. Nurse surveyors are in multiple facilities over the course of their careers and can often be of help on how to operationalize goals and objectives related to the standards.

When all the JCAHO preparedness plan objectives have been met and the last minute details have been resolved, relax and approach the visit as a learning experience. Let the members of the executive team and those who have played a role in preparing for the visit, by accepting additional responsibility, know how much you appreciate their efforts. During the actual survey try and keep department heads informed about the surveyors timetable. There is nothing more demoralizing than to have a department head anticipate a visit from a member of the survey team that never comes. Schedule updates should be communicated to the affected parties on a frequent basis.

When the survey is concluded and the summation conference is over, the nurse executive group may want to plan a celebration of their own for a job well done. If no recommendations were made at the summation conference so much the better, but regardless, the organization of the group's work plan and their execution thereof should be acknowledged.

The nurse executive should prepare a preliminary report to the staff of the nursing department, identifying probable recommendations included in the summation conference, if any, and an expression of appreciation to them for their efforts on behalf of the department and the organization. The staff should be advised that there is usually a 4- to 6-month period between the actual visit and receipt of the written report. A commitment should be made to brief the staff on the written report when it is received and analyzed.

There is understandably a let-down period that follows any surveillance activity, the satisfaction that comes from the skilled management of a well-developed plan is one of the most satisfying experiences a nurse executive and members of her executive team have during an administrative career, enjoy— you've earned it.

BIOGRAPHICAL SKETCH

Mary S. Tilbury, Ed.D., RN, CNAA, received her baccalaureate degree in Nursing from Duke University, her master's degree in Nursing Service Administration from the University of Maryland, and her doctorate in higher education administration from Virginia Tech. Dr Tilbury is currently Vice President-Administration/Director of Nursing at Rochester General Hospital in Rochester, New York. Previously she was Vice President for Nursing and Support Services, The Alexandria Hospital. She has held faculty appointments at the University of Maryland, Marymount University, and Georgetown University Schools of Nursing, and has precepted graduate students from multiple institutions including George Mason University, Catholic University of America, and the University of Pittsburgh.

Index

Absolute privilege, 33
Accounting equations, basic, 265–266f
Accounts, major classes of, 266–267
Accounts receivable, 275–276
Accreditation model of evaluation, 451
Accretion, 45
Accrual accounting
  asset valuation and, 279
  vs. cash accounting, 269–270
Accrued liabilities, 276
Act deontology, 7, 9t, 10
Activity ratios, 272t
Act utilitarianism, 5–6, 9t, 10
Administrative competence, of women administrators, 111–112
Administrative law, 40–43
Admissions, recording of, 37–38
Adult learning theory, 390–391
Advancement of nursing practice, 18
Adverse patient occurrences (APOs), 64
Advertising, 202–203
Affective educational objectives, 388

Age Discrimination Employment Act, 50
Aggregative decision techniques, 142–143
AIDS, 79
American Medical Association (AMA), 74
American Nurses' Association (ANA)
  Commission on Nursing Services, 17
  health care policy and, 74
  legislative reform of nursing homes and, 92–97
  Social Policy Statement, 71
  standards for organized nursing services, 17–18t
Anarchy, organizational, 139
Androgogy, assumptions of, 391
Androgynous management, 111
APOs (adverse patient occurrences), 64
Applications software, 306–307
Appraisal system, for quality assurance program, 452
Arbitration, binding, 49

Assault, 31
Assessment model, for management development programs, 249, 250f
Asset(s)
  contra, 265–266
  current, 275–276
  equity and, 265–266
  fixed or long-term, 265
  valuation, 278–279
Assistant vice president management role, 346
Attribution theory, 100–101
Automation. See also Computers
  division of labor and, 307–308
  effect on health care delivery systems, 358–359
  nurse-vendor collaboration and, 316–328f
  associate administrators role, 317
  task force role, 317–318
  of routine work, 304–308
Autonomy
  definition of, 332
  organizational change and, 242

Autonomy (*cont.*)
in professional bureaucracy, 238–239
respect for, 11–12
Avoidable or escapable costs, 280

Balance sheet, 263–265*f*, 269
Bargaining
collective, 43–44
good faith, 46–47
incrementalism and, 140–141
power
of health care service buyers, 160–161
of suppliers, 161
BARS (behavioral anchored rating scale), 419*f*
Battery, 31
Behavioral anchored rating scale (BARS), 419*f*
Behavioral assessment of nursing staff productivity, 341
Behavioral process approach, to market segmentation, 197
Behavior modification, 100
Beneficence, components of, 12–13
Benefit-cost analysis, 144
Bentham, Jeremy, 5
Binding arbitration, 49
Biological clock theory, 390
Birth position, of women executives, 107–108
Boards of Nursing examiners, 29–30
Bookkeeping, double entry, 267–268*f*
Breach of duty, 34
Breakeven analysis, 282*t*–283*t*
Budget(s)
capital, 284
cash, 284

for clinical nursing research program, 403
flexible, 286
nursing cost methods for, 364–366
operating, 284
as standards, 286–287
static or fixed, 286
variances, 286–287*t*
Budgeting
process of, 284–285
purposes of, 283–284
types of, 283–284
Buyers, bargaining power of, 160–161

Capital, net working, 274–275
Capital budget, 284
Case by case analysis, in risk identification, 63–66*t*
Case load, 359
Case management
advantages of, 379
description of, 337–338
health care restructuring and, 361–362
Case manager, 361–362
Cash accounting
asset valuation in, 279
vs. accrual accounting, 269–270
Cash budget, 284
Cash flow
analysis, 274, 275
importance of knowing, 270–271
Centralization, vs. decentralization of professional development departments, 392–394
Central processing unit (CPU), 305
Central tendency, 423
Certificate of need, 162, 277
Charting errors, corrections of, 37

Chart of accounts, nurse administrators and, 268
Checklists, 417–418*t*
CIPP model, evaluation types in, 447–448
Clinical ladder program, 292, 338
Clinical nurse specialist, 81
Clinical nursing research program
acceptance of, 406–407
conduction of, 406
evaluation of, 407–408
financial resources for, 403
goals and objectives of, 403
guidelines
establishment of, 402–408
for leadership of program, 404
for protocols for review of research proposals, 404–405
for research utilization, 405–406
Cognitive educational objectives, 388
Cognitive style, 389–390
Cognitive theory of motivation, 100
Collaboration, to enhance nursing, 394–398
Collaborative practice committee, 292
Collective bargaining, 43–44
Commitment, to common philosophy, 158
Common law, 29
Communication system, within nursing division, 425–426*f*
Community health agencies, organizational structure of, 358
Community hospital, case study of head nurse preceptor program, 116–123

Compensation, performance appraisal and, 411
Compensatory damages, 33
Competence
administrative, of women administrators, 111–112
clinical, 387
personal, of women administrators, 110–111
professional, of women administrators, 111
promotion of, 158
Competition in health care, direct and indirect, 194f
Competitive analysis, for strategic planning, 159–162f
Competitors
analysis of, 193–195f
rivalry among, 161–162
potential, treat of entry by, 159
Computer-based management information systems. *See* Management information systems
Computer literature personnel, 312
Computers. *See also* Automation
effect on health care delivery, 358–359
management information systems and, 305–306t
selection of, nurse-vendor collaboration and, 316
Conduct, unprofessional, 30
Confidentiality, 31–32
Conflict, between needs of work group and individual, 24
Congruence model, 234–235f
Consent, informed, 39–40
Consequentialist theory, 5–6

Consistency, 158
Constituents, classification of, 191
Construct validity, 421–422
Consultant, 248
Consultation process
establishing consultant-client relationships, 249
evaluation and replanning, 253
implementing action plan, 252–253
problem solving phases, 249–253f
relationship conditions, 248–249
in strategic planning, 169
Consumer satisfaction, 196–197
Content, moral justification and, 3
Context evaluation, 447
Contingency model, 239–241f
Contingency theory of decision-making methods, 145
Continuity of care, responsibility of, 32
Contra assets, 265–266
Contract courses, 397
Contributory negligence, 34–35
Coordination, 239, 252
Corporate culture, 157–158
Corporate liability, 30
Corporate strategy, 356
Corporate vs. professional culture conflict, 354–355
Corporate women, traits of, 108–109
Cost(s)
avoidable or escapable, 280
budgeted/actual, 279–280
committee/noncommitted, 279
concepts
categories of, 278t

and controls, 277–283t
for volume category, 281
controllable/noncontrollable, 279
direct/indirect, 279
fixed, 281
health care, factors contributing to increases in, 77–78
opportunity, 280
semifixed or semivariable, 281
step, 281
variable, 281
Cost-analysis models, 449–450
Cost-benefit analysis, 137, 449
Cost containment, 22, 76–77
Cost-effectiveness
analysis, 449
of team vs. primary nursing, 360–361
Cost-feasibility analysis, 449–450
Cost leadership, 86
Cost management, managerial control of, 279–280
Cost-utility analysis, 450
Countenance model, 446–447
Countersigning, 37, 38
County health department, initiation of marketing in, 219–224t
CPU (central processing unit), 305
Credentials, nursing, 42
Credibility, strategy development and, 177–178
Criteria for attainment, 443
Critical incident performance appraisal, 420t
Critical success factor approach, 167
Cultural networks, 158
Curriculum
design, content in, 388–389

Curriculum (*cont.*)
    financial, 295*f*

Damages, 33–34
Data, changing to information, 165–166
Data abstract, for analysis of risk management indicators, 63–66*t*
Data bases, 304, 308
"Death with dignity" statutes, 39
Decentralization
    of decision making, 358
    of nursing system, 344–350
    vs. centralization of professional development departments, 392–394
Decertification petitions, 48–49
Decision-facilitative models, 447–448
Decision making
    cost concepts in, 280
    decentralization of, 358
    in decentralized professional structure, 238
    levels
        business, 354
        in corporations, 353–354
        functional, 354
    management information systems and, 312
    methods of, 134–143
        aggregative techniques, 142–143
        garbage can approach, 138–139
        incrementalism, 140–141
        multidimensional, case study of, 148–152
        rational-policy analysis, 136–138
        routine or bureaucratic procedures, 134–136
    moral, 3–4
    moral reasoning in, 21–27
    study of, 133–134

systems
    comparisons of, 143–145*t*
    recommendations for, 143–145
Decision rules, 135
Decision support systems (DSS), 301
Defamation, 32–33
Deinstitutionalization, 85
Delphi technique, 142, 145
Deontology, 6–8, 9*t*
Deunionization, 48–49
Devices and material, defective or malfunctioning, 36
Diagnostic-related groups (DRGs), 81, 317, 364, 365
Differentiation in health care system, 86–87
Director of Nursing Management Systems, 293
Direct work, in health organizations, 239, 240
Discharges, hospital, 37–38
"Discovery" rule, 34
Discrepancy evaluation model, 451–452*t*
Discrimination
    employment, legal bases for, 51
    against pregnant women, 50–51
    related to age, 50
Divisional organizational structure, 357*f*, 358. *See also* Product line management
Division of labor, 329
DNR orders, 39
Documentation, software, 310
Documentation system, 455
Double entry bookkeeping, 267–268*f*
DSS (decision support systems), 301
Due dates, for budgeting process, 284

Durable power of attorney, 40
Duty, fiduciary, 34

Economic man approach, to decision making, 136–138
Economic strike, 48
Education. *See also* Professional development
    within community health clinic, 126–127
    programs, to increase job satisfaction, 292
    for research, 405–406
    of women executives, 108
Educational objectives, 388–389
EEOC (Equal Employment Opportunity Commission), 50–52
Efficiency
    models, for program evaluation, 448–450
    of routine decision-making process, 134–135
Egalitarian perspective, of justice, 14
EIS (executive information systems), 301–302
Emotional reactions, influence of cognitive processes on, 101
Employees. *See* Personnel
Employer, unfair labor practices of, 47
Employment discrimination, legal bases for, 51
Empowerment, within community health clinic, 127–129
Endorsement, professional, 208
Environment
    assessment, for strategic plan, 174–175
    in congruence model, 234, 235*f*

consultative process and, 250

external, assumptions about in budget, 285

for learning experience for nurses, 391–392

nursing standards and, 18

in systems model, 233–234

Equal Employment Opportunity Commission (EEOC), 50–52

Equal Employment Opportunity Law, 50–51

Equal Pay Act, 51

Equipment, defective or malfunctioning, 36

Equity, 265–266

Escapable or avoidable costs, 280

Essay performance appraisal, 420

Ethical dilemmas

assessment based on prima facie duties, 8–9

and legal dilemmas, 15–16

in personnel management, 22–27

Ethics

interrelationship with law 15–17

of marketing of health care, 190

politics and, 78

principles of

beneficence, 12–13

justice, 13–15

respect for autonomy, 11–12

standards of care and, 17–19t

theories, classical, 4–11t

Evaluation specialist, 452

Evaluator, internal vs. external, 439

Exchange transactions, 186f

Executive information systems (EIS), 301–302

Exit interview, 291–292

Expectancy, 101

Expenses, 266, 267

Expert systems, 312

Externships, 396

Fairfax Hospital System, Virginia

financial control of, assumption by nursing administration, 289–297t

table of organization, 372f

Fair Haven Community Health Clinic, feminist mangagment of, 124–130

Fair Labor Standards Act, 51

False imprisonment, 33

Federal Civil Rights Act of 1964, Title VII, 50–51

Federal Mediation and Conciliation Services (FMCS), 49

Feedback

as job dimension, 332

loop, in systems model, 233

in supervisor-employee relationship, 414

Feminist management, at community health clinic, 124–130

Fiduciary duty, 34

Field methods of data collection, 442

Field review evaluation, 420

Financial analyses, 271–277

Financial curriculum, 295f

Financial management, assumption by nursing staff, 289–297

Financial managers, 271

Financial statements, interpretation of, 263–271f

Financial systems, nursing assuming financial control in tertiary hospital, 289–297

Fiscal period, 268–269

Fixed costs, 281

Fixed or long-term assets, 265

Flexible budgets, 286

FMCS (Federal Mediation and Conciliation Services), 49

Forced checklist, 418t

Forced distribution performance appraisal, 417

For profit financial statements, 269, 270t

"Functional nursing," 81

Functional organizational structure, 356f, 358

Functional or task method, 359

Fund balance, 266

Garbage can decision making model, 138–140, 144t

General damages, 33

Generalization effect, 423

General systems theory

application to organizations, 229–231f

models of, standard elements in, 235

Geographic catchment area system, 359

Gestalt theory, 389

Goal attainment models, 445–446

Goal-free evaluation, 446

Goals

for job functions, performance appraisal and, 412–413f

organizational, examination of, 153. See also Strategic planning

setting of, by staff nurses in community hospital, 424–435f

vs. objectives, in program evaluation, 443

Good, promotion of, 12

Good faith bargaining, 46–47
Good will, in deontology, 7
Goodwin House, strategic implementation for, 179–184f
Grievances, 48, 59–60
Guaranteed access, 76

Halo effect, 422
Harassment, sexual, 51–52
Hardware, selection of, 309
Harm, prevention or removal of, 12
Head nurse
  assistant, job redesign of, 347–348
  job redesign of, 346–347
  NLRA and, 45–46
  preceptor program, case study of, 116–123
Health care agencies, 358
Health care behavioral segments, 197
Health care competition, direct and indirect, 194f
Health care costs, increased, factors contributing to, 77–78
Health care delivery systems
  alternative, 84, 160
  changes and current restructuring, 84–85
  reorganization of, 79–81
  traditional, 82
  transformation of, 358
Health care employment laws, 49–52
Health care expenditures, 88
Health care marketing, vs. packaged goods marketing, 200–201
Health care policy. See Health policy
Health care program managers, 452
Health care services, buyers of, bargaining power of, 160–161

Health care system
  competitive advantage, strategies for, 86–87
  future of, 85–89
  realities, current, 88
Health care transactions, multiple exchanges in, 187f
Health expenditures, national, 77f
Health insurance, for aged, 74
Health maintenance organizations (HMOs), 84, 160
Health policy
  description of, 71–72
  federal government and, 72–73
  historical review, 72–75
  private sector and, 73–74
  shaping of, forces involved in, 75–79
  state government and, 73
Health workers, types of, 80–81
High exit barriers, 161–162
HMOs (health maintenance organizations), 84, 160
Holding self out doctrine, 36, 42
Home health agency, impact of changes in Medicare reporting, 254–260f
Horn effect, 422
Hospital(s)
  administrative change, 102–104
  approaches to attract patients, 195–196
  discharges from, 37–38
  length of stay per DRG, 365
  organizational structure of, 358
  reimbursements for, 80
Human resource manage-

ment, performance appraisal and, 409, 410f
Hume, David, 5
Hygiene factors, 333

ICF (intermediate care facilities), 96
Imprisonment, false, 33
Incident reports, 41–42
Incompetency, 30
Incremental adjustments, 284
Incremental costs, 280
Incrementalism, 140–141, 144t, 145
Information, from data, 165–166
Information systems, in health care, 299
Informed consent, 39–40
Informed refusal, 40
INOVA, 289–290
Inputs
  consultative process and, 250–251
  as emphasis in judgmental model, 446
  evaluation of, 447
Institute of Medicine, study on quality of care in nursing homes, 93–94
Instructors, 42
Intermediate care facilities (ICF), 96
Internships
  advantages of, 396
  description of, 118
  purposes of, 386–387
Interpersonal approach, 166
Interpersonal component of job, 329–330
Interview
  exit, 291–292
  for performance appraisal, 414–416
Inventories, 276

JCAHO. *See* Joint Commission on Accreditation of Healthcare Organizations
Job
  core dimensions of, 332, 333*f*
  dissatisfaction and satisfaction, 332
  enlargement, 331
  performance
    performance appraisal and, 414
    supervision and, 414
  performance criteria for staff nurse, 426–429*t*
  qualifications statement and description, 426
  simplification, 330–331
Job analysis, 329–330
Job content, 329
Job design
  change, perceiving need for, 340
  implementation of, 339–343
    evaluation stage, 342–343
    implementation stage, 342
    planning stage, 340–342
  job characteristics and, 329
  in nursing, 336–339
  systematic, history of, 330–335*f*
Job enrichment, 331–332
Job functions, 329
Job productivity, performance appraisal and, 411–412
Job redesign, in community hospital, 344–350
Job rotation, 331
Job satisfaction
  evaluation of, 291
  increasing, 292
  motivational factors and, 332

of newly employed nurses, 386
for team and primary nurses, 360
Joint Commission on Accreditation of Healthcare Organizations (JCAHO)
  accreditation visit, 374
  ideal goal of, 455
  organizational approaches to, 459–461
  preparation for, 455–456
  educational seminars of, 457
  judgmental models and, 446
  maintenance of accreditation, 455–461
  manual, standards in, 456
  publications of, 456
  quality assurance and, 451
  telephone number, toll-free, 457
Judgmental models of program evaluation, 446–447, 451
Justice
  description of principle, 13–14
  distributive, 14, 17
  egalitarian perspective, 14
  libertarian perspective, 14
  materials principles of, 13
  need based perspective, 15
  utilitarian perspective, 14

Kant, Immanuel, 6–7
Key indicator approach, 167

Labor contracts
  administration of, 48, 57–58
  good faith bargaining and, 46–47
  negotiation of, 56–57
  subject of bargaining, 47

unfair labor practices and, 47
Labor-management laws, 43–49
Labor organizations
  for hospital employees, 43
  legal organizing efforts for, 44–45
  union recognition process, 44–45
LAN (local area networks), 305
Law. *See also specific legal concepts*
  administrative, 40–43
  interrelationship with ethics, 15–17
  labor-management, 43–49
Leaders, role models, mentors and networks, 112–114
Learning experience, 391–392
Learning style, 389–390
Learning theories, 389
Leverage ratios, 272–273*t*
Liabilities
  corporate, 30
  current, 276–277
  definition of, 267
  equity and, 266
  short-term, 276
  vicarious, 30
Libel, 32
Libertarians, perspective of justice, 14
Licensing of nurses, 29–30
Life cycle theory, 390
Likert rating scale, 418–419*f*
Liquidity ratios, 271–272*t*
"Living wills," 39
Local area networks (LAN), 305
Loss control, 41
LOTUS 123, 306
Loyalty, in health care services, 201

Make-or-buy decisions, 280
Malpractice, 30–31
Management
    consultation, 247–254f
    decisions, 144
    development programs,
        planning for, 117,
        253–254
    by exception, 304
    literature on professional
        development pro-
        grams, organiza-
        tional structures of,
        392–393
    by objectives, 413, 421, 445
    strategic, need for, 163–165
Management information
        systems
    automation revolution
        and, 304–305
    benefiters of, 301
    cost effectiveness of, 300–
        301f
    future organizational ob-
        jectives, 311–313
    growth cycle, 302, 303t
    microcomputers and, 305–
        306t
    new trends in, 301–302
    in nursing, 312–313
    selection of, 308–311
Managerial control, 279–280
Managers, benefits of man-
        agement informa-
        tion system and, 301
Manpower predictors, estab-
        lishment of, 292–293
Marginality, 110
Marketable securities, 275
Market identity, 189
Marketing
    application to recruitment
        and retention, 203–
        204
    of health care, 192–193
    ethics of, 190
    incorporation into health
        care organization,
        190–191

restructuring and, 191–
        192
    initiation in county health
        department, 219–224t
    as organization-wide is-
        sue, 188
    overview of, 185–188
    plan, 202–203
    principles
        application of in work
            setting, 220, 222
        application to nurses in
            outpatient psychiatric
            service, 208–211
        applied by nurses in out-
            patient psychiatric
            service, 208–218t
    role in strategic planning,
        193–202f
    strategies, recognition of
        service industries,
        189
    support of strategic plan-
        ning
        by competitor analysis,
            193–195f
        by consumer satisfac-
            tion, 196–197
        by market segment anal-
            ysis, 196
        by potential consumer
            analysis, 195–196
Market segmentation, 196
Material risks, 39–40
Matrix organizations, 236,
        358
McKinsey Seven-S frame-
        work, 179–184f
Measurement contamina-
        tion, 422
Measurement deficiency, 422
Mediation, 49
Medicaid legislation, 74, 75,
        82–83
Medical records
    changes, corrections and
        countersigning, 37
    legal aspects of, 37–39

legal importance of, 37
    patient access to, 37
Medicare
    legislation for, 74, 75, 82–
        83
    opposition against, 74
    reimbursement, changes
        in, 277
    reporting, changes in, 254–
        260f
Medication error analysis,
        67t
Men, stereotypical traits of,
        99–100f
Mentoring, 112–113, 397
Microcomputers. See Com-
        puters
Middle line management,
        237–238
Mill, John Stuart, 5
Mission strategy and objec-
        tives, in systems
        model, 233
Mixed scanning method, for
        decision making, 145
Modems, 305
Modular catchment area sys-
        tem, 359
Modular information cen-
        ters, 311
Montgomery County Health
        Department, delinea-
        tion of nursing ser-
        vices in, 378–383
Moral justification, 3–4t
Moral reasoning
    definition of, 3–4
    in personnel decisions, 21–
        27
Mount Vernon Hospital
    nursing service organiza-
        tion of, 374, 375f
    product line management
        at, 371

Narrative description, 419–
        421t

National Health Insurance, proposals for, 75, 76t
National health policy, 72, 88
National Joint Practice Commission (NJPC), 102
National Labor-Management Relationship Act (NLRA), 43–46, 49
National Labor Relations Board (NLRB), 44
National League for Nursing (NLN), 74
"Natural death" statutes, 39
Naturalistic models, 448
Need-based perspective of justice, 15
Negligence, 34–36t
Negotiation, of labor contract, 56–57
Neo-behaviorist theory, 389
Net funds, 275
Networking, informal, 394
Net working capital, 274–275
Networks, 114
NGT (nominal group technique), 142, 143, 145
Nightingale, Florence, 74, 99
Nightingale School of Nursing model, 334, 335f
NJPC (National Joint Practice Commission), 102
NLN (National League for Nursing), 74
NLRA (National Labor-Management Relationship Act), 43–46, 49
NLRB (National Labor Relations Board), 44
No-code orders, 39
Nominal damages, 33
Nominal group technique (NGT), 142, 143, 145
Nonconsequentialism, 5, 6–8
Nonmaleficence, 12
Not-for-profit financial statements, 269, 270t
No treatment orders, 39

Nurse administered unit model, 339
Nurse administrators. *See also* Nursing administration
  assistant, responsibilities of, 373
  associate, role in vendor selection process, 317
  chart of accounts and, 268
  collaboration with graduate faculty, 379
  dilemma between corporate and professional culture, 354
  ethical decision making in personnel matters, 21–27
  health policy shaping and, 89
  readiness for JCAHO accreditation, 457
  standards of care and, 17–18
  women, successful, 105–114
Nurse executives
  advantages/disadvantages of product line management, 376–377
  as corporate team member, 354
Nurse extender model, 336–337
Nurse managers, financial management skills for, 295
Nurse practice acts, 29
Nurse practitioners, 81, 82
Nurse recruiter, 291
Nurses. *See also under specific nursing staff titles*
  as adult learners, 388–392
  as instructor and supervisor, 42–43
  questionable behavior of, 23–24
  restructuring of responsibilities, 293, 295–296

staff
  job redesign of, 348–349
  performance criteria for, 426–429t
  work roles of, 334–335t
Nursing administration. *See also* Nurse administrators
  attitudes of, relationship to union, 60
  feminist, at Fair Haven Clinic, 129–130
  interface with ethics and law, 15–16
  legal aspects of, 29–69
  in product line environment, 370–377
  roles in, 362–363
  sources of information for JCAHO accreditation, 456–457
  support structures, 363
Nursing assistant, 349
Nursing care delivery
  costing of nursing resources, 363–366
  delineation of services in community health agency, 378–383
  modes of, 359
  organization at unit level, 359–362
  organization of, 353–383
  structure for, 366
Nursing consultants, 457
Nursing cost methods, 364–366
Nursing director, 457–458
Nursing homes
  legislative reform of, ANA role in, 92–97
  registered nurse-staffing in, 96
Nursing manager, characteristics and function of, 296–297
Nursing profession
  collaboration between ser-

Nursing profession (*cont.*)
  vice and education,
    394–398
  interface with ethics and
    law, 15–16
  management information
    systems and, 312–313
  professional practice and,
    102
  scope of, 29
  as sex-segregated occupa-
    tion, 101–102
Nursing recruitment, 290–
    292
Nursing research. *See* Re-
    search
Nursing resource coordina-
    tor, 349
Nursing resources, costing
    of, 363–366
Nursing risk managment
    system, design of,
    61–69*t*
Nursing shortage
  ethical decision making
    and, 23–24
  recruitment and, 204
  use of alternate health
    workers, 80–81
Nursing specific indicators,
    63, 64*t*
Nursing staff problems
  development of methods
    to reduce or remedy
    problems, 341
  diagnosis of, 341
  turnover, 290–291
Nursing students, 42
Nursing supervisor, 349–350
Nursing system, decentral-
    ization of, 344–350
Nurturing, within commu-
    nity health clinic, 129

Objectives, vs. goals, in pro-
    gram evaluation, 443
Occupational Safety and
    Health Act of 1970, 50

Omnibus Budget Reconcilia-
    tion Act of 1987, 97
Open systems models
  description of, 229–231*f*
  use of, 244–245
Operating budget, 284
Operating core, 238
Operating decisions, in bud-
    get, 285
Operational managers, 354
Operations, assumptions of
    in budget, 285
Opportunity costs, 280
Orders
  legal aspects of, 38
  not to resuscitate, 39
Organizational anarchy, 139
Organizational change
  criteria, 244–245
  nurse administrator and,
    340
  resistance to, 248
Organizational development
  congruence model, 234–
    235*f*
  contingency model, 239–
    241*f*
  open systems models, 229–
    231*f*
  performance appraisal
    and, 412
  professional bureaucracy
    model, 236–239*f*
  systems model, 231–234*f*
Organizational development
    consultants, 245
Organizational goals, exam-
    ination of, 153. *See
    also* Strategic planning
Organizational history, in
    congruence model,
    234
Organizational processes,
    233
Organizational strike, 48
Organizational structures
  alternative, 356–359*f*
  centralized functional,
    242–243

  customer-centered ap-
    proach, 191, 192*f*
  functional approach, 191,
    192*f*
  implementation of differ-
    ent strategies, effects
    of, 355–356
  mixed approach, 191–192*f*
  multiple division, 243
  open systems models, 229–
    231*f*
  for orientation goals, 386
  product/service line man-
    agement approach,
    191, 192*f*
  simple, 241
  simple, functional, 242
Organizations
  career development
    within, 103
  as decision making sys-
    tems, 133–145
  duty to employee, 24–25
  equity of, 266, 267
  expanding or adding new
    services, 273–274
  growth
    by contracts, mergers,
      acquisitions, 243
    horizontal or vertical,
      243
  health care
    market-driven, 187*f*
  indicators for, 188–190*t*
    production-driven, 188
    strategic planning in,
      153–184
  life cycle stages of, 241–
    244*f*
  matrix, 236, 358
  moral responsibility to em-
    ployee, 25
  perspective of women ad-
    ministrators, 109–110
  restructuring of, 236
  sex structuring of, 103
  standard operating proce-
    dures, 134–135
  success of, based on pro-

vider/market relationship, 189
supporting health insurance for aged, 74
Orientation period, for head nurse preceptor program, 120–122
Orientation programs
 centralized vs. decentralized approach, 393–394
 for new nurse employees, 386
Outpatient psychiatric service nurses, application of marketing principles, 208–211
Outputs
 as emphasis in judgmental model, 446
 in systems model, 233
Outreach continuing education programs, 397

PACs (Political Action Committees), 75
Paraprofessionals, 80–81
Paternalism, justification of, 12–13
Patient classification systems
 automated
  development process, 319–321
  features of, 318–319
  planning for implementation, 321–322
  integration into nursing management information system, 317
  nursing cost methods and, 364–365
  proposal form for, 292–293, 294f
Patient fall analysis, 68t–69t
Patient rights
 to privacy and confidentiality, 31–32
 to refuse treatment, 39

Patient satisfaction
 marketing program and, 196–197
 in team vs. primary nursing, 360
Patient welfare, endangerment of, 36
Peer preceptors, 117–118
People, in systems model, 233
Performance appraisal
 compensation and, 411
 components of, 412–416f
 critical incident, 420t
 in employee relations process, 409
 evaluation methods, 416–421t
  checklists, 417–418t
  narrative description, 419–421t
  rating scale, 418–419f
 form, objective of, 416
 interview, 414–416
 job productivity and, 411–412
 job-related, 411
 methods, historical perspective, 409–410
 productivity-oriented, 411
 purposes of, 410–412
 reliability, 422–423
 trait-oriented, 411–412
 validity, 421–422
Performance standards, 443
Personal competence, of women administrators, 110–111
Personal selling, 203
Personal work stations, availability of, 311–312
Personnel. See also specific personnel
 decisions
  moral reasoning in, 21–27
  performance appraisal and, 409

termination, promotion, demotion and transfer, 412
 evaluation system, example of, 424–425
 paraprofessionals, 80–81
 professional development programs, purposes of
  for continuing nurse employees, 387–388
  for new nurse, 386
 professional staff and administrators, internal assessment of, 157
 selection, appointment and assignment of, 43
 staff development programs, 26, 177–178
 staffing, performance appraisal and, 412
Petitioning, by labor organization, 44
Petitions, decertification, 48–49
Physician, relationship to nurse, 336
Physician assistants, 82
Physician extenders, 81, 82
Physician orders, legal aspects of, 38
Physician-patient relationship, privileged communications, 32
Pigeonholing, 238
Planning cell, 142
Policy
 change, implementation of, 148–152
 definition of, 71
 formulation, 356
Policy analytic approach, to decision making, 136–138
Political Action Committees (PACs), 75
Political forces, shaping health policy, 76–78

Political systems, incremental, 141

Politics, relationship to public policy, 71

Position description, 413–414

Positioning, 201–202

Potential consumer analysis, 195–196

Power of attorney, durable, 40

Preceptorships
advantages of, 396
at community hospital, example of, 116–123
limitations of, 396
purposes of, 386–387

Preference aggregation decision model, 144t, 145

Preference ranking techniques, 142

Preferred provider organizations (PPOs), 84, 160

Pregnant women, prohibition of discriminatory treatment of, 50–51

Presurvey conferences, 457

Prices, based on value to customers, 190

Prima facie duties, 8–11

Primary care nursing model, 337–338

Primary nursing
development of, 81
research findings on, 360–361

Primary providers, new, 82

Primitive organizational structure, 356f, 358

Privacy, 31–32

Private sector, health policy and, 73–74

Privilege, qualified or absolute, 33

Privileged communications, 32

Problem, working on, in consultative process, 251–252

Procedures, standardized, 35–36

Process, moral reasoning and, 3

Process evaluation, 443–444, 447

Product evaluation, 443–444, 447

Product line development, 177

Product line management
assessment of, 373–377
description of, 357f, 358, 370
implementation of, 371, 372f
integration of nursing services in, 373

Product managers, 371

Professional bureaucracy model, 236–239f

Professional competence, of women administrators, 111

Professional development.
See also Education
adult learning and, 388–392
departments, centralization vs. decentralization, 392–394
guidelines for establishing a clinical nursing research program, 402–408
for nurse clinicians, 397
purposes of programs, 385–388

Professional misconduct, 30–31

Professional nursing organizations, 395

Professional socialization, 387–388

Profitability ratios, 272t

Profit contributions, 243

Pro forma statements, 273–274

Program evaluation
decision-making process and, 438–439
field of, historical development of, 439–441
forms of, 438
funding and, 439
models
decision-facilitative, 447–448
efficiency, 448–450
formative vs. summative distinction, 443
goal attainment, 445–446
goals, objectives and criteria for attainment, 443
judgmental, 446–447
major characteristics of, 441–444
major classes of, 444–448t
naturalistic, 448
process vs. product distinction, 443–444
qualitative vs. quantitative approach, 442
overview, 440t
qualitative vs. quantitative, 442
quality assurance, 450–453t
techniques of, 438
vs. research, 437–438

Promotion, marketing, 190, 202

Proposal rating form, 293, 294f

Prospective payment system, 83–84, 277

Protection, of patients and public from harm, 36

Provider choice, 190

Psychomotor educational objectives, 388

Public Law 89-97, 82–83

Public Law 98-21, 83

Public policy, 71, 93

Public relations, 203

Punitive damages, 34

Qualified privilege, 33
Qualitative evaluation, 442
Quality assurance, 41, 450–452
Quality care concerns, 17
Quality control, 450
Quantitative evaluation, 442
Queen Bee Syndrome, 109–110

Ranking, of performance appraisal, 416–417
Rating scale, 418–419f
Rational decision model, 144t
Rational method, for decision making, 136–138
Rational-policy analysis, for decision making, 136–138
Reality shock, 335, 394
Recency effect, 423
Referral agents, 197
Refusal
    informed, 40
    of treatment, 39
Relevance, in collaborative teaching, 397–398
Reliability factor, in patient classification system, 364–365
Replacement cost basis, for asset valuation, 278–279
Request for proposals (RFP), 293
Research
    conduct of, 406
    and development, 437–438
    education for, 405–406
    enhancement of, need for collaboration and, 394–396
    facilitation of, 404–405
    proposals, review protocol for, 404–405
    vs. program evaluation, 437–438

Res ipsa loquitur, 31
Resources, in congruence model, 234
Respect for persons concept, 11–12, 18
Respondent superior, 30
Retained earnings, 266
Retirement, mandatory, 50
Return on investment, 243
Revenues, 266, 267
Reward system for managers, 243
RFP (request for proposals), 293
Right to work laws, 47
Risk avoidance, 66–67
Risk control, 66–67, 69
Risk management
    case by case analysis, 63–66t
    legal aspects of, 41–42
    medication error analysis, 67t
    nursing specific indicators, 63, 64t
    patient fall analysis, 68t–69t
    plan, 62–63
    quality assurance and, 41
    risk identification aspect of, 63–64, 66
    system
        accountability, increasing, 61–62
        environment and, 61
Risks
    material, 39–40
    prevention of, 41
Rituals and rites, 158
Role models, 112
Ross, W.D., 8
Routine decision model, 144t
Rule deontology, 7–8, 9t, 10
Rule utilitarianism, 6, 9t, 10

Scientific management theory, 330–331, 392
Second-generation primary nursing, 338

Segmentation analysis, 196–197
Self-assessment
    for head nurse preceptor program, 119–120
    internal, 198
Self-determining actions, 11
Self-reflection, 423
Semifixed or semivariable costs, 281
Service-line management, 357f, 358. See also Product line management
Service-line manager model, 337
Service portfolio analysis, 198–200f
Services, as solutions to customers' problems, 189–190
Sexist attitudes, organizational sex structuring and, 103–104
Sex role stereotypes, expectations and, 101
Sexual harassment, 51–52
Shared governance, 338–339
Short-term liabilities, 267, 276
Simple checklist, 417t
Situation audit, 157
Skilled nursing facilities (SNF), 96
Skill variety, 332
Slander, 32
SNF (skilled nursing facilities), 96
Social forces, shaping health care policy, 78–79
Socialization, women executives and, 106–107
Social policy, 71
Social Security Amendments of 1982, 83
Sociotechnical arrangements, 233
Software
    applications, 306–307

Software (*cont.*)
  cost of, 309
  for report writing, 320
  selection considerations, 311–312
  variables, related to selection, 309
Special damages, 33
Sports, in socialization of women executives, 107
Spreadsheet software programs, 306–307
Staff development programs, 26, 177–178
Staffing, performance appraisal and, 412
Standardization, 134
Standardized procedures, 35–36
Standard of care, 17–19*t*, 35
Standards of practice, 22
State government, role in health care policy, 73
Statement of revenues and expenses, 263–265*f*, 269
Static or fixed budgets, 286
Statute of limitations, 34
Step costs, 281
Stereotyping, 101, 103–104
Stereotyping theory, 99–100*f*
Straight ranking performance appraisal, 416–417
Strategic apex, 236–237
Strategic business unit structure, 357*f*, 358
Strategic indicators
  elicitation during interview, 169
  sources of, 167–168
Strategic management, need for, 163–165
Strategic managers
  description of, 354
  internal focus of, 157–158
  management information systems and, 301

Strategic objectives, 189
Strategic options, 162
Strategic plan
  decisions in, 193
  feasibility, evaluation of, 162
  implementation of, 179–184
  purpose of, 355
Strategic planning
  assessing internal strategic capacities, 157–158
  competitive analysis and, 159–162*f*
  definition of, 153
  effectiveness of, 154
  evaluation and control, 165–169
  financial ratios for, 271–273*t*
  formulation and implementation of plan, 162
  implementation
    avoidance of pitfalls, 163–169
    pitfalls in, 165
  management information systems and, 312
  marketing's role in, 193–202*f*
    positioning and, 201–202
    self-assessment, 198
    service portfolio analysis, 198–200*f*
  for nursing education department, case study of, 172–178
  pitfalls in, 163–165*t*
  process of, 154–156*f*
  questions for, 155*f*
  success
    low incidence of, 163
    need for top management involvement, 163
Strategy
  in congruence model, 234
  corporate, 356

definition of, 355–356
development of, 176–178, 200–201
formulation of, 356
Strategy-structure sequence, 355
Strikes, 48
Substitution, treat of, 160
Success, sex role stereotypes and, 101
Successive developmental crises, 390
Sunk costs, 280
Supervision
  job performance and, 414
  of subordinates and students in nursing practice, 42
Supervisors
  NLRA definition of, 45–46
  nurses as, 42–43
  status, determination of, 45–46
Suppliers, bargaining power of, 161
Support staff, 237
Surprise strike, 48
SWOT Analysis, 155
Sympathy strike, 48
Syntax errors, 310
Systems model
  description of, 231–234*f*
  vs. congruence model, 235

Tactical managers, 301, 354
Taft-Hartley Act, 1974 amendment to, 43–44, 48
Target markets, 188–189
Task identity, 332
Task significance, 332
Tax Equity and Fiscal Responsibility Act (TEFRA), 83
Teaching
  collaborative, 396–398
  strategies for, 392
Team leader, 359

Team nursing
advantages of, 378–379
description of, 359
nursing shortages and, 81
research findings on, 360–361
Technostructure, 237
Telephone orders, legal aspects of, 38
Terminals, comparison of, 305, 306t
Timetable, for budgeting process, 284
Tokenism, 109
Top management, 301
Tort law, 31, 33
Transactional report approach, 166
Transfers, recording of, 37–38
Transformation
process of, 229–230f
in systems model, 233
Treatment refusal, 39
Trend analysis, 66

Unfair labor practices, 47, 48, 58
Union
administrative attitudes and relationships, 60
organization of, 55–56
recognition process for, 44–45t
Union security clause, 47
Unit directors, advantages of product line management and, 374

United States government
agencies of, involved in health care policy, 73
departments of, involved in health care policy, 73
involvement in health care, 72–73
regulations affecting health facilities and programs, 40–41
Unit manager, 295
Unit secretary, 295
Unity, stages of, 395–396t
Utilitarianism, 5–6, 9t, 14

Validity
in patient classification system, 364–365
of performance appraisal, 421–422
Values, 157–158
Variable costs, 281
VDT (video display terminals), 304
Verbal orders, legal aspects of, 38
Vicarious liability, 30
Video display terminals (VDT), 304
Vision, 153
Visiting Nurse Association of Northern Virginia (VNA), 254
Volume of services
cost concepts and, 281
effect on unit cost per service, 300–301f

Washington Hospital center, automation of patient classification system, 316–322
Weighted checklist, 417–418t
Wildcat strikes, 48
Women
executives, personal profiles of, 106–109
as managers, 103–104
stereotypical traits of, 99–100f
as successful administrators, characteristics of, 110–112
Word processing software, 307
Work
attitudes, measurement of, 341
changes in division and flow of, 307–308
direct and managerial, 239
setting, application of marketing principles in, 220, 222
Workers compensation legislation, 49–50
Work group design, 333–334
Working capital analyses, 274–277
Work standard, 414

Zero-based budget approach, 284